The Metabolic Syndrome

Henning Beck-Nielsen
Editor

The Metabolic Syndrome

Pharmacology and Clinical Aspects

Springer

Editor
Henning Beck-Nielsen
Department of Endocrinology
Odense University Hospital
Odense C, Denmark

ISBN 978-3-7091-1330-1 ISBN 978-3-7091-1331-8 (eBook)
DOI 10.1007/978-3-7091-1331-8
Springer Wien Heidelberg New York Dordrecht London

Library of Congress Control Number: 2013934531

Printed on acid-free paper

Springer is a part of Springer Science+Business Media (www.springer.com)

Contents

1 **Introduction and Definition of the Metabolic Syndrome** 1
Henning Beck-Nielsen

2 **Epidemiology of the Metabolic Syndrome** 7
Knut Borch-Johnsen

3 **Pathophysiology of the Metabolic Syndrome** 17
John J. Nolan and Donal J. O'Gorman

4 **The Metabolic Syndrome and Cardiovascular Disease** 43
Frank Pistrosch, Frank Schaper, and Markolf Hanefeld

5 **The Metabolic Syndrome and Cancer** 55
Frank Pistrosch and Markolf Hanefeld

6 **Lifestyle Intervention: Prevention of Complications to the Metabolic Syndrome** 63
Pirjo Ilanne-Parikka and Jaakko Tuomilehto

7 **Low-Carbohydrate Diets in the Treatment of the Metabolic Syndrome** 87
Marc-Andre Cornier and Boris Draznin

8 **Treatment with Metformin** 99
Clifford J. Bailey

9 **Treatment with Thiazolidinediones** 117
Seda Suvag, Kristina M. Utzschneider, and Steven E. Kahn

10 **The Role of Statins in the Metabolic Syndrome** 147
Peter M. Nilsson

11 **The Indication for Antithrombotic Primary Prophylaxis and Treatment in Case of Thromboembolic Complications in Patients with Metabolic Syndrome** 155
Steen Husted

12 The Role of Glucagon-like Receptor-1 Agonists in the Metabolic Syndrome 165
Tina Vilsbøll, Salvatore Calanna, and Filip K. Knop

13 Treatment of Hypertension in the Metabolic Syndrome 185
Michael Hecht Olsen

14 Treatment of the Metabolic Syndrome by Bariatric Surgery 191
Sten Madsbad

15 Treatment of the Metabolic Syndrome in Daily Clinical Practice: Algorithms 221
Henning Beck-Nielsen

Index 227

Abbreviations

A	Late/atrial ventricular filling velocity
ACEi	Angiotensin-converting enzyme inhibitors
ACS	Acute coronary syndrome
ACT NOW	ACTos NOW for prevention of diabetes
ADA	American Diabetes Association
ADOPT	A diabetes outcome progression trial
ADP	Adenosine diphosphate
AHA	American Heart Association
AHEI	Alternative healthy eating index
ALLHAT	Antihypertensive and lipid-lowering treatment to prevent heart attack trial
AMIGO	AC2993: diabetes management for improving glucose outcome
AMP	Adenosine monophosphate
AMPK	Adenosine monophosphate kinase
AP1	Activator protein-1
APOA5	Apolipoprotein A-V
ARB	Angiotensin II-AT1 receptor blockers
ARIC	Atherosclerosis risk in communities
ATP	Adenosine triphosphate
AusDiab	Australian diabetes obesity and lifestyle
BCAA	Branched chain amino acids
BIGPRO	Biguanides and prevention of the risk of obesity
BMI	Body mass index
CABG	Coronary artery bypass grafting
CAD	Coronary artery disease
CANOE	CAnadian normoglycemia outcomes evaluation
CAPRIE	Clopidogrel versus aspirin in patients at risk of ischaemic events
CCK	Cholecystokinin
CETP	Cholesterol ester transfer protein
CHARISMA	Clopidogrel for high atherothrombotic risk and ischaemic stabilization, management, and avoidance
CI	Confidence interval
COX-1	Cyclo-oxygenase-1

CRP	C-reactive protein
CT	Computerised axial tomography
CVD	Cardiovascular disease
DAG	Diacylglycerol
DASH	Dietary approaches to stop hypertension
DEXA	Dual-energy X-ray absorptiometry
DIG	Diabetes in Germany
DNA	Deoxyribonucleic acid
DPP	Diabetes Prevention Program
DPP-4	Dipeptidyl peptidase-4
DPS	Diabetes prevention study
DREAM	Diabetes REduction assessment with ramipril and rosiglitazone medication study
DURATION	Diabetes therapy utilisation: researching changes in HbA1c, weight, and other factors through intervention with exenatide once-weekly
E	Early ventricular filling velocity
EASD	European Association for the Study of Diabetes
EGIR	European Group for the Study of Insulin Resistance
ELIXA	Evaluation of cardiovascular outcomes in patients with type 2 diabetes after acute coronary syndrome during treatment with AVE0010 (Lixisenatide)
ELSA	English longitudinal study of ageing
EMA	European Medicines Agency
EXSCEL	Exenatide study
FDA	United States Food and Drug Administration
FFA	Free fatty acids
FIELD	Fenofibrate intervention and event lowering in diabetes
FPG	Fasting plasma glucose
GCKR	Glucokinase receptor
GI	Glycaemic index
GIP	Glucose-dependent insulinotropic polypeptide
GLP-1	Glucagon-like peptide-1
GLP-1R	Glucagon-like peptide-1 receptor
GLUT4	Glucose transporter type 4
GP	Glycoprotein
GWAS	Genome wide association studies
HDL	High-density lipoprotein
HMGCoA	3-Hydroxy-3-methyl-glutaryl-CoA
HOMA-IR	Homeostasis assessment model for insulin resistance
HPS	Heart protection study
HR	Hazard ratio
i.v.	Intravenous
ICAM-1	Intracellular cell adhesion module 1
IDF	International Diabetes Federation

IDPP	Indian Diabetes Prevention Program
IFG	Impaired fasting glucose
IGF	Insulin-like growth factor
IGT	Impaired glucose tolerance
IL	Interleukin
IMPROVE-IT	Improved reduction of outcomes: vytorin efficacy international trial
IMT	Intima-media thickness
IOM	Institute of Medicine
IRS-1	Insulin receptor substrate-1
JNK	c-Jun N-terminal kinase
JUPITER	Justification for the use of statin in prevention: an intervention trial evaluating rosuvastatin
LAGB	Laparoscopic adjustable gastric banding
LDL	Low-density lipoprotein
LEAD	Liraglutide effect and action in diabetes
LEADER	Liraglutide effect and action in diabetes: evaluation of cardiovascular outcome results—a long term evaluation
LIPC	Lipase hepatic
LKB1	Liver kinase B1
LMWH	Low-molecular-weight heparin
LPL	Lipoprotein lipase
LTPA	Leisure time physical activity
LV	Left ventricular
LVDD	Left ventricular diastolic dysfunction
MCP-1	Monocyte chemotactic protein-1
MDRD	Modification in diet in renal disease
MI	Myocardial infarction
MMP-9	Matrix metalloproteinase-9
MR	Magnetic resonance
MTNR1B	Melatonin receptor 1B
mTOR	Mammalian target of rapamycin
MUFA	Monounsaturated fat
NAD	Nicotinamide adenine dinucleotide
NAFLD	Non-alcoholic fatty liver disease
NASH	Non-alcoholic steatohepatitis
NCEP ATP III	National Cholesterol Education Program Adult Treatment Panel III
NEAT	Non-exercise activity thermogenesis
NFκB	Nuclear factor of kappa light polypeptide gene enhancer in B-cells 1
NHANES	National Health and Nutrition Examination Survey
NIMA	Non-invasive measurements of atherosclerosis
NO	Nitric oxide
NSTE	Non-ST-elevation

NYHA	New York Heart Association
OCT1	Organic cation transporter-1
OGTT	Oral glucose tolerance test
ORIGIN	Outcome reduction with an initial glargine intervention
PAD	Peripheral arterial disease
PAI	Plasminogen activator inhibitor
PATO	Platelet inhibition and patient outcomes
PCI	Percutaneous coronary intervention
PCOS	Polycystic ovary syndrome
PERISCOPE	Pioglitazone effect on regression of intravascular sonographic coronary obstruction prospective evaluation
PGC-1α	Peroxisome proliferator-activated receptor γ coactivator-1α
PKC	Protein kinase C
POPADAD	Progression of arterial disease and diabetes
PPAR	Peroxisome proliferator-activated receptor
PPREs	Peroxisome proliferator response elements
PROACTIVE	Prospective pioglitazone clinical trial in macrovascular events
PRoFESS	Prevention regimen for effectively avoiding second strokes
PUFA	Polyunsaturated fat
PYY	Peptide YY
RBP-4	Retinol-binding protein-4
REWIND	Researching cardiovascular events with a weekly incretin in diabetes
RISC	Relationship between insulin sensitivity and cardiovascular disease
RQ	Respiratory quotient
RR	Relative risk
RYGB	Roux-en-Y gastric bypass
SAA	Serum amyloid A
SAFA	Saturated fatty acids
SCORE	Systematic coronary risk evaluation
SIROCCO	The effects of simvastatin and rosiglitazone combination in patients with the metabolic syndrome
SIRT1	Sirtuin-1
SNPs	Single nucleotide polymorphisms
SOS	Swedish Obesity Study
STAR	The study of trandolapril/verapamil SR and insulin resistance
STEMI	ST-elevation
STOP-NIDDM	Study to prevent non-insulin dependent diabetes mellitus
SU	Sulphonylurea
TFAP2B	Transcription factor AP-2 beta
TIDE	Thiazolidinedione intervention with vitamin D evaluation
TNFα	Tumour necrosis factor α
TNT	Treat to target

TOD	Target organ damage
TODAY	The treatment options for type 2 diabetes in adolescents and youth
t-PA	Tissue plasminogen activator
TRIMS	Reversal intervention for metabolic syndrome
TRIPOD	Troglitazone in the prevention of diabetes
TRITON-TIMI	Trial to Assess Improvement in Therapeutic Outcomes by Optimizing Platelet InhibitioN with Prasugrel-Thrombolysis in Myocardial Infarction
TZDs	Thiazolidinediones
UFH	Unfractionated heparin
UKPDS	United Kingdom Prospective Diabetes Study
USDA	United States Department of Agriculture
VALUE	Valsartan antihypertensive long-term use evaluation
VCAM-1	Vascular cell adhesion module 1
VLDL	Very low-density lipoprotein
vWF	von Willebrand factor
WHI-OS	Women's Health Initiative Observational Study
WHO	World Health Organization
WLM	Weight loss maintenance trial
ZNF259	Zinc Finger Protein 259

Introduction and Definition of the Metabolic Syndrome

1

Henning Beck-Nielsen

1.1 Introduction

The metabolic syndrome is a common syndrome affecting about 20 % of the adult population without known diabetes and cardiovascular disease (CVD) in Europe, and probably the prevalence is of the same magnitude in other industrialised countries worldwide. This syndrome, which is linked to leisure lifestyle and overeating/obesity, can develop into type 2 diabetes, CVD, cancer, gout, non-alcoholic fatty liver disease (NAFLD), polycystic ovary syndrome (PCOS), sleep apnoea and dementia and may result in increased mortality.

The metabolic syndrome is mainly caused by western lifestyle resulting in abdominal obesity but also a genetic predisposition plays a role. Abdominal obesity leads to insulin resistance and hyperinsulinaemia, further resulting in glucose intolerance and dyslipidaemia (high plasma triglyceride and low high-density lipoprotein (HDL) cholesterol values) and arterial hypertension. These are all risk factors for the diseases mentioned above. Around 50 % of subjects suffering from the metabolic syndrome develop type 2 diabetes, including the problems and complications connected with this disease. Figure 1.1 describes our model for the pathophysiology of the metabolic syndrome and its consequences.

As clinicians, we need to be aware of the syndrome and be able to treat the individual components in order to avoid the complications.

The treatment should of course be based on the pathophysiology in order to change the lifestyle by reducing calorie intake (especially saturated fat and sugar) by an increase in physical activity (interval training seems to be effective) and by reduction of mental stress and tobacco use. However, pharmacological treatment

H. Beck-Nielsen (✉)
Department of Endocrinology, Odense University Hospital, Kloevervaenget 6, 4th floor, 5000 Odense C, Denmark
e-mail: henning.beck-nielsen@ouh.regionsyddanmark.dk

H. Beck-Nielsen (ed.), *The Metabolic Syndrome*,
DOI 10.1007/978-3-7091-1331-8_1, © Springer-Verlag Wien 2013

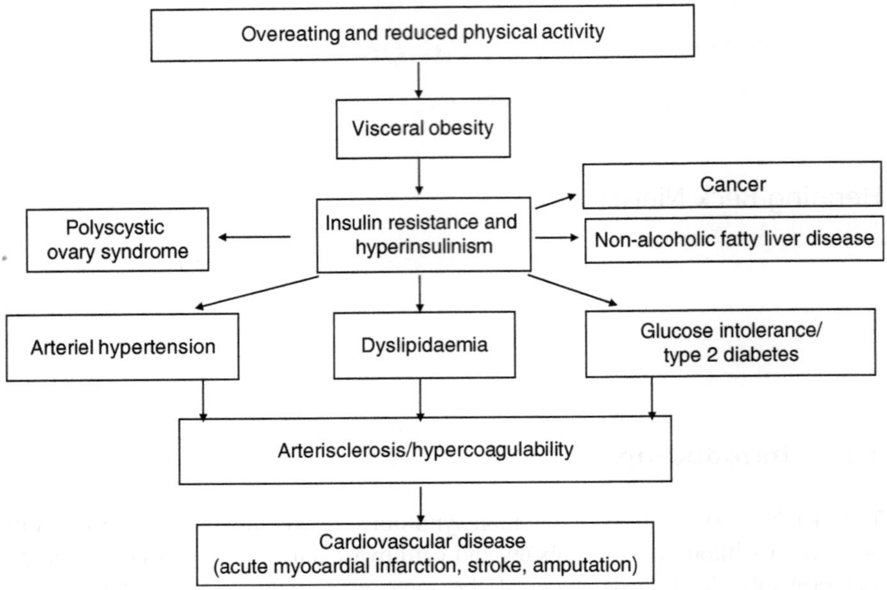

Fig. 1.1 The pathophysiology of the metabolic syndrome

may be necessary in most subjects in order to avoid the consequences of the syndrome and therefore treatment of these components seems obligatory.

Insulin resistance can be treated by metformin, which also seems to reduce the risk for CVD and cancer development. This drug seems to be a logic basis for treating the metabolic syndrome since it affects specifically insulin resistance. Also, thiazolidinediones (TZDs) seem to be specifically effective in subjects with metabolic syndrome since they improve peripheral insulin sensitivity, specifically in skeletal muscle, and reduce ectopic fat disposition e.g. in liver and muscle cells, which seems to play an important role for the development of insulin resistance. Fat liver itself is a variable for subjects with metabolic syndrome. Despite therapeutic preference of TZDs based on their mechanisms, the drugs on the market have serious side effects, which should be taken into account.

Statins have proven to be effective in specifically patients with metabolic syndrome suffering from type 2 diabetes and CVD and therefore they are the first drug of choice in most subjects in order to treat dyslipidaemia. Fibrates may specifically be an option in patients with increased triglyceride levels.

In time, the metabolic syndrome results in "exhaustion" of beta-cells further resulting in reduced insulin secretion, which causes hyperglycaemia—therefore, beta-cell stimulation may be recommended. Glucagon-like peptide 1 (GLP-1) agonists, which also reduce body weight and blood pressure, therefore, seem to be an obvious choice in many subjects with metabolic syndrome—perhaps also in the prediabetic state in order to reduce body weight.

Recently, gastric bypass surgery has been shown to be an alternative to pharmacological treatment in specifically very obese subjects.

Finally, about 80 % of subjects with metabolic syndrome suffer from arterial hypertension, which is an important factor for the development of CVD and stroke. Therefore, a proper treatment of blood pressure is necessary and inhibition of the angiotensin system seems obligatory.

All these aspects will be covered in this book, and based on that an algorithm will be proposed for proper treatment of the metabolic syndrome in clinical practice.

1.2 History

The relationship between obesity, specifically abdominal obesity and metabolic abnormalities, such as increased lipid, glucose and urate values together with arterial hypertension, has been known and described for decades. It has also been described that patients suffering from this dysmetabolism have a higher risk for developing type 2 diabetes and CVD. Professor Vague was in 1952 the first to describe the syndrome linking masculine fat disposition (abdominal obesity) to metabolic disturbances, CVD and gout [1]. Short after, Professor Crepaldi described the "plurimetabolic syndrome", which is close to what we today consider to be the metabolic syndrome [2]. In 1981, Professor Hanefeld further evaluated the hypothesis and presented the first tentative definition of the syndrome [3]. However, the interest for the syndrome really grew in 1988 when Professor Reaven in his Banting lecture defined the syndrome X, which was later named "the insulin resistance syndrome" and today is called "the metabolic syndrome" [named by the World Health Organization (WHO)] [4]. The syndrome also has a WHO diagnostic code: ICD9. However, the term metabolic syndrome is in a way misleading since metabolism is a phenomenon taking place in normal subjects. What, however, characterises these patients is dysmetabolism and therefore "the dysmetabolic syndrome" would be a more correct and meaningful name.

1.3 Dysmetabolism

Subjects with metabolic syndrome are characterised by dysmetabolism showing increased levels of plasma glucose, free fatty acids, triglyceride, alpha hydroxybutyrate, branched chain amino acids and urate in the fasting state. Plasma-free fatty acids would normally be suppressed by a meal, but not in these subjects, while both free fatty acids and triglycerides are severely increased during the entire 24-h period in patients with metabolic syndrome. Intracellularly insulin-mediated glycogen storage in both liver and muscles is reduced together with a reduction in glucose oxidation, whereas lipid oxidation is relatively increased (due to increased substrate supply), as is glycolysis. The last may result in an increase in plasma lactate and consequently an increase in gluconeogenesis. The increase in lipid intake results in abdominal obesity and consequently ectopic lipid disposition in both liver, skeletal muscles and beta-cells. Thus, subjects with metabolic syndrome seem to have a defect in glycogen storage, whereas lipid storage is increased

Table 1.1 Newest criteria defined by the International Diabetes Federation (IDF) for clinical diagnosis of the metabolic syndrome

Measure	Categorical cut-points
Elevated waist circumference[a]	Population- and country-specific definitions
Elevated triglycerides (drug treatment for elevated triglycerides is an alternate indicator[b])	≥150 mg/dL (1.7 mmol/L)
Reduced HDL cholesterol (drug treatment for reduced HDL cholesterol is an alternate indicator[b])	<40 mg/dL (1.0 mmol/L) in males <50 mg/dL (1.3 mmol/L) in females
Elevated blood pressure (antihypertensive drug treatment in a patient with a history of hypertension is an alternate indicator)	Systolic ≥130 and/or diastolic ≥85 mmHg
Elevated fasting glucose[c] (drug treatment of elevated glucose is an alternate indicator)	≥100 mg/dL (5.6 mmol/L)

Three components must be fulfilled to make the diagnosis
HDL indicates high-density lipoprotein
[a]It is recommended that the IDF cut-points are used for non-Europeans and either the IDF or the American Heart Association/National Heart, Lung, and Blood Institute cut-points are used for people of European origin until more data are available
[b]The most commonly used drugs for elevated triglycerides and reduced HDL cholesterol are fibrates and nicotinic acid. A patient taking one of these drugs can be presumed to have high triglycerides and low HDL cholesterol. High-dose ω-3 fatty acids presumes high triglycerides
[c]Most patients with type 2 diabetes mellitus will have the metabolic syndrome by the proposed criteria
Alberti KG, Eckel RH, Grundy SM, Zimmet PZ, Cleeman JI, Donato KA, Fruchart JC, James WP, Loria CM, Smith SC Jr; International Diabetes Fedration Task Force on Epidemiology and Prevention; National Heart, Lung, and Blood Institute; American Heart Association; World Heart Federation; International Atherosclerosis Society; International Association for the Study of Obesity. Harmonizing the metabolic syndrome: a joint interim statement of the International Diabetes Federation Task Force on Epidemiology and Prevention; National Heart, Lung and Blood Institute; American Heart Association; World Heart Federation; International Atherosclerosis Society; and International Association for the Study of Obesity. *Circulation 2009*; *120*: *1640*

both abdominally and intracellularly in liver and muscles [5–7]. Protein oxidation seems normal, but branched chain amino acids seem to accumulate [8].

It is difficult to tell what the primary and secondary factors of these events are, but environmental factors such as leisure lifestyle and overeating seem to play a central role, and also a genetic susceptibility seems to be important.

To understand the metabolic syndrome is to understand the dysmetabolism, and this understanding is also important for the diagnosis of the syndrome as used in clinical practice.

1.4 Definition and Diagnosis

The International Diabetes Federation (IDF) has recently formulated a new operational definition of the metabolic syndrome to be used in clinical practice worldwide (Tables 1.1 and 1.2) [9]. The definition is based on visceral obesity as the

Table 1.2 Current recommended waist circumference thresholds for abdominal obesity by organisation

Recommended waist circumference thresholds for abdominal obesity			
Population	Organisation (Ref)	Men (cm)	Women (cm)
Europid	IDF	≥94	≥80
Caucasian	WHO	≥94 (Increased risk) ≥102 (Still higher risk)	≥80 (Increased risk) ≥88 (Still higher risk)
United States	AHA/NHLBI ATP III[a]	≥102	≥88
Canada	Health Canada	≥102	≥88
European	European Cardiovascular Societies	≥102	≥88
Asian (including Japanese)	IDF	≥90	≥80
Asian	WHO	≥90	≥80
Japanese	Japanese Obesity Society	≥85	≥90
China	Cooperative Task Force	≥85	≥88
Middle East, Mediterranean	IDF	≥94	≥88
Sub-Saharan Africa	IDF	≥94	≥88
Ethnic Central and South America	IDF	≥90	≥88

[a]Recent AHA/NHLBI guidelines for the metabolic syndrome recognise an increased risk for cardiovascular disease and diabetes at waist circumference thresholds of ≥94 cm in men and ≥80 cm in women and identify these as optional cut-points for individuals or populations with increased insulin resistance

IDF International Diabetes Federation, *WHO* World Health Organization, *AHA* American Heart Association, *NHLBI* National Heart, Lung, and Blood Institute

primary factor of the syndrome. The most optimal measurement of visceral obesity is obtained by a magnetic resonance (MR) scan, which is able to accurately measure visceral fat without including subcutaneous fat. For several reasons, MR scans are, however, not always usable in clinical practice, whereas waist circumference has shown to be a useful surrogate measurement and is therefore recommended in all patients showing signs of the metabolic syndrome. Waist circumference is defined as the circumference of abdomen measured in the middle of the rib curvature and the *crista iliaca* when the patient is standing up. Waist-to-hip ratio has previously been suggested as a preferable measurement, but this measurement is a poorer measurement for visceral fat than waist circumference. The limit values for waist circumference are different depending on ethnicity and gender. In Europe, the normal limit of waist circumference is lower than 94 cm for men and lower than 80 cm for women. Higher values than these are associated with increased morbidity and mortality. In addition to waist circumference, IDF recommends measuring blood pressure, which must be done when the patient is sitting down after 10 min resting, as well as measuring fasting plasma triglyceride, HDL cholesterol and fasting plasma glucose. If the patient's waist circumference is too high and if the pathological values for two of the four additional factors are present, the patient suffers from the metabolic syndrome, as defined by IDF. The weakness of this and other syndrome definitions is that the definitions do not always include the same factors, and different phenotypes with the same diagnosis may therefore be presented. This, however, does not change the fact that the diagnosis is operational.

As mentioned, the metabolic syndrome has been linked to CVD and the degrees of the syndrome have been used as a risk engine for development of CVD. However, only about 20–30 % of patients with metabolic syndrome develop CVD, and better risk engines than the metabolic syndrome exist. Therefore, the metabolic syndrome should today be diagnosed in order to draw the attention to the clustering of the metabolic abnormalities (dysmetabolism). If one of the components in the syndrome is diagnosed, the other components must be measured. Thereby, diagnosing of the metabolic syndrome may lead to a reduced risk of developing the clinical consequences: type 2 diabetes, CVD, cancer, NAFLD, PCOS, sleep apnoea and dementia.

Based on these arguments, diagnosis of the metabolic syndrome makes sense mainly in premorbid state (before development of the diseases) in order to characterise the risk factors.

References

1. Vague J (1956) The degree of masculine differentiation of obesities: a factor determining redisposition to diabetes, atherosclerosis, gout, and uric calculous disease. Am J Clin Nutr 4(1):20–34
2. Avagaro P et al (1967) Association of hyperlipidemia, diabetes mellitus and obesity. Acta Diabetol Let 4:572–590
3. Hanefeld M, Leonhardt W (1981) Das Metabolische Syndrom. Deutsche Gesundheit Wesen 36 (13):545–552
4. Reaven GM (1988) Banting lecture 1988. Role of insulin resistance in human disease. Diabetes 37:1595–1607
5. Befroy DE, Petersen KF, Dufour S, Mason GF, de Graaf RA, Rothman DL, Shulman GI (2007) Impaired mitochondrial substrate oxidation in muscle of insulin-resistant offspring of type 2 diabetic patients. Diabetes 56:1376–1381
6. Giebelstein J, Poschmann G, Hojlund K, Schechinger W, Dietrich JW, Levin K, Beck-Nielsen H, Podwojski K, Stuhler K, Meyer HE, Klein HH (2012) The proteomic signature of insulin-resistant human skeletal muscle reveals increased glycolytic and decreased mitochondrial enzymes. Diabetologia 55:1114–1127
7. Kelley DE, Mandarino LJ (2000) Fuel selection in human skeletal muscle in insulin resistance: a reexamination. Diabetes 49:677–683
8. Newgard CB, An J, Bain JR, Muehlbauer MJ, Stevens RD, Lien LF, Haqq AM, Shah SH, Arlotto M, Slentz CA, Rochon J, Gallup D, Ilkayeva O, Wenner BR, Yancy WS, Eisenson H, Musante G, Surwit RS, Millington DS, Butler MD, Svetkey LP (2009) A branched-chain amino acid-related metabolic signature that differentiates obese and lean humans and contributes to insulin resistance. Cell Metab 9:311–326
9. Alberti KGMM, Zimmet P, Shaw J (2006) Metabolic syndrome—a new world-wide definition. A consensus statement from the International Diabetes Federation. Diabet Med 23:469–480

Epidemiology of the Metabolic Syndrome 2

Knut Borch-Johnsen

2.1 Introduction

Insulin resistance—an essential component of the metabolic syndrome—has been known for nearly 70 years. Himsworth [1] suggested the existence of two different types of diabetes: one characterised by high levels of insulin sensitivity (what we now know as type 1 diabetes, characterised by beta-cell destruction) and another characterised by insulin insensitivity (what we now know as type 2 diabetes, characterised by insulin resistance). Detailed, explanatory studies in this field were impossible until the introduction of the radioimmunoassay for insulin in 1960 [2]. This technology opened the door for larger studies of the role of insulin resistance in relation to diabetes as well as to cardiovascular disease (CVD). Throughout the following 25 years the association between hypertension, dyslipidaemia, glucose intolerance and hyperinsulinaemia was established through first smaller case–control studies and subsequently through large, population-based studies [3–6].

In 1988 Reaven reviewed the existing knowledge around the association between insulin resistance and a variety of metabolic risk factors for diabetes and CVD in his paper "Role of insulin resistance in human disease" [7]. Reaven had a background in physiology, and he concludes his review by elegantly proposing a hypothesis offering the suggestion that insulin resistance could be the common denominator underlying a syndromic clustering of metabolic risk factors explaining the clustering of CVD risk factors in selected groups. By doing so, he offered a pathophysiological model that could be tested, confirmed or rejected. The scientific community rather uncritically accepted his suggestion of a new "syndrome", and rather than designing studies that could test his hypothesis, a plethora of studies confirming the basic associations or proposing new markers that were also

K. Borch-Johnsen (✉)
Holbæk Hospital, Smedelundsgade 60, 4300 Holbaek, Denmark
e-mail: knbo@regionsjaelland.dk

H. Beck-Nielsen (ed.), *The Metabolic Syndrome*,
DOI 10.1007/978-3-7091-1331-8_2, © Springer-Verlag Wien 2013

associated with insulin resistance were published. Through this process, epidemiology contributed more to confusion than to clarity and understanding. The observational evidence of association was all too often taken as evidence of causality. The literature proliferation popularised the concept of the "metabolic syndrome", and from being hypothesised in 1988 it became fully established by the World Health Organization (WHO) in 1999 [8]. The underlying rationale was reviewed by the American Diabetes Association (ADA) and the European Association for the Study of Diabetes (EASD) in 2005 [9], and they concluded that: "the criteria are ambiguous and incomplete; the rationale for thresholds are ill defined; the value of including diabetes in the definition is questionable; the role of insulin resistance as the unifying aetiological factor is uncertain; there is no clear basis for including or excluding other CVD risk factors; the CVD risk value is variable and dependent on the specific risk factors present; the CVD risk associated with the "syndrome" appears to be no greater than the sum of its parts; the treatment of the syndrome as a whole is no different from that of each of its components and the medical value of diagnosing the syndrome is unclear".

Despite this rather harsh criticism, the "metabolic syndrome" demonstrated its capacity to survive even in a hostile scientific environment. Definitions of the syndrome were disputed (Chap. 1), but the name survived. Most importantly the rationale changed from being a hypothetical, explanatory physiological model into being that the metabolic syndrome represents an easy risk prediction model identifying individuals at risk of developing CVD (and diabetes) and as such we have learned to live with the term. Many clinicians have found the risk tool easy to use, despite the fact that other risk prediction programmes may be more sensitive and specific in separating those at high risk from those at low risk.

The first section of this chapter will be devoted to classical epidemiological characteristics of the syndrome including global variation in the prevalence of the metabolic syndrome and will focus on the impact of age, gender and ethnicity. The second section of the chapter will focus on the clinical, epidemiological aspects of the syndrome focusing on the ability of the syndrome to predict the risk of developing diabetes and CVD. The concluding section of the chapter will be devoted to reflections on the future of the metabolic syndrome in relation to risk prediction and public health.

2.2 Epidemiology of the Metabolic Syndrome

The rapid changes in the definition over time make it very difficult to compare studies and therefore also to evaluate temporal trends and regional variations in the prevalence of the metabolic syndrome. The most recent definitions have introduced region-specific cut-points for the level of obesity (waist circumference) defining the metabolic syndrome. The introduction of region-specific cut-points is rational from the point of view that the association between obesity and glucose intolerance [10],

Table 2.1 Prevalence of the metabolic syndrome in population-based surveys

Country	Age (year)	Number	Prevalence (%)	Diagnostic criteria	Study
Saudi Arabia	10–18	1,231	10 (M) 8 (F)	NCEP	[15]
Oman	20+	1,419	20 (M) 23 (F)	NCEP	[16]
Turkey	49 ± 13	2,398	27 (M) 39 (F)	NCEP	[17]
Finland	42–60	1,005 males	14 21	NCEP WHO	[18]
India	20+	1,091	8 (M) 18 (F)	NCEP	[19]
United States	12–17	2,014	7 (M) 2 (F)	IDF	[20]
United States	30–79	Framingham offspring 3,224 San Antonio Heart S. 1,081 (white) 1,656 (Mexican Hispanic)	15 (M) 14 (F) 9 (M) 13 (F) 14 (M) 21 (F)	NCEP	[21]
China (urban)	15+	1,206	26 (M) 28 (F)	NCEP	[22]
China (rural)	18–74	13,505 females	22 17 23	IDF NCEP ATP-III modified	[23]

blood pressure [11] and dyslipidaemia [12] varies between ethnic groups. On the other hand, the use of the region-specific cut-points may also mask some of the true regional differences in the prevalence of the syndrome.

2.2.1 Regional Variation in the Metabolic Syndrome

Most epidemiological studies have used definitions that did not include region-specific cut-points for obesity like the National Cholesterol Education Program Adult Treatment Panel III (NCEP ATP-III) [13], European Group for the Study of Insulin Resistance (EGIR) [14] or WHO [8]. Using these definitions, population-based studies have demonstrated marked regional differences in the prevalence of the metabolic syndrome. The highest prevalence is found in the Middle East region (Table 2.1), where more than every third person above the age of 20 fulfils the criteria for having the metabolic syndrome.

Within countries, the prevalence also varies by ethnicity. In the National Health and Nutrition Examination Survey III (NHANES III) [24], the age-adjusted prevalence was 30–40 % higher in people of Mexican–American origin than in persons of White and African–American origin.

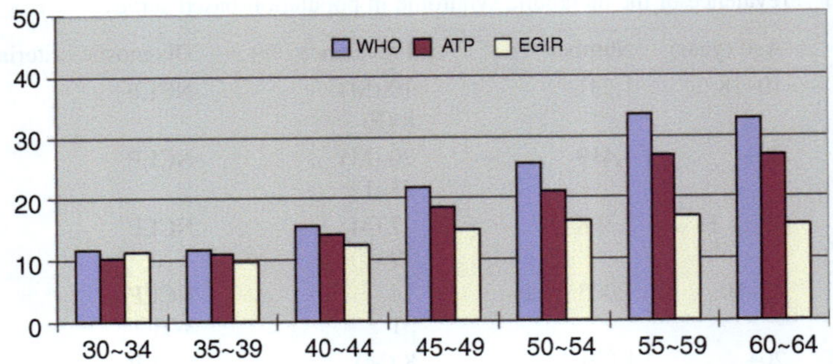

Fig. 2.1 Prevalence of the metabolic syndrome in a population-based sample of 6,667 non-diabetic Danes aged 30–60 years (Inter-99 study). The prevalence increases by age with the diagnostic criteria from the World Health Organization (WHO) [8], the National Cholesterol Education Program Adult Treatment Panel III (NCEP-ATP-III) [13] and the European Group for the Study of Insulin Resistance (EGIR) [14] although the EGIR criteria are less age dependent

2.2.2 Ageing and the Metabolic Syndrome

The prevalence of obesity, hypertension, dyslipidaemia and hyperglycaemia all increase with age (Fig. 2.1), and thus it is not surprising that the prevalence of the metabolic syndrome also increases by age. In a large, collaborative European study [25–27] including 11 population-based cohorts, the prevalence increased markedly from the age of 30, and similar observations have been made in the United States and China [24, 28]. The prevalence peaks around the age of 60–75 years, whereafter it decreases. This decrease is likely to be explained by differential survival of those with and without the metabolic syndrome.

2.2.3 Gender and the Metabolic Syndrome

Data regarding gender effect are conflicting with the majority of the studies finding the highest prevalence in women compared to men [28, 29] while the collaborative European analysis found no gender difference [26, 27]. The conflicting results with respect to gender effect may partly be explained by the application of different definitions for the metabolic syndrome. When applying the NCEP ATP III and the International Diabetes Federation (IDF) criteria respectively to an Asian Indian population, the gender difference was higher using the NCEP-ATP III definition than when applying the IDF criteria [30].

2.3 Consequences of the Metabolic Syndrome

One important argument for maintaining the concept of the metabolic syndrome has been the assumption that presence or absence of the syndrome predicts the future risk of developing diabetes and CVD, respectively. This assumption is natural as the definition of the metabolic syndrome includes important risk factors for both diabetes and CVD. Consequently, the rational question is not whether the presence of the metabolic syndrome predicts development of diabetes or CVD, but rather whether the presence of the syndrome predicts these diseases over and above the predictive value of the individual components of the syndrome.

2.3.1 Prediction of Diabetes by the Metabolic Syndrome

Several epidemiological studies have shown that presence of the metabolic syndrome increases the probability of developing type 2 diabetes three to fourfold, and that the risk increases with the number of elements of the syndrome present. This has been shown using several different definitions of the metabolic syndrome [51, 18, 52–54, 31]. Some very strong risk factors for development of type 2 diabetes are not included in the definition, the most important being age and family history. These factors are among the strongest predictors of diabetes in diabetes risk scores like the FINDRISK [32] and the Danish diabetes risk score [33].

In 2004 Stern et al. [34] published an analysis where they compared the NCEP ATP-III definition of the metabolic syndrome [13] with the San Antonio Heart Study risk score for diabetes [35] with respect to ability to predict future development of diabetes. Their analysis was based on two population-based cohorts: the San Antonio Heart Study [36], including 3,301 Mexican Americans and 1,857 non-Hispanic whites, aged 25–64 years at baseline and followed for a median of 7 years and the Mexico City Diabetes Study [55], including 2,282 persons aged 35–64 years followed for a median of 6.3 years. As shown in Table 2.2, both the metabolic syndrome and the diabetes risk score predicted incident diabetes (as expected), but if the effect of the metabolic syndrome was adjusted for the effect of the diabetes risk score, then the odds ratio was reduced from 6.3 to 1.9. In contrast, when the effect of the diabetes risk score was adjusted for the effect of the components of the metabolic syndrome, then this only markedly reduced the odds ratio from 6.5 to 5.2. Consequently, diabetes risk scores appear to be of greater value in identifying those at risk of developing diabetes and therefore at need of lifestyle intervention [38–40].

2.3.2 Prediction of CVD by the Metabolic Syndrome

Numerous studies have confirmed that presence of the metabolic syndrome increases the risk of subsequent development of CVD [18, 26, 27, 41–43]. Unfortunately, some of the definitions of the metabolic syndrome have included individuals with diabetes, and consequently some studies of the association of the syndrome with incident CVD may have been confounded by the strong association between diabetes and CVD.

As was the case for the prediction of diabetes, several important and very strong risk factors for CVD are not included in the metabolic syndrome. The two most

Table 2.2 Odds ratio (95 % confidence interval (CI)) for prediction of diabetes and cardiovascular disease using the metabolic syndrome (NCEP ATP-III), the San Antonio Diabetes Risk Score [35] and the Framingham Risk Score [37]

	Univariate	Multivariate
Prediction of diabetes in the San Antonio heart study		
Metabolic syndrome	6.32 (4.61–8.65)	1.94 (1.34–2.82)
Diabetes risk score	6.46 (4.97–8.40)	5.18 (3.89–6.91)
Prediction of diabetes in the Mexico City diabetes study		
Metabolic syndrome	2.63 (1.80–3.85)	1.15 (0.74–1.77)
Diabetes risk score	4.22 (3.11–5.72)	4.03 (2.87–5.65)
Prediction of CVD in the San Antonio heart study		
Metabolic syndrome	4.28 (3.08–5.94)	1.50 (1.03–2.18)
Framingham risk score	9.41 (6.53–13.6)	7.87 (5.29–11.7)

The multivariate model for prediction of diabetes combined the metabolic syndrome and the diabetes risk score in a stepwise model. The multivariate model for prediction of cardiovascular disease combined with the metabolic syndrome and the Framingham risk score (From [34])
NCEP ATP-III National Cholesterol Education Program Adult Treatment Panel III

important are not only age and smoking but also family history and physical activity are generally included in CVD risk scores.

The previously mentioned study by Stern et al. [34] based on the San Antonio Heart Study and the Mexico City Diabetes Study also analysed whether presence or absence of the metabolic syndrome improved the identification of individuals at risk of developing CVD when risk prediction was based on the Framingham Risk Score for incident CVD [37]. In the analysis of prediction of CVD, only data from the San Antonio Heart Study were included. As shown in Table 2.2, the odds ratio for CVD based on the univariate analysis using the Framingham Risk Score was 9.4 compared with 4.3 for the metabolic syndrome. In the multivariate analysis, where the effect of the metabolic syndrome was adjusted for the effect of the Framingham Risk Score and vice versa, the results were even clearer. In the multivariate analysis, the odds ratio using the metabolic syndrome decreased from 4.3 to 1.5, while for the Framingham Risk Score decreased from 9.4 to 7.9. Similar conclusions were drawn by Eddy et al. [44] and Sattar et al. [31] based on other CVD risk scores.

2.4 The Future of the Metabolic Syndrome in Epidemiology, Risk Prediction and Clinical Practice

While the definition of the syndrome has been disputed, and while its relevance as risk predictor for diabetes and CVD is still controversial, there is still no doubt that the term has been established and is likely to stay. Unless the definition of the syndrome continues to change, it may also be a simple tool for monitoring the future societal risk diabetes and CVD based on risk factors that can easily be monitored. This type of monitoring at regional or country level may guide health authorities in prioritising and targeting their preventive efforts.

At the individual level, presence or absence of the metabolic syndrome appears to create a tool for guiding the clinician and the patient with respect to the risk of developing diabetes. For diabetes, other risk assessment tools are available. Most of these can be self-administered and most do not require blood sampling or measurements by health professionals [32, 33, 45–48]. The challenge when using risk scores, however, seems to be sure they are implemented rather than choosing the right test [49].

For prediction of CVD, the problem is even greater. Although the metabolic syndrome predicts the development of CVD, it is still by far outperformed by other, very well-validated CVD risk scores like the Framingham Risk Score and by the European correspondent, the Systematic Coronary Risk Evaluation (SCORE) [50].

The real importance of the syndrome may well be reverting to the hypothesis formulated by Reaven in [7]. Although nearly 25 years have passed since his Banting lecture, many of his questions regarding the role of insulin resistance in human disease remain unanswered. If these are answered, they may guide us in our efforts to prevent the development of diabetes and CVD.

References

1. Himsworth H (1936) Diabetes mellitus: a differentiation into insulin-sensitive and insulin-insensitive types. Lancet 1:127–130
2. Yalow RS, Berson SA (1960) Plasma insulin concentrations in nondiabetic and early diabetic subjects: determinations by a new sensitive immunoassay technique. Diabetes 9:254–260
3. Avogaro P, Crepaldi G, Enzi G, Tiengo A (1967) Associazione di iperlidemia, diabete mellito e obesita di medio grado. Acto Diabetol Lat 4:36–41
4. Orchard TJ, Becker DJ, Bates M, Kuller LH, Drash AL (1983) Plasma insulin and lipoprotein concentrations: an atherogenic association? Am J Epidemiol 188:326–337
5. Stern MP, Haffner SM (1986) Body fat distribution and hyperinsulinemia as risk factors for diabetes and cardiovascular disease. Atherosclerosis 6:123–130
6. Ferrannini E, Buzzigoli G, Bonadornna R, Giorico MA, Oleggini M, Graziadei L, Pedrinelli R, Brandi L, Bevilacqua S (1987) Insulin resistance in essential hypertension. N Engl J Med 317:350–357
7. Reaven GM (1988) Banting lecture 1988. Role of insulin resistance in human disease. Diabetes 37:1595–1607
8. World Health Organization (1999) Definition, diagnosis and classification of diabetes mellitus and its complications. Part 1: diagnosis and classification of diabetes mellitus. WHO, Geneva
9. Kahn R, Buse J, Ferrannini E, Stern M (2005) The metabolic syndrome: time for a critical appraisal. Diabetologia 48:1684–1699
10. Nakagami T, Qiao Q, Carstensen B, Nøhr-Hansen C, Hu G, Tuomilehto J, Balkau B, Borch-Johnsen K (2003) The DECODE-DECODA Study Group. Age, body mass index and Type 2 diabetes—associations modified by ethnicity. Diabetologia 46:1063–1070
11. Saad MF, Lilloja S, Nyomba BL et al (1991) Racial differences in the relation between blood pressure and insulin resistance. N Eng J Med 324:733–739

12. Lee CM, Huxley RR, Woodward M et al (2008) The metabolic syndrome identifies a heterogeneous group of metabolic component combinations in the Asia-Pacific region. Diabetes Res Clin Pract 8:377–380
13. NCEP (2001) Third report of the national cholesterol education program (NCEP) expert panel on detection, evaluation and treatment of high blood cholesterol in adults (Adult Treatment Panel III). JAMA 285:2486–2497
14. Balkau B, Charles MA (1999) Comment on the provisional report from the WHO consultation. European Group for the Study of Insulin Resistance (EGIR). Diabet Med 16:442–443
15. Al-Daghri NM (2010) Extremely high prevalence of metabolic syndrome manifestations among Arab youth: a call for early intervention. Eur J Clin Invest 40:1063–1066
16. Al-Lawati JA, Mohammed AJ, Al-Hinai HQ, Jousilahti P (2003) Prevalence of the metabolic syndrome among Omani adults. Diabetes Care 26:1781–1785
17. Onat A, Ceyhan K, Basar O, Erer B, Toprak S, Sansoy V (2002) Metabolic syndrome: major impact on coronary risk in a population with low cholesterol levels—a prospective and cross sectional evaluation. Atherosclerosis 165:285–292
18. Lakka HM, Laaksonen DE, Lakka TA, Niskanen LK, Kumpusalo E, Tuomilehto J, Salonen JT (2002) The metabolic syndrome and total and cardiovascular disease mortality in middle-aged men. JAMA 288:2709–2716
19. Gupta A, Gupta R, Sarna M, Rastogi S, Gupta VP, Kothari K (2003) Prevalence of diabetes, impaired fasting glucose and insulin resistance syndrome in an urban Indian population. Diabetes Res Clin Pract 61:69–76
20. Ford ES, Li C, Zhao G, Pearson WS, Mokdad AH (2008) Prevalence of the metabolic syndrome among US adolescents using the definition from the international diabetes federation. Diabetes Care 31:587–589
21. Meigs JB, Wilson PWF, Nathan DM, D'Agostino RB, Williams K, Haffner SM (2003) Prevalence and characteristics of the metabolic syndrome in the San Antonio Heart and Framingham Offspring Studies. Diabetes 52:2160–2167
22. Li JB, Wang X, Zhang JX, Gu P, Zhang X, Chen CX, Guo R, Wu M (2010) Metabolic syndrome: prevalence and risk factors in southern China. J Int Med Res 38:1142–1148
23. Cai H, Huang J, Xu G, Yang Z, Liu M, Mi Y, Liu W, Wang H, Qian D (2012) Prevalence and determinants of metabolic syndrome among women in Chinese rural areas. PLoS One 7(5): e36936
24. Ford ES, Giles WH, Dietz WH (2002) Prevalence of the metabolic syndrome among US adults: findings from the third National Health and Nutrition Examination Survey. JAMA 287:356–359
25. Qiao Q, Tuomilehto J, Balkau B, Borch-Johnsen K, Heine R, Wareham NJ, DECODE Study Group (2005) Are insulin resistance, impaired fasting glucose and impaired glucose tolerance all equally strongly related to age? Diabet Med 22:1476–1481
26. Hu G, Qiao Q, Tuomilehto J et al (2004) Prevalence of the metabolic syndrome and its relation to all-cause mortality in non-diabetic European men and women. Arch Intern Med 164:1066–1076
27. Hu G, Qiao Q, Tuomilehto J, Eliasson M, Feskens EJ, Pyörälä K, DECODE Insulin Study Group (2004) Plasma insulin and cardiovascular mortality in non-diabetic European men and women: a meta-analysis of data from eleven prospective studies. Diabetologia 47:1245–1256
28. Gu D, Reynolds K, Wu X et al (2005) Prevalence of the metabolic syndrome and overweight among adults in China. Lancet 365:1398–1405
29. Ford ES, Giles WH, Mokdad AH (2004) Increasing prevalence of the metabolic syndrome among US adults. Diabetes Care 27:2444–2449
30. Wasir JS, Misra A, Vikram NK, Pandey RM, Gupta R (2008) Comparison of definitions of the metabolic syndrome in adult Asian Indians. J Assoc Physicians India 56:158–164
31. Sattar N, McConnachie A, Shaper AG, Blauw GJ, Buckley BM, de Craen AJ, Ford I, Forouhi NG, Freeman DJ, Jukema JW, Lennon L, Macfarlane PW, Murphy MB, Packard CJ, Stott DJ, Westendorp RG, Whincup PH, Shepherd J, Wannamethee SG (2008) Can metabolic syndrome

usefully predict cardiovascular disease and diabetes? Outcome data from two prospective studies. Lancet 371:1927–1935
32. Lindström J, Tuomilehto J (2003) The diabetes risk score: a practical tool to predict type 2 diabetes risk. Diabetes Care 26:725–731
33. Glümer C, Carstensen B, Sandbæk A, Lauritzen T, Jørgensen T, Borch-Johnsen K (2004) A Danish diabetes risk score for targeted screening. Diabetes Care 27:727–733
34. Stern MP et al (2004) Does the metabolic syndrome improve identification of individuals at risk of type 2 diabetes and/or cardiovascular disease. Diabetes Care 27:2676–2681
35. Stern MP, Williams K, Haffner SM (2002) Identification of individuals at high risk of type 2 diabetes: do we need the oral glucose tolerance test? Ann Intern Med 136:575–581
36. Haffner SM, Miettenen H, Gaskill SP, Stern MP (1990) Metabolic predictors of hypertension: the San Antonio Heart Study. Arch Intern Med 156:1994–2000
37. Wilson PWF, D'Agostino RB, Levy D, Belanger AM, Silbershatz H, Kannel WB (1998) Prediction of coronary heart disease using risk factor categories. Circulation 97:1837–1847
38. Tuomilehto J, Lindström J, Eriksson JG, Valle TT, Hämäläinen H, Ilanne-Parikka P, Keinänen-Kiukaanniemi S, Laakso M (2001) Prevention of type 2 diabetes mellitus by changes in lifestyle among subjects with impaired glucose tolerance. N Eng J Med 344:1343–1350
39. Pan X, Li G, Hu Y et al (1997) Effects of diet and exercise in preventing NIDDM in people with impaired glucose tolerance: the Da Qing IGT and diabetes study. Diabetes Care 20:537–44
40. The Diabetes Prevention Program Research Group (2002) Reduction in the incidence of type 2 diabetes with life style intervention or metformin. N Engl J Med 346:393–403
41. Pyörälä M, Miettinen H, Halonen P, Laakso M, Pyörälä K (2000) Insulin resistance syndrome predicts the risk of coronary heart disease and stroke in healthy middle-aged men: the 22-year follow-up results of the Helsinki Policemen Study. Arterioscler Thromb Vasc Biol 20:538–544
42. Isomaa B, Almgren P, Tuomi T, Forsén B, Lahti K, Nissén M, Taskinen MR, Groop L (2001) Cardiovascular morbidity and mortality associated with the metabolic syndrome. Diabetes Care 24:683–689
43. Girman CJ, Rhodes T, Mercuri M, Pyörälä K, Kjekshus J, Pedersen TR, Beere PA, Gotto AM, Clearfield M, S Group and the AFCAPS/TexCAPS Research Group (2004) The metabolic syndrome and risk of major coronary events in the Scandinavian Simvastatin Survival Study (4S) and the Air Force/Texas Coronary Atherosclerosis Prevention Study (AFCAPS/TexCAPS). Am J Cardiol 93:136–141
44. Eddy DM, Schlessinger L, Heikes K (2008) The metabolic syndrome and cardiovascular risk: implications for clinical practice. Int J Obes 32(Suppl 2):S5–S10
45. Herman WH, Smith PJ, Thomson TJ, Engelgau MM, Aubert RE (1995) A new and simple questionnaire to identify people at increased risk of undiagnosed diabetes. Diabetes Care 18:382–387
46. Ruige JB, Neeling JND, Kostence PJ, Bouter LM, Heine RJ (1997) Performance of an NIDDM screening questionnaire based on symptoms and risk factors. Diabetes Care 20:491–496
47. Baan CA, Ruige JB, Stolk RP, Witteman JC, Dekker JM, Heine RJ, Feskens EJ (1999) Performance of a predictive model to indentify undiagnosed diabetes in a health care setting. Diabetes Care 22:213–219
48. Griffin SJ, Little PS, Hales CN, Kinmonth AL, Wareham NJ (2000) Diabetes risk score: towards earlier detection of Type 2 diabetes in general practice. Diabetes Metab Res Rev 16:164–171
49. Christensen JO, Sandbaek A, Laurtizen T, Borch-Johnsen K (2004) Population-based stepwise screening for unrecognised type 2 diabetes ineffective in general practice despite reliable algorithms. Diabetologia 47:1566–1573
50. Conroy RM, Pyörälä K, Fitzgerald AP et al (2003) Estimation of 10-year risk of fatal cardiovascular disease in Europe: the SCORE project. Eur Heart J 24:987–1003
51. Hanson RL, Imperatore G, Bennett PH, Knowler WC (2002) Components of the "metabolic syndrome" and incidence of type 2 diabetes. Diabetes 51:3120–3127

52. Ford ES (2005) Risk for all-cause mortality, cardiovascular disease and diabetes associated with the metabolic syndrome: a summary of the evidence. Diabetes Care 28:1769–1778
53. Wilson PW, D'Agostino RB, Parise H, Sullivan L, Meigs JB (2005) Metabolic Syndrome as a precursor of cardiovascular disease and type 2 diabetes mellitus. Circulation 112:3066–3072
54. Meigs JB (2006) Metabolic Syndrome and risk for type 2 diabetes. Expert Rev Endocrinol Metab 1:57–66
55. Burke JP, Williams K, Haffner SM, Villalpando CG, Stern MP (2001) Elevated incidence of type 2 diabetes in San Antonio, Texas, compared with that of Mexico City, Mexico. Diabetes Care 24:1573–1578

Pathophysiology of the Metabolic Syndrome

3

John J. Nolan and Donal J. O'Gorman

3.1 Introduction

The metabolic syndrome is an increasingly prevalent clinical syndrome, closely related to the risk of progression to type 2 diabetes, to cardiovascular disease (CVD) and to several cancers [1–4]. Despite its prevalence (at about 20 % of many western populations and much higher in several high risk populations), it has been a controversial topic since it was first described, largely because of lack of agreement about criteria for definition and diagnosis [5–7]. This has been further compounded by lack of clarity about how the syndrome should be treated. In this chapter, we focus on the pathophysiology of the metabolic syndrome. At the core of this pathophysiology is a gradual and progressive distortion of normal metabolic homeostasis, affecting all of the major metabolically active organs and tissues. Here we will describe these abnormalities in physiology, with the aim of providing a basis on which the treatment of this syndrome can be addressed in a scientifically and medically rational manner.

3.2 Clinical Phenotype and Pathophysiology

3.2.1 Obesity and Disorders of Adipose Tissue

Failure of weight regulation and the onset of obesity, particularly abdominal obesity, is central to the pathophysiology of the metabolic syndrome [8]. This is clear from the various iterations in recent years of the definition of the syndrome, all

J.J. Nolan (✉)
Steno Diabetes Center A/S, Niels Steensens Vej 2-4, 2820 Gentofte, Denmark
e-mail: jjnl@steno.dk

D.J. O'Gorman
Centre for Preventive Medicine, Dublin City University, Health and Human Performance, Dublin 9, Ireland
e-mail: donal.ogorman@dcu.ie

H. Beck-Nielsen (ed.), *The Metabolic Syndrome*,
DOI 10.1007/978-3-7091-1331-8_3, © Springer-Verlag Wien 2013

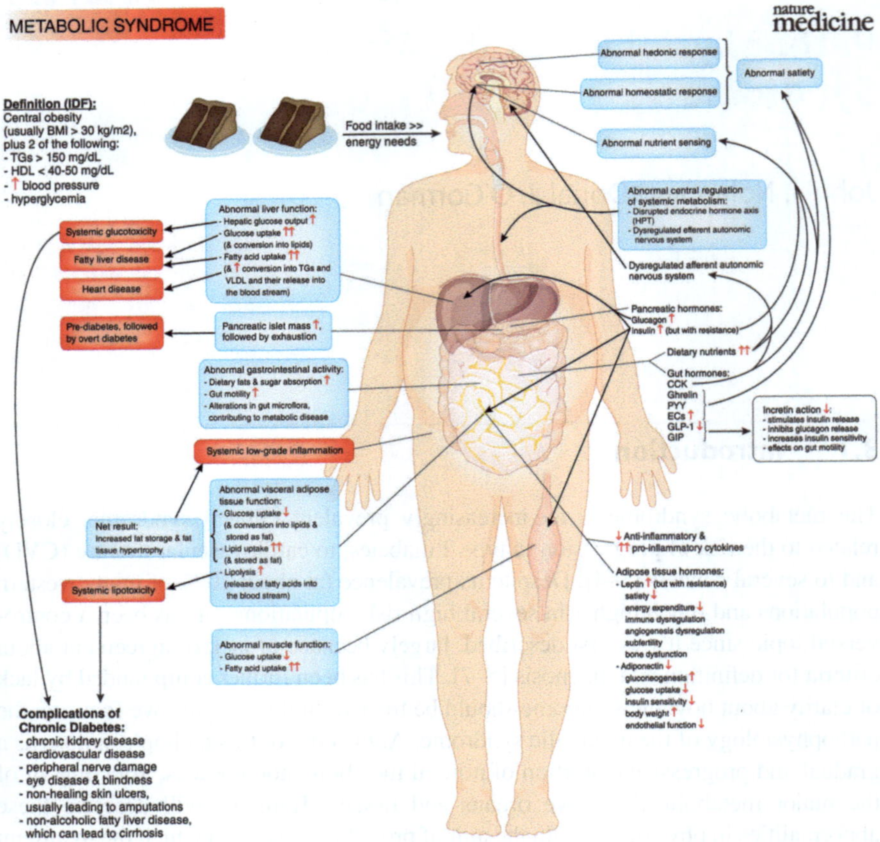

Fig. 3.1 An overview of the aetiology of the metabolic syndrome (Nature Medicine: http://www.nature.com/nm/poster/eposter_full.html)

of which have included some measure of central obesity. The modern pandemic of obesity has been the driving force behind the increasing prevalence of the metabolic syndrome and its later progression to both type 2 diabetes and CVD [8–12].

Weight gain, whether due to increased caloric intake or reduced expenditure in physical activity, can lead to an alteration of normal visceral adipose tissue function (see Fig. 3.1). This is the key element in the pathogenesis of the metabolic syndrome. Weight gain is not always associated with this progressive syndrome. Healthy individuals may experience fluctuations in weight without the associated metabolic perturbations. In the metabolic syndrome, visceral adipose tissue metabolism is altered, with decreased glucose uptake (due to insulin resistance), increased lipid uptake and increased storage of fat as well as increased lipolysis (also due to tissue insulin resistance), and, crucially, increased release of non-esterified ("free") fatty acids (FFA) into the circulation. Hypertrophied intra-abdominal adipocytes are resistant to the antilipolytic effects of insulin [13]. This leads to an increased flux of FFA from the visceral adipose tissue compartment to the liver, resulting in increased liver fat, increased hepatic glucose output and decreased overall liver function. Consistent with these abnormalities, the obesity pandemic has been associated with a dramatic and rapid increase in the prevalence of non-alcoholic hepatic steatosis, a serious chronic liver disease in its own right, with risk of progression to end stage liver disease and death [14]. Insulin resistance in the liver is associated with decreased apolipoprotein B degradation and increased production of triglyceride-rich lipoproteins. In obesity, adipose tissue is infiltrated by macrophages, contributing to an increased state of chronic inflammation. Many of the cytokine products of adipose tissue are altered in character and concentration in viscerally obese subjects. Typically C-reactive protein (CRP), Interleukin (IL)-6 and tumour necrosis factor α (TNFα) are increased, while adiponectin is decreased. The overall effect of the increase in visceral adipose tissue is an alteration of FFA metabolism coupled with a proinflammatory profile, both of which are associated with insulin resistance and altered glucose homeostasis typical of pre-diabetes and progression to type 2 diabetes [15]. Thus, the impact of changes in visceral adipose tissue can be described as a state of systemic lipotoxicity associated with low-grade systemic inflammation, mediated through changes in liver metabolism of both carbohydrate and fat.

3.2.2 Insulin Resistance

The metabolic syndrome since its first description has been intimately associated with insulin resistance. However, unlike previous definitions, the current definition of the syndrome does not include a specific reference to insulin resistance. A very practical fact underlies this issue: insulin resistance is difficult to measure in clinical practice and still remains a clinical research measurement. The gold standard measurement technique using the hyperinsulinaemic glucose clamp is time-consuming (several hours minimum), expensive and completely unrealistic in clinical practice. A wide range of surrogate measurements are possible, many of which are validated against the clamp, all of which involve some expense and investigation beyond what is available in routine clinical practice. Without specifically requiring a measurement of insulin resistance, the current definition of the metabolic syndrome comprises the most common clinical features of insulin resistance: central obesity, a characteristic classic dyslipidaemia, hypertension and elevation in fasting glucose. The importance of insulin resistance as the underlying metabolic milieu is that insulin resistance is a major risk factor for the development of diabetes, and thus for the later complications of diabetes especially CVD, chronic kidney disease, retinopathy and neuropathy. As already described above, insulin resistance is the best unifying hypothesis for the pathophysiology of the metabolic syndrome. A major contributor to the development of insulin resistance is the alteration in fat metabolism, with an excess of circulating FFA originating either from adipose tissue triglyceride stores (released by hormone sensitive lipase) or from triglyceride-rich lipoproteins [by the action of lipoprotein lipase (LPL)] [16, 17]. Insulin plays a key role in the suppression of lipolysis by both these routes, and a very early sign of impaired insulin action is the failure of this mechanism. Increased circulating FFA further impairs the anti-lipolytic effect of insulin, exacerbating this effect. Excess FFA contribute to insulin resistance in insulin target tissues such as skeletal muscle and liver, through several cellular mechanisms [18]. In addition to these effects, it has also been shown that insulin-resistant subjects display abnormalities of mitochondrial oxidative phosphorylation that correlate with the accumulation of triglycerides and other related fat molecules in muscle tissue [19], [20]. More recently, the field of metabolomics has begun to demonstrate a completely new profile of the metabolic "signature" of insulin resistance at a more fundamental level. Characteristic of this signature is a preponderance of branched chain amino acids (BCAA), along with the expected higher circulating concentrations of total and various species of FFA [21, 22]. What is important about these new insights from metabolomics is that amino acid data have been shown to provide information on the future risk of diabetes beyond what could be known from standard risk factors (such as body mass index (BMI), diet pattern and fasting glucose). Thus, metabolomic patterns can be correlated with standard measures of insulin resistance and beta-cell function, but amino acid concentrations have been shown also to be accurately predictive of diabetes progression even among individuals with similar fasting insulin and glucose concentrations. The more that can be understood concerning the underlying metabolic basis of insulin resistance, the better will be the capacity to use specific metabolic or metabolomic measurements to assess risk (of later diabetes and complications). One of the ongoing clinical challenges is that not all obese individuals are insulin resistant nor do all obese subjects progress to develop diabetes. Some lean individuals are insulin resistant and develop type 2 diabetes, in spite of an apparently low risk phenotype.

3.2.3 Metabolic Flexibility

Another approach to understand the biological basis of the metabolic syndrome is the concept of metabolic flexibility, which is the capacity of the organism to adapt fuel oxidation to fuel availability. For example, the inability to modify fuel oxidation in response to changes in nutrient availability has been implicated in the accumulation of intramyocellular lipid and insulin resistance in skeletal muscle [23]. The epidemiology of the metabolic syndrome could be explained by the change in the dietary habits of modern populations to an energy-dense diet high in fats. Following on from these sustained (if even minor) changes in nutrient intake, an impaired capacity to up-regulate muscle lipid oxidation in the face of high lipid supply in some subjects may lead to increased muscle fat accumulation and insulin resistance. As outlined previously, the chronic accumulation of lipids as triglycerides and other molecular species including ceramides and diglycerides (lipotoxicity) can impair insulin action through a variety of mechanisms [18]. Conversely, the ability to adjust and increase lipid oxidation in response to increased availability (or metabolic flexibility) reduces the formation of harmful lipid products such as ceramides and diglycerides, and thus protects against changes in insulin sensitivity. The term "metabolic flexibility" was first termed by Kelley and Mandarino as "the capacity to switch from predominantly lipid oxidation and high rates of fatty acid uptake during fasting conditions to the suppression of lipid oxidation and increased glucose uptake, oxidation, and storage under insulin-stimulated conditions" [24]. Consistent with this description, the switch from carbohydrate to lipid oxidation during an overnight fast or in response to high-fat diets [measurable by a reduction in respiratory quotient (RQ)] are examples of normal metabolic flexibility. An underlying component of the metabolic syndrome is the maladaptation of modern man to increased fat availability in typical western diets. Individuals who are metabolically inflexible are prone under these conditions to the accumulation of harmful lipid species in metabolically active tissues such as muscle, adipose tissue and liver, where these compounds may contribute to reduced insulin sensitivity. An important corollary to this is that lifestyle changes (reduction in dietary fat intake coupled with physical activity and weight loss) can restore or improve metabolic flexibility in skeletal muscle, thereby contributing to improved insulin action and prevention of diabetes.

3.2.4 Blood Pressure

The relationship between elevated blood pressure and insulin resistance has been extensively studied. High blood pressure is a classical feature of the metabolic syndrome. It has been reported that up to one-third of hypertensive subjects have a clinical phenotype of the metabolic syndrome. A number of potential physiological mechanisms for this association have been documented [25]. Insulin has vasodilatory effects in healthy subjects and also contributes to sodium retention in the kidney [26]. There are important differences between white people, Africans and Asians in these mechanisms. In insulin-resistant subjects, the vasodilatory effect of insulin is lost [27], while the sodium retention is maintained, which may contribute to elevation of blood pressure. Another potential mechanism of blood pressure elevation is the effect of insulin to stimulate the sympathetic nervous system. Further possible mechanisms include oxidative stress, endothelial dysfunction and an activated renin–angiotensin system, all pro-hypertensive effects and all of which have been shown to be more common in subjects with the metabolic syndrome. However, large scale studies suggest that the overall contribution of insulin resistance per se to elevated blood pressure is modest [28]. The mechanistic relationship between hypertension and the metabolic syndrome has been outlined in a recent review by Yanai and colleagues [29].

3.2.5 Lipids

As already outlined, the metabolic syndrome is fundamentally a disorder of lipid metabolism. In clinical practice, the metabolic syndrome is associated with a "classic" dyslipidaemia phenotype of elevated triglycerides (and FFA), together with reduced high-density lipoprotein (HDL)-cholesterol and changes in the low-density lipoprotein (LDL) particle to a smaller, denser and more atherogenic variant. This classical plasma lipoprotein phenotype results from increased FFA flux to the liver, leading to increased production of apo B-containing triglyceride-rich very low-density lipoproteins (VLDL). Under conditions of normal physiology, insulin inhibits the secretion of VLDL into the circulation. In the setting of insulin resistance, this homeostasis is lost, and hypertriglyceridaemia results, becoming a central component of the criteria for diagnosis of the metabolic syndrome. In the presence of hypertriglyceridaemia, a decrease in the cholesterol content of HDL results from decreases in the cholesteryl ester content of the lipoprotein core, with variable increases in triglyceride making the particle small and dense [30]. This alteration of the composition of the lipoprotein leads to increased clearance of HDL from the circulation. LDL is also changed in composition in the setting of insulin resistance and the metabolic syndrome. Subjects in whom triglycerides (in the fasting state) exceed 2.0 mmol/l usually have a predominance of small dense LDL circulating [31, 32]. In this modified LDL particle, unesterified cholesterol, esterified cholesterol and phospholipid are depleted, while LDL triglyceride is either unchanged or increased. Small dense LDL is considered to be more atherogenic than buoyant LDL, for a number of possible reasons, including: it is more toxic to the endothelium, it has a greater ability to transit through the endothelial basement membrane, it adheres to glycosaminoglycans, it is more susceptible to oxidation, it is more selectively bound to scavenger receptors on monocyte-derived macrophages [33, 34]. Taken together, the combined altered lipid phenotype, which is typical for the metabolic syndrome, constitutes an increased risk phenotype for CVD and is a key clinical characteristic of the syndrome.

3.3 Genetic and Environmental Contributors

The development of the metabolic syndrome is associated with positive energy balance that results in lipid accumulation and weight gain. The outcomes of energy imbalance are quantified by changes in waist circumference and BMI. However, the underlying physiology is more complex and represents a multi-system change in metabolic regulation that results in insulin resistance, increased sympathetic nervous system activity, endothelial dysfunction, hypertension and an increase in circulating triglycerides. The environmental and genetic contributors to the aetiology of the metabolic syndrome are presented below.

3.3.1 Environment

3.3.1.1 Physical Inactivity

Energy expenditure is not only required to sustain life by supporting the function of body tissues but is also necessary to conduct voluntary movements of daily living.

Man has evolved to support physical activity as a necessary means of hunting and gathering food based primarily on the production of energy by aerobic means [35, 36]. Modern living is associated with lower levels of occupational and recreational physical activity due to technological advances. When energy expenditure is decreased and energy intake stays the same, or increases, the excess energy is stored in adipose and other body tissues. Physical inactivity is associated with more than 30 chronic diseases and despite the known benefits of living an active life, a significant proportion of the population still do not meet the recommended targets.

Daily energy expenditure can be broadly classified into exercise or non-exercise activity thermogenesis (NEAT). Those who exercise, or perform structured physical activity, have a lower risk of cardiovascular and all-cause mortality as well as the metabolic syndrome and type 2 diabetes [35, 36]. The impact of NEAT accounts for all other activities and has great potential as a contributor to daily energy expenditure as we are awake for approximately 16 h per day. The impact of modern lifestyle and technology has been to reduce NEAT to the point where adults in the United States are sedentary for approximately 55 %, or 7.7 h, of their non-sleep time [37].

Sedentary time, defined as sitting or lying while awake, is associated with an increased risk of type 2 diabetes, CVD as well as all-cause and cardiovascular mortality [38]. Sitting time confers a twofold increased risk of the metabolic syndrome and is related to other risk factors including weight and adipose tissue gain. Television viewing, often used as a surrogate marker of sedentary time, is associated with a dose-dependent increase in the prevalence of the metabolic syndrome as well as increased risk of obesity, type 2 diabetes, hypertension, high triglycerides and low HDL cholesterol [39–41]. Therefore, physical inactivity is likely to be an important contributor to the development of the metabolic syndrome and may offset the benefits of recommended levels of physical activity.

It is reasonable to question whether a 30 min bout of exercise, 5 days per week, is enough to offset the impact of 7–8 h of daily sedentary time. The 1st Stock Conference on obesity reported that daily energy expenditure should be approximately 500 kcal/day more than energy expenditure in sedentary activities [42]. The Institute of Medicine report also found that those who remained lean throughout their life had daily energy expenditure approximately 70 % greater than their basal metabolic rate. Both of these reports suggest that a sedentary individual would require 45–60 min of physical activity to attain this target [42, 43]. Sedentary time predicts the development of the metabolic syndrome independent of exercise, BMI or other indices of adiposity [39]. This suggests that metabolic risk factors cannot be offset by current physical activity recommendations and reducing sedentary time has to become a key element of future strategies. Sedentary time has a strong inverse relationship with light physical activity, but not with moderate to vigorous activity associated with exercise training [38]. Therefore, the replacement of light physical activity accrued from daily occupational and recreational activities by sedentary activities such as TV viewing could be the major factor contributing to increase the risk of metabolic syndrome.

While most of these findings are based on association studies, the more controlled and extreme model of bed rest has provided direct evidence of metabolic alterations due to physical inactivity [44, 45]. With as little as 3–5 days of reduced activity, there are marked changes in glucose tolerance and insulin sensitivity [46]. Skeletal muscle accounts for approximately 80 % of insulin-mediated glucose disposal and a decrease in glucose uptake and glycogen synthesis has been reported from 7 days of bed rest [47, 48]. Many of the original bed rest studies provided a nutrient intake to maintain body mass. However, the inactivity associated loss of muscle mass meant fat mass increased during these studies to maintain body mass. Subsequent studies that have controlled fat mass during bed rest have shown that inactivity per se leads to a greater postabsorptive and postprandial insulin response, without a change in plasma glucose concentrations. In addition to, or as a consequence of insulin resistance, bed rest studies have shown an increase in postprandial lipids due to a decrease in plasma clearance. This has been confirmed by a decrease in lipid oxidation and an increase in ectopic fat accumulation [44].

In conclusion, physical inactivity is a major contributor to the development of the metabolic syndrome due to the decrease in daily energy expenditure and the reduction in the physiological stimuli required to maintain normal metabolic function. The strategy of promoting daily physical activity of at least 30 min, while based on evidence of decreased cardiovascular risk, is unlikely to offset the time spent engaged in sedentary activities. The dramatic increase in sedentary time in recent years, at the expense of light daily activities, has removed a significant portion of daily energy expenditure. These studies have demonstrated strong links between inactivity and risk factors of the metabolic syndrome, while bed rest studies have shown that the physiology of inactivity promotes insulin resistance, hyperlipidaemia and ectopic lipid accumulation.

3.3.1.2 Nutrition

The relationship between energy intake, body mass and the metabolic syndrome is well established. In the past few decades, daily energy intake has increased and this change is positively associated with metabolic syndrome risk factors [49, 50]. Excessive nutrient intake, in itself, confers greater risk, but recent data suggest that specific nutrients can accelerate the development of the metabolic syndrome.

Dietary carbohydrate: Most common carbohydrates, once ingested, are metabolised to glucose. Glucose stimulates insulin secretion from the pancreatic beta-cells to facilitate glucose transport into cells and tissues of the body. The industrialisation of food production has resulted in greater processing and preservation. One of the consequences of these steps has been a dramatic increase in fructose consumption. Fructose is a naturally occurring monosaccharide, commonly found in fruit, but can be produced cheaply as a sweetener or preservative. The most common form is sucrose, a disaccharide of glucose and fructose, that is enzymatically produced from cornstarch and present in many foods linked to risk factors of the metabolic syndrome including soft drinks [49, 51].

There are a number of differences between fructose and glucose that increase the risk of the metabolic syndrome when excessively consumed. Unlike glucose, fructose does not stimulate insulin secretion and is almost completely metabolised in the liver. While the metabolic pathways are distinct from glucose, the substrates of fructose metabolism can be oxidised or stored as glycogen within the liver or else converted to glucose and lactate and released into circulation [49, 51]. Glucose metabolism is regulated by the cellular energy status and in particular by negative feedback from enzymes such as adenosine monophosphate kinase (AMPK) as well as metabolic substrates such as citrate and adenosine diphosphate (ADP). However, fructose is not regulated in the same way and, to a certain extent, by-passes many of the usual glucose regulatory processes, including possibly those related to appetite control. Of greatest consequence is the fact that fructose is more lipogenic than glucose and is associated with greater circulating triglycerides, total cholesterol and LDLs [49, 51, 52].

The contribution of fructose ingestion to the metabolic syndrome is difficult, if not impossible, to quantify given that it is ingested as part of a nutrient mix, often including glucose. Association studies have found positive relationships between fructose ingestion, excess energy intake, body weight and the increasing trends in type 2 diabetes, CVD or renal disease [51]. While it is difficult to attribute the metabolic syndrome to one particular nutrient, the physiological data suggests that a high fructose diet can induce metabolic changes. The greater *de novo* lipogenesis can contribute to intrahepatic, visceral and ectopic lipid accumulation, all of which are associated with insulin resistance. So while fructose does not stimulate insulin secretion, it can have an indirect impact on insulin action and circulating blood glucose levels. A high fructose diet has been shown to increase blood pressure in animals, possibly by increased sympathetic nervous system activity, and tissue specific inflammation by a variety of proinflammatory cascades including uric acid, cytokine production and oxidative stress [49]. Therefore, fructose can directly or indirectly contribute to each of the risk factors for the metabolic syndrome.

Dietary fat: The digestion, absorption and metabolism of dietary fat increase the concentration of circulating lipids that are broadly classified as (1) saturated fatty acids, (2) unsaturated fatty acids and (3) *trans*-fatty acids. These lipids have important physiological functions, including the structure and fluidity of cell membranes, as substrates for energy production and for the retention of body heat. When the supply of dietary fat exceeds physiological requirements, lipid accumulates in plasma, subcutaneous and visceral adipose tissue as well as most tissues that regulate metabolism. The accumulation of adipose and ectopic fat is associated with most risk factors for the metabolic syndrome. A high fat diet, where greater than 30 % of total energy intake comes from fat sources, will promote excess fat storage when energy expenditure is not adequate. However, it is primarily the content and action of saturated and *trans*-fatty acids that confer the risk of metabolic syndrome [50].

It is recommended that saturated fat should comprise less than 10 % of daily energy intake. Excessive saturated fat consumption increases circulating triglycerides, total cholesterol and LDL cholesterol and may also contribute to hepatic *de novo* lipogenesis and ectopic fat accumulation [50]. *Trans*-fatty acids have a different metabolic action, decreasing HDL cholesterol and increasing insulin resistance possibly by indirectly increasing FFA. Both saturated and *trans*-fatty acids trigger inflammatory processes in adipocytes by increasing the production of pro-inflammatory cytokines that contribute to insulin resistance and the metabolic syndrome [53, 54].

Unsaturated fatty acids are classified as either polyunsaturated or monounsaturated. These fatty acids are generally viewed as having a positive impact on metabolic regulation by decreasing hepatic VLDL production, HDL cholesterol and lipogenesis while increasing hepatic lipid oxidation and plasma membrane fluidity [50]. The impact of polyunsaturated fatty acids on insulin sensitivity is not clear and requires further investigation. At this time it does not appear that these fatty acids impact significantly on insulin sensitivity [55]. Total fat intake, irrespective of lipid composition, will increase the risk of metabolic syndrome. In conclusion, while total energy intake is an important factor in creating a positive energy balance and promoting ectopic lipid accumulation, the composition of individual nutrients also play an important role. These data suggest that a diet high in saturated and *trans*-fatty acids coupled with high fructose ingestion confers a very strong risk of developing the metabolic syndrome.

3.3.1.3 Diurnal Rhythms

The quantity and quality of nutrient ingestion and the amount of daily physical activity are the most common aetiological factors, but it has become clear that many physiological processes occur in rhythmical or cyclical patterns that also have a profound impact on risk factors for the metabolic syndrome. Circadian rhythms and sleep have been linked with the regulation of hunger, carbohydrate and lipid metabolism, as well as hormonal signalling and their disruption are associated with obesity, type 2 diabetes and CVD [56]. The central neural regulator of circadian rhythm, or "*clock*", is the suprachiasmatic nucleus of the hypothalamus [56, 57]. It receives input from environmental cues such as light and nutrients and maintains biological rhythms in peripheral tissues by neuroendocrine modulation. In most tissues the biological "*clock*" regulates up to 20 % of total gene expression [56, 57] including nutrient sensors (sirtuin 1 (SIRT1) and AMPK), nuclear receptors (peroxisome proliferator-activated receptor (PPAR)γ, PPARα, REV-ERBα), metabolites (nicotinamide adenine dinucleotide $(NAD)^+$, heme) and rate limiting enzymes [nicotinamide phosphoribosyltransferase (Nampt), 3-hydroxy-3-methylglutaryl-CoA reductase (Hmgcr), aminolevunilate, delta-, synthase 1 (Alas1)] [57, 58].

The key components of central and peripheral circadian rhythm are also involved in the regulation of energy metabolism, including glucose/lipid metabolism, thermogenesis, feeding behaviour and sleep–wake cycles [56, 57, 59]. When the clock gene is disrupted in animal models, nutrient digestion and absorption are affected, resulting in weight gain, hyperphagia, hyperlipidaemia and hypoinsulinaemic hyperglycaemia [56]. In adipose tissue the release of leptin and adiponectin are altered and the disruption may also influence the distribution of adipose tissue in visceral and subcutaneous compartments. There is also an impact on blood pressure, glucose tolerance, insulin action and hepatic lipid metabolism.

It is difficult to quantify the contribution of circadian disruption to the development of metabolic abnormalities in humans. Sleep continuity has been identified as a risk factor for CVD while short and long sleep duration increases the risk of diabetes and the metabolic syndrome [60]. Studies examining the impact of shift work on metabolic risk factors have found evidence of increased risk of obesity, diabetes and CVD [60]. The increased risk may be associated with delayed or altered sleep patterns, irregular meal times or nocturnal eating. However, there is a lot of variation in the experimental design of published studies, including the type of shift work as some, but not all, is nocturnal. In conclusion, while it is difficult to demonstrate cause and effect relationships in humans, it is likely that a disruption of circadian rhythm by altering the day–night cycle or weight gain is an important interacting variable in the development of metabolic risk factors.

3.3.2 Genetics, Epigenetics and Early Developmental Biology

Metabolic processes are also regulated by genes, and the variation in their sequences, as they are used to produce the proteins and enzymes necessary to carry out biochemical reactions. However, genes alone do not fully explain the variation in gene expression. Recently, it has been shown that methyl groups on deoxyribonucleic acid (DNA) nucleotides and modification to histones that surround DNA, collectively referred to as the epigenome, provide an important contribution to the regulation of gene expression. While the epigenome can be modified, many of the methylation patterns are inherited or influenced during early development. The contribution of genetic and epigenetic factors to the metabolic syndrome is not fully understood, but their regulation of gene expression and is likely to play a very important role.

3.3.2.1 Genetics

Advances in technology have allowed the human genome to be comprehensively analysed to quantify the genes and sequence variations that might account for the onset and progression of human diseases. In some cases, these approaches have identified monogenic determinants that result in extreme metabolic phenotypes [61]. In other cases, candidate gene approaches have been used to associate clinical phenotypes with variation in specific genes. For example, a polymorphism in the *FTO* gene is associated with fat mass, obesity and more recently with the metabolic syndrome [62]. These approaches have greatly assisted our understanding of the genetic contribution to individual components of the metabolic syndrome, such as insulin resistance and obesity, but are more limited when trying to determine if there is a specific genetic contribution to accumulated risk factors.

It is now possible to associate multiple gene sequence variations, typically called single nucleotide polymorphisms (SNPs), with a specific clinical outcome in case-controlled studies. The genome-wide association studies (GWAS) have identified hundreds of potential genetic variants that may contribute to disease pathophysiology. One of the major challenges is to conduct studies that are sufficiently powered to overcome individual variation, but have well-characterised clinical outcome measures to perform the association analysis. The metabolic syndrome has an additional level of complexity as it comprises a constellation of risk factors that each have their own genetic determinants.

At this point only a limited number of studies have addressed the genetic contribution to the metabolic syndrome. Using a systems biology approach, Sookoian and Pirola [63], identified 58 molecular pathways that were significantly related to the metabolic syndrome. The 15 highest ranked pathways and 50 genes (Table 3.1) included many of those expected to be associated with the metabolic syndrome, such as reverse cholesterol transport, the leptin system, lipoprotein metabolism, adipocytokine signalling, obesity and visceral fat. However, the analysis identified other pathways of interest including tryptophan metabolism and nuclear receptors in lipid metabolism, strengthening the link with circadian rhythm. As individual and small clustering of gene variants only account for a minor proportion of phenotypic variance, it is more likely that genetic networks influence physiological processes and the risk of developing the metabolic syndrome.

The likely contribution of common genetic variants to the metabolic syndrome or combinations of metabolic syndrome traits was investigated using a bivariate GWAS analysis on seven epidemiological data sets [64]. This study found 29 common variants associated with the metabolic syndrome or pairs of traits. Metabolic syndrome was associated with genetic variance in *BUD13* (BUD13 homolog), *ZNF259* (Zinc Finger Protein 259), *APOA5* (apolipoprotein A–V), *LPL* and *CETP* (cholesterol ester transfer protein). A number of other genes including *GCKR* (glucokinase receptor), *MTNR1B* (melatonin receptor 1B), *LIPC* (lipase hepatic) and *TFAP2B* (transcription factor AP-2 β) were associated with pairs of traits. None of the 29 unique SNPs were significantly associated with three or more metabolic syndrome traits. A cluster of the top 16 SNPs accounted for 9 % of the variance in triglycerides, 5.8 % for HDL cholesterol, 3.6 % for glucose, 2.3 % for waist circumference and 1.4 % for systolic blood pressure. These results support a polygenic involvement in the metabolic syndrome that is likely to result in numerous interacting pathways contributing to phenotypic alterations.

This is supported by another recent study that used a bivariate (multivariate) linear mixed-effects model to estimate narrow-sense heritability and heritability explained by common SNPs to quantify the genetic information for single and shared traits of the metabolic syndrome [65]. This study found that the narrow-sense heritability accounted for by common SNPs explained approximately 39 % of heritability across metabolic syndrome traits, 41 % for BMI, 46 % for waist-to-hip ratio, 30 % for glucose, 39 % for insulin, 34 % for triglycerides, 25 % for HDL cholesterol and 80 % for systolic blood pressure. The findings suggest that many common genetic variants, with small effect, are likely to contribute to the phenotypic variation of the metabolic syndrome.

However, not all studies report evidence of common genetic variants linking metabolic syndrome traits. Kristiansson et al. [66] conducted a GWAS study on

Table 3.1 Genes influencing the risk of metabolic syndrome components

Gene symbol	Approved gene name	Overall *P*-value
Nuclear receptors		
NR1H4	Nuclear receptor subfamily 1, group H, member 4	8.14×10^{-14}
RXRA	Retinoid X receptor, alpha	1.41×10^{-13}
THRB	Thyroid hormone receptor, beta	2.00×10^{-13}
THRA	Thyroid hormone receptor, alpha	4.35×10^{-13}
RARA	Retinoid acid receptor, alpha	1.22×10^{-12}
RXRB	Retinoid X receptor, beta	3.27×10^{-12}
PGR	Progesterone receptor	3.98×10^{-12}
ESRRA	Estrogen-related receptor alpha	4.06×10^{-12}
RARG	Retinoic acid receptor, gamma	1.21×10^{-11}
NR5A2	Nuclear receptor subfamily 5, group A, member 2	2.19×10^{-11}
NR1H2	Nuclear receptor subfamily 1, group H, member 2—LXR-b	3.68×10^{-11}
HNF1B	HNF1 homeobox B	1.77×10^{-10}
NR1I2	Nuclear receptor subfamily 1, group I, member 2-PXR	3.15×10^{-10}
Cytochrome P450 family		
CYP11A1	Cytochrome P450, family 11, subfamily A, polypeptide 1	4.08×10^{-13}
CYP11B1	Cytochrome P450, family 11, subfamily B, polypeptide 1	1.38×10^{-11}
Immune response, inflammatory related genes, and chemokine receptors		
CTLA4	Cytotoxic T-lymphocyte-associated protein 4	2.98×10^{-10}
CD44	CD44 molecule (Indian blood group)	2.09×10^{-10}
CD40LG	CD40 ligand	8.86×10^{-12}
NFKB1	Nuclear factor of kappa light polypeptide gene enhancer in B-cells 1	1.08×10^{-11}
TLR4	Toll-like receptor 4	1.04×10^{-10}
PTGS2	Prostaglandin-endoperoxide synthase 2-cyclooxygenase 2	1.14×10^{-14}
STAT3	Signal transducer and activator of transcription 3	4.44×10^{-11}
CXCR4	Chemokine (C–X–C motif) receptor 4	4.46×10^{-11}
CCR5	Chemokine (C–C motif) receptor 5	5.53×10^{-11}
C5AR1	Complement component 5a receptor 1	4.47×10^{-11}
Growth factors		
TGFB2	Transforming growth factor, beta 2	3.33×10^{-11}
PDGFRA	Platelet-derived growth factor receptor, alpha polypeptide	1.14×10^{-10}
GHRHR	Growth hormone releasing hormone receptor	1.18×10^{-10}
PDGFRB	Platelet-derived growth factor receptor, beta polypeptide	1.85×10^{-10}
EGFR	Epidermal growth factor receptor	9.78×10^{-12}
Miscellanea		
NOS1	Nitric oxide synthase 1	1.29×10^{-13}
ALB	Albumin	1.66×10^{-11}
SLC2A4	Solute carrier family 2 (facilitated glucose transporter), member 4	1.01×10^{-12}
KNG1	Kininogen 1	1.78×10^{-11}
EDNRB	Endothelin receptor type B	1.84×10^{-11}
PDX1	Pancreatic and duodenal homeobox 1	2.15×10^{-11}

(continued)

Table 3.1 (continued)

Gene symbol	Approved gene name	Overall *P*-value
THBS1	Thrombospondin 1	2.41×10^{-11}
LHCGR	Luteinizing hormone/choriogonadotropin receptor	3.10×10^{-11}
JUN	Jun oncogene	4.54×10^{-11}
PLAT	Plasminogen activator, tissue	1.01×10^{-10}
APOF	Apolipoprotein F	1.16×10^{-10}
CHRM1	Cholinergic receptor, muscarinic 1	1.58×10^{-10}
BCL2	B-cell CLL/lymphoma 2	1.58×10^{-10}
ERBB2	v-erb-b2 erythroblastic leukaemia viral oncogene homolog 2	1.58×10^{-10}
PIK3R1	Phosphoinositide-3-kinase, regulatory subunit 1 (alpha)	5.14×10^{-12}
HSPD1	Heat shock 60 kDa protein 1 (chaperonin)	2.40×10^{-10}
ADORA2A	Adenosine A2a receptor	1.14×10^{-14}
ITGB2	Integrin, beta 2	8.14×10^{-14}
LRP1	Low density lipoprotein receptor-related protein 1	1.15×10^{-11}
EP300	E1A-binding protein p300	3.85×10^{-10}

Adapted from Sookoian and Pirola [63]

four Finnish cohorts and found a strong lipid gene contribution to the metabolic syndrome, but none of the susceptibility loci were associated with more than one trait. In addition, a GWAS study of the metabolic syndrome in Indian Asian men found similar genetic variants, as reported in other populations, including *LPL* and *CETP*, but found little evidence of a common genetic basis for the metabolic syndrome [67].

3.4 Epigenetics and Early Developmental Biology

It is now clear that gene expression has multiple cellular regulators that act co-operatively or competitively to control protein content and cell function. Epigenetic regulation refers to the changes that occur in gene transcription that are not associated with changes in the DNA sequence. There are two main types of epigenetic modification (1) the methylation of DNA nucleotides and (2) the covalent modification of histone proteins surrounding the DNA double helix. DNA methylation and histone modifications are important because they are both heritable and under environmental regulation and can help explain inter-individual variation. Epigenetic modifications can be passed from parent to offspring during cell division, thereby retaining a "memory" of parental gene expression patterns. DNA methylation patterns can change during ageing, with younger monozygotic twins having indistinguishable epigenetic markings, but older twins have substantial epigenetic variation and further differences in gene expression [68]. It is therefore likely that the inherited epigenetic profile influences gene expression patterns and the long-term risk of disease.

The relationship between foetal development and metabolic disease in adulthood, hypothesised as the thrifty phenotype, has been espoused for some time. According to this hypothesis, in utero stress caused by an inadequate nutrient availability results in a lower birth weight and initiates an adaptive response that predisposes energy storage and increased susceptibility to CVD [69–71]. Low birth weight has also been associated with increased risk of hypertension, impaired glucose tolerance and type 2 diabetes later in life [70]. However, low birth weight caused by dietary restriction or inadequate placental nutrient supply is not the only contributor to foetal stress. Maternal obesity and high fat feeding have also been linked with changes in appetite, altered lipid metabolism and insulin resistance [71]. The tissue-specific changes, including decreased skeletal muscle mass and insulin sensitivity, increased fat storage, decreased insulin secretion, leptin resistance and altered renin–angiotensin system, are consistent with the metabolic syndrome.

In addition to heritable regulation of the epigenome, there is emerging evidence of lifestyle-related modification of DNA methylation. An acute bout of exercise has been shown to decrease metabolic gene promoter methylation in an intensity-dependent manner with a corresponding increase in gene transcription [72]. In addition, a deficiency in dietary folate, methionine or choline can induce DNA hypomethylation [73]. These data suggest that some forms of DNA methylation can be transiently affected, are responsive to lifestyle choices and reinforce the importance of appropriate dietary intake and physical activity to maintain normal physiological function. It is premature to suggest that epigenetic modifications account for the increased susceptibility to the metabolic syndrome, but, as a key regulator of gene expression and a potential link between environment and genes, there is considerable interest in furthering the understanding of the epigenome.

3.5 Gut Microbiota and the Metagenome

A new and very important (both genetic and environmental contributor) to human metabolism is the so-called intestinal microbiome. Bacteria that reside in the human gut constitute a new organ system with more than three million genes. This is a completely new area of metabolic and genetic research. There is good evidence already that the gut microbiome can transfer metabolic disease from one animal to another. There is growing interest in the potential mechanisms by which this might occur, and several mechanisms have been mooted, some of which have been shown to lead to low-grade inflammation, alteration in adipose tissue plasticity, hepatic steatosis, insulin resistance and cardiovascular changes—all consistent with the typical metabolic syndrome. This important new topic is a subject of very active investigation now and is coming into the field of clinical investigation in human subjects. A recent review by Burcelin and colleagues provides an up to date perspective [74].

3.6 Underlying Mechanisms

3.6.1 Intracellular Lipid Accumulation and Insulin Resistance (Muscle, Liver, Pancreas, Brain)

Insulin resistance in skeletal muscle is associated with abnormalities in both glucose and lipid metabolism [75]. In relation to lipid metabolism, there is increased intramyocellular storage of triglycerides and other lipid intermediates and dysregulation of the beta-oxidation of fatty acids [76]. A number of mechanisms have been suggested that could explain the association between cytosolic lipid accumulation and insulin resistance in skeletal muscle. The accumulation of lipids in muscle tissue could result from increased fatty acid delivery, reduced utilisation or the combination of both [77, 78]. The composition of dietary lipids is also a factor in determining the contribution of ectopic lipid accumulation to insulin resistance and metabolic dysfunction.

Palmitate, the most abundant dietary lipid, can lead to the formation of cellular ceramide [79]. The accumulation of this lipid intermediate activates protein kinase C zeta (PKCζ) and protein phosphatase 2A leading to a decrease in Akt/PKB activation and subsequent impairment of insulin action [79]. Insulin-resistant obese subjects have twice the amount of intramuscular ceramide and a corresponding decrease in Akt/PKB activation [80]. Muscle ceramide levels are correlated with insulin resistance [81] and decrease in response to exercise training that improves insulin sensitivity [82]. Saturated fatty acids can also lead to ceramide accumulation by the activation of inflammatory cascades following binding with the toll-like receptor-4 [79]. A decrease in cellular ceramide can impact on adipokine production and has been shown to decrease leptin and TNF-α. Another adipokine, adiponectin, may play an important regulatory role in ceramide formation. Adiponectin has been shown to improve insulin sensitivity, and circulating levels of this hormone are positively correlated with insulin sensitivity. There is some evidence to suggest that adiponectin activates an intracellular cascade that lowers ceramide formation and thus mediates an improvement in insulin action. Ceramide accumulation also contributes to the development of mitochondrial dysfunction, a factor that has been strongly associated with insulin resistance [79]. When ceramide production is impaired in mice fed with a high fat diet, there is an increase in oxygen consumption and the activity of citrate synthase, a key enzyme in the mitochondria [83].

However, ceramide formation is not the only mediator of lipid-induced metabolic dysfunction. The accumulation of diglycerol is the result of an increase in intracellular triglycerides. Diglycerols activate protein kinase C epsilon and theta (PKCε & PKCθ) that increase the serine phosphorylation of the insulin receptor and insulin receptor substrate 1 (IRS-1). This effect appears to be independent of the ceramide inhibition of Akt/PKB though both result in a decrease in insulin action. The source of diglycerols is not clear with evidence to suggest that saturated and/or polyunsaturated are the main sources of lipid in the diet [79]. The decreased utilisation of intracellular triglycerides has been proposed as the main reason for diglycerol accumulation and this has increased the focus on mitochondrial function as a regulator of insulin resistance and the metabolic syndrome.

3.6.2 Mitochondrial Function

Skeletal muscle mitochondria could contribute to the pathogenesis of type 2 diabetes, according to one hypothesis, if a primary defect in mitochondrial functional capacity could lead to intramyocellular accumulation of "toxic" lipid intermediates, which would then disrupt insulin signalling leading to insulin resistance [19, 20]. However, it remains contentious whether altered mitochondrial biology itself contributes to insulin resistance or merely reflects the consequence of other systemic factors and is not a primary contributor to the pathophysiology of insulin resistance. A number of studies using a variety of techniques have shown that skeletal muscle of insulin-resistant, obese or type 2 diabetes subjects have reduced mitochondrial oxidative capacity as compared with lean, healthy controls [84–90]. However, it has not been definitively established whether the reduced oxidative capacity present in insulin-resistant states is a result of reduced mitochondrial mass, deficiency in mitochondrial function or both. There is evidence that the mitochondrial dysfunction associated with insulin resistance actually precedes the development of obesity and diabetes. It has been shown that lean but insulin-resistant offspring of patients with type 2 diabetes have increased intramyocellular lipid content, reduced baseline activity of mitochondrial oxidative phosphorylation, and decreased skeletal muscle mitochondrial density and content [87, 88]. These observations support the theory that skeletal muscle mitochondrial dysfunction is heritable. Thus, mitochondrial dysfunction could contribute to the primary pathology underlying insulin resistance and the progression to diabetes.

Taken together, a number of studies of skeletal muscle from obese and type 2 diabetes patients suggest a disruption in mitochondrial biology as evidenced by reduced concentrations of oxidative enzymes [90–92], reduced mitochondrial size and altered mitochondrial morphology [85, 93]. Studies of skeletal muscle mitochondrial respiration provide conflicting evidence. One study using high resolution respirometry performed in isolated myofibrils suggests that the function of skeletal muscle mitochondria in type 2 diabetes is normal, and that the reduced skeletal muscle oxidative capacity of these patients is due to a reduction in mitochondrial content [84]. Other studies provide evidence that at least some parts of electron transport chain have decreased functional capacity, resulting in diminished mitochondrial respiration [94, 95].

Mitochondrial biogenesis requires the concordant activation of both the mitochondrial and the nuclear genomes to generate electron transport chain subunits and other proteins that are necessary for mitochondrial function. Insulin resistance in muscle of individuals with obesity or type 2 diabetes is associated with reduced expression of nuclear genes responsible for oxidative metabolism such as peroxisome proliferator-activated receptor γ coactivator-1α (PGC-1 α) [96]. Remarkably, insulin-resistant muscle has been shown to display a coordinated reduction in the expression of a cluster of genes encoding proteins of the mitochondrial inner membranes, respiratory chain complexes, adenosine triphosphate (ATP) synthesis, fatty acid oxidation, Krebs cycle and pyruvate kinase [91]. The expression of the transcriptional co-activators PGC-1α and PGC-1β has been shown to be downregulated in non-diabetic individuals who have a positive family history of diabetes [91]. Proteomic studies have also recently demonstrated a reduction in mitochondrial proteins in insulin-resistant muscle [97]. In parallel, reduced expression of mitofusin-2, a key protein essential for mitochondrial fusion and the regulation of inner membrane potential, has been described in patients with type 2 diabetes [98].

Lifestyle and behavioural interventions have the potential to affect both mitochondrial biogenesis and mitochondrial dysfunction. It has been long established that the content of the mitochondria in skeletal muscle depends directly on the level of physical activity and that skeletal muscles have metabolic plasticity and can enhance oxidative phosphorylation in response to exercise. Therefore, some researchers advocate that the reduced skeletal muscle oxidative phosphorylation in states of insulin resistance is a reflection of sedentary lifestyle leading to obesity and type 2 diabetes. Several studies have investigated the effect of weight loss and exercise interventions on mitochondrial function in obesity and type 2 diabetes. These have shown that both mitochondrial content and electron transport chain activity improve in skeletal muscle in both obese and type 2 diabetes patients in response to weight loss and exercise training [86, 99, 100]. This effect is paralleled by improvements in insulin sensitivity. Interestingly, although both are insulin-sensitising interventions, exercise training results paradoxically in *increased* intramyocellular lipid content, in contrast to the effect of diet-induced weight loss [86, 99]. The net effect of combined dietary and exercise interventions may therefore be expected to result in unchanged intramyocellular lipid content pre- and post-intervention. It has been shown that diet-induced weight loss has no effect on mitochondrial capacity, despite reducing intramyocellular lipid content in subjects with type 2 diabetes [86]. These observations suggest that interplay between muscle cytosolic lipid content and muscle mitochondrial function contribute to insulin sensitivity. Very recently, new data have been published suggesting that there are regional anatomical differences in skeletal muscle mitochondrial respiration, and that locomotor muscles play an important metabolic role [101].

Thus the role of mitochondrial dysfunction in the pathogenesis of the metabolic syndrome is not yet completely understood. Future studies will probably focus on identifying specific sub-phenotypes of patients who have distinct mitochondrial biology and who have accordingly lesser or greater potential to respond to lifestyle intervention. In parallel with efforts to improve the drug treatment of diabetes, this avenue of research supports the ultimate goal of personalised medicine and the design of a tailored approach to lifestyle interventions. In addition to this, the output from studying the molecular pathways leading to mitochondrial dysfunction may also facilitate the development of new pharmacotherapeutic interventions for this growing population of patients.

3.6.3 Inflammation

Obesity and the metabolic syndrome are characterised by chronic low grade inflammation, particularly in adipose tissue. The cause of the inflammatory response is not fully known, but macrophage infiltration could be triggered by hypoxia following adipocyte hypertrophy [102, 103]. The excess energy stored as triglycerides in adipocytes causes them to get bigger and activate signalling cascades that promote inflammatory processes. What begins as local tissue inflammation can develop into low grade systemic inflammation and cause insulin resistance and metabolic dysfunction. Inflammation is associated with increased lipolysis in the muscle, liver and adipose tissue resulting in higher circulating lipid levels. In the liver cholesterol and lipid biosynthesis are increased, there are greater levels of ceramide formation and fatty acid oxidation is decreased [104].

The mechanisms responsible are not completely understood, but consist of an increase in the production of pro-inflammatory cytokines and the recruitment and infiltration of macrophages [102–104]. The production of pro-inflammatory cytokines, such as TNF-α, IL-1 and IL-6, is driven by the nuclear factor kappa-light-chain-enhancer of activated B cells (NFκB) and activator protein 1 (AP1) gene expression pathways [102–104]. These cytokines can act in a paracrine manner or be released into circulation where they bind to receptors on other tissues including skeletal muscle and liver. They can then activate intracellular stress responsive signalling cascades such as c-Jun N-terminal kinases (JNK) and protein kinase C phi (PKCφ) that inhibit IRS-1 by increasing serine phosphorylation [104]. In addition to the action of pro-inflammatory cytokines, the inflammatory response can also be initiated by saturated fatty acids, possibly by binding the toll-like receptor-4, increasing NFκB-mediated gene expression and ceramide production. Nutrient regulation of inflammation can also be inhibitory as polyunsaturated fatty acids can activate anti-inflammatory cascades.

3.6.4 Amino Acid Metabolism

Fatty acids and lipid-derived metabolites have for many years been regarded as central players in the pathogenesis of insulin resistance and type 2 diabetes, as has already been outlined in this chapter. Recent advances in the field of mass spectrometry and metabolomic analysis have led to the description of several new associations between small molecules and insulin resistance as well as type 2 diabetes. Surprisingly, BCAA and related metabolites are more strongly associated with insulin resistance than are many common lipid species. Among the new associations that have recently been described are those between branched chain and aromatic amino acids (leucine, isoleucine, valine, tyrosine, phenylalanine) and type 2 diabetes [105, 106], between branched chain amino acids and obesity [21, 22], between neutral amino acids and insulin resistance [107, 108] and between alpha-hydroxybutyrate, glycine, and urate and insulin sensitivity [107, 109]. A recent analysis of the Relationship between Insulin Sensitivity and

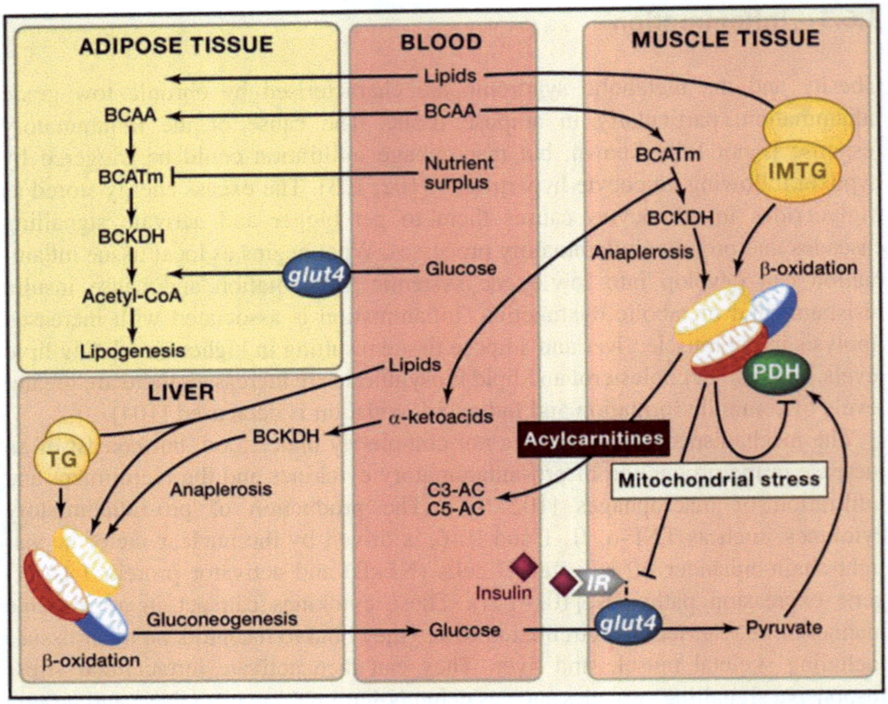

Fig. 3.2 Schematic working model of the potential interaction between lipids and BCAA in the pathogenesis of obesity-related insulin resistance (from Newgard [21])

Cardiovascular Disease (RISC) study [110] identified novel associations between insulin sensitivity and small molecules including amino acids glycine, cysteine, isoleucine and creatine, and the organic acids alpha-hydroxybutyrate and alpha-ketobutyrate [107]. Alpha-hydroxybutyrate was identified as the small molecule most strongly associated with decreased insulin sensitivity (measured by the hyperinsulinaemic euglycaemic clamp). Glycine was the amino acid most strongly associated with increased insulin sensitivity. While some of these metabolites may represent important biomarkers of early diabetes processes, including insulin resistance and the metabolic syndrome, the question remains whether these molecules play a causative role in disease progression or whether they represent a secondary phenomenon due to other elements of the underlying pathology of the disease.

The field of metabolomics remains in its early stages of development and will require a longer period of translational studies to secure the foundations of how intermediary metabolites contribute to disease processes. Important progress has been made with respect to insulin resistance, and this has been reviewed in recent years by Chris Newgard [21, 22]. Newgard has proposed a hypothesis of BCAA overload, which can result from overnutrition and a relative deficiency of insulin-like growth factor-1 (IGF-1), in which circumstances the metabolic milieu is distorted towards excess of BCAA and downstream metabolites including C5 and C3 acyl-CoA and acylcarnitines (Fig. 3.2). This milieu leads to further alterations in insulin signalling eventually resulting in insulin resistance. Based on this type of observation, another experimental approach to this same question has been to study common genetic variants that are associated with metabolites in the glutathione and glycine biosynthesis pathways. A recent analysis conducted in the RISC study, and later replicated in the Botnia study, used a genome-wide association investigation of insulin sensitivity-related metabolites including those involved in the synthesis of glutathione and glycine (Xie et al. unpublished data). A number of associations were confirmed by this analysis, between genetic variants linked to various combinations of amino acid metabolites and insulin resistance.

In addition to the above associational evidence (for correlation between BCAA and metabolic disease), there is recent evidence that these metabolites can be predictive of both disease progression and the response to intervention. For example, in an analysis of the responses to a weight loss diet in the weight loss maintenance trial (WLM), the improvement in insulin sensitivity over 6 months was strongly predicted by a BCAA-related principal component factor score, and not at all by lipid-related factors [111]. Similarly, a metabolomic profile including Leu, Ile, Val, Phe and Tyr has been shown to be the best predictor of incident diabetes in a sample of 189 subjects from the Framingham cohort (followed over an interval up to 12 years), in comparison with a matched cohort of 189 subjects (matched for weight, lipid profile and other clinical variables), who did not progress [106]. Furthermore, it has been shown that changes in BCAA levels may track with response to interventions aiming at improving metabolic control. Newgard and colleagues have shown that obese subjects undergoing gastric bypass surgery have a much more pronounced decline in circulating BCAA, C3 and C5 acylcarnitines, Phe and Tyr than observed in those treated by dietary intervention, despite similar weight loss [112]. This is an important observation, as there is increasing evidence that bariatric surgery (such as gastric bypass surgery in this case) leads to greater improvement in glucose homeostasis than dietary intervention.

Conclusion

The metabolic syndrome is increasingly prevalent, driven by the progressive changes in physical activity and diet that have come with modern living and driven by the pandemic of obesity. Notwithstanding controversies about how to define the metabolic syndrome, the syndrome is very much in focus at the centre of a growing urgency to design effective preventive measures to halt progression to type 2 diabetes, CVD and cancer. The clinical pathophysiology of this syndrome arises from a gradual distortion of metabolic homeostasis, with an increase in central adiposity and sustained increase in lipolysis. Insulin resistance is at the centre of the clinical phenotype, in skeletal muscle, liver and adipose tissue. A characteristic dyslipidaemia and elevation of blood pressure accompany these metabolic alterations and provide the high risk milieu for progression to diabetes, CVD and certain cancers.

It has proved difficult to identify any single and distinct cause for the metabolic syndrome. An insidious and progressive change in environmental factors associated with modern living is currently the best available explanation. Both diet and physical activity habits have changed markedly in the past decades and have clearly contributed to the modern obesity pandemic and to the expression of the insulin-resistant phenotype in those who are at risk because of yet unknown combinations of genetic or epigenetic risk factors. This field of research is developing rapidly and has led to a much better understanding of underlying cellular and biological mechanisms. Metabolomics has opened a new vista of biochemical abnormalities underlying insulin resistance, particularly in the area of amino acid and fatty acid metabolism as well as mitochondrial function. Inflammation and altered coagulation add to this milieu, providing a complex combination of disease risk factors, none of which are simple to treat in isolation, outside of a concerted effort at smart prevention of this modern threat to public health.

References

1. DeFronzo RA, Ferrannini E (1991) Insulin resistance: a multifaceted syndrome responsible for NIDDM, obesity, hypertension, dyslipidemia, and atherosclerotic cardiovascular disease. Diabetes Care 14(3):173–194
2. Eckel RH, Grundy SM, Zimmet PZ (2005) The metabolic syndrome. Lancet 365 (9468):1415–1428
3. Lakka HM et al (2002) The metabolic syndrome and total and cardiovascular disease mortality in middle-aged men. JAMA 288(21):2709–2716
4. Reaven GM (1988) Banting lecture 1988. Role of insulin resistance in human disease. Diabetes 37(12):1595–1607
5. Alberti K, Zimmet P (2008) Should we dump the metabolic syndrome? No. Br Med J 336 (7645):641–641
6. Gale EAM (2008) Should we dump the metabolic syndrome? Yes. Br Med J 336(7645):640
7. Reaven GM (2005) The metabolic syndrome: requiescat in pace. Clin Chem 51(6):931–938
8. Després JP, Lemieux I (2006) Abdominal obesity and metabolic syndrome. Nature 444 (7121):881–887
9. Astrup A, Finer N (2000) Redefining type 2 diabetes: 'diabesity'or 'obesity dependent diabetes mellitus'? Obes Rev 1(2):57–59
10. Mokdad AH et al (2003) Prevalence of obesity, diabetes, and obesity-related health risk factors, 2001. JAMA 289(1):76–79
11. Pincock S (2006) Paul Zimmet: fighting the "diabesity" pandemic. Lancet 368(9548):1643
12. Zimmet P, Alberti K, Shaw J (2001) Global and societal implications of the diabetes epidemic. Nature 414(6865):782–787
13. Mittelman SD et al (2002) Extreme insulin resistance of the central adipose depot in vivo. Diabetes 51(3):755–761
14. Chiang DJ, Pritchard MT, Nagy LE (2011) Obesity, diabetes mellitus, and liver fibrosis. Am J Physiol Gastrointest Liver Physiol 300(5):G697–G702
15. Berg AH, Scherer PE (2005) Adipose tissue, inflammation, and cardiovascular disease. Circ Res 96(9):939–949
16. Eckel RH (1989) Lipoprotein lipase. A multifunctional enzyme relevant to common metabolic diseases. N Engl J Med 320(16):1060–1068
17. Jensen M et al (1989) Insulin regulation of lipolysis in nondiabetic and IDDM subjects. Diabetes 38(12):1595–1601

18. Moro C, Bajpeyi S, Smith SR (2008) Determinants of intramyocellular triglyceride turnover: implications for insulin sensitivity. Am J Physiol Endocrinol Metab 294(2):E203–E213
19. Hirabara SM, Curi R, Maechler P (2010) Saturated fatty acid induced insulin resistance is associated with mitochondrial dysfunction in skeletal muscle cells. J Cell Physiol 222(1):187–194
20. Koves TR et al (2008) Mitochondrial overload and incomplete fatty acid oxidation contribute to skeletal muscle insulin resistance. Cell Metab 7(1):45–56
21. Newgard CB (2012) Interplay between lipids and branched-chain amino acids in development of insulin resistance. Cell Metab 15(5):606–614
22. Newgard CB et al (2009) A branched-chain amino acid-related metabolic signature that differentiates obese and lean humans and contributes to insulin resistance. Cell Metab 9(4):311–326
23. Krssak M et al (1999) Intramyocellular lipid concentrations are correlated with insulin sensitivity in humans: a 1H NMR spectroscopy study. Diabetologia 42(1):113–116
24. Kelley DE, Mandarino LJ (2000) Fuel selection in human skeletal muscle in insulin resistance: a reexamination. Diabetes 49(5):677–683
25. Ferrannini E et al (1987) Insulin resistance in essential hypertension. N Engl J Med 317(6):350–357
26. Steinberg H et al (1994) Insulin-mediated skeletal muscle vasodilation is nitric oxide dependent. A novel action of insulin to increase nitric oxide release. J Clin Invest 94(3):1172
27. Tooke J, Hannemann M (2000) Adverse endothelial function and the insulin resistance syndrome. J Intern Med 247(4):425–431
28. Hanley AJG et al (2002) Factor analysis of metabolic syndrome using directly measured insulin sensitivity. Diabetes 51(8):2642–2647
29. Yanai H et al (2008) The underlying mechanisms for development of hypertension in the metabolic syndrome. Nutr J 7:10
30. Murakami T et al (1995) Triglycerides are major determinants of cholesterol esterification/transfer and HDL remodeling in human plasma. Arterioscler Thromb Vasc Biol 15(11):1819–1828
31. De Graaf J et al (1993) Identification of multiple dense LDL subfractions with enhanced susceptibility to in vitro oxidation among hypertriglyceridemic subjects. Normalization after clofibrate treatment. Arterioscler Thromb Vasc Biol 13(5):712–719
32. Manzato E et al (1993) Levels and physicochemical properties of lipoprotein subclasses in moderate hypertriglyceridemia. Clin Chim Acta 219(1):57–65
33. Krauss RM (1995) Dense low density lipoproteins and coronary artery disease. Am J Cardiol 75(6):53B–57B
34. Packard C (1996) LDL subfractions and atherogenicity: an hypothesis from the University of Glasgow. Curr Med Res Opin 13(7):379–390
35. Booth FW et al (2002) Waging war on physical inactivity: using modern molecular ammunition against an ancient enemy. J Appl Physiol 93(1):3–30
36. Booth FW et al (2000) Waging war on modern chronic diseases: primary prevention through exercise biology. J Appl Physiol 88(2):774–787
37. Matthews CE et al (2008) Amount of time spent in sedentary behaviors in the United States, 2003–2004. Am J Epidemiol 167(7):875–881
38. Wilmot EG et al (2012) Sedentary time in adults and the association with diabetes, cardiovascular disease and death: systematic review and meta-analysis. Diabetologia 55(11):2895–2905
39. Hamilton MT, Hamilton DG, Zderic TW (2007) Role of low energy expenditure and sitting in obesity, metabolic syndrome, type 2 diabetes, and cardiovascular disease. Diabetes 56(11):2655–2667
40. Hu FB et al (2003) Television watching and other sedentary behaviors in relation to risk of obesity and type 2 diabetes mellitus in women. JAMA 289(14):1785–1791
41. Katzmarzyk PT (2010) Physical activity, sedentary behavior, and health: paradigm paralysis or paradigm shift? Diabetes 59(11):2717–2725

42. Saris WH et al (2003) How much physical activity is enough to prevent unhealthy weight gain? outcome of the IASO 1st stock conference and consensus statement. Obes Rev 4(2):101–114
43. Brooks GA et al (2004) Chronicle of the Institute of Medicine physical activity recommendation: how a physical activity recommendation came to be among dietary recommendations. Am J Clin Nutr 79(5):921S–930S
44. Bergouignan A et al (2011) Physical inactivity as the culprit of metabolic inflexibility: evidence from bed-rest studies. J Appl Physiol 111(4):1201–1210
45. Blanc S et al (2000) Fuel homeostasis during physical inactivity induced by bed rest. J Clin Endocrinol Metab 85(6):2223–2233
46. Mikus CR et al (2012) Lowering physical activity impairs glycemic control in healthy volunteers. Med Sci Sports Exerc 44(2):225–231
47. Mikines KJ et al (1989) Effect of 7 days of bed rest on dose–response relation between plasma glucose and insulin secretion. Am J Physiol 257(1 Pt 1):E43–E48
48. Mikines KJ et al (1991) Seven days of bed rest decrease insulin action on glucose uptake in leg and whole body. J Appl Physiol 70(3):1245–1254
49. Ferder L, Ferder MD, Inserra F (2010) The role of high-fructose corn syrup in metabolic syndrome and hypertension. Curr Hypertens Rep 12(2):105–112
50. Lottenberg AM et al (2012) The role of dietary fatty acids in the pathology of metabolic syndrome. J Nutr Biochem 23(9):1027–1040
51. Tappy L et al (2010) Fructose and metabolic diseases: new findings, new questions. Nutrition 26(11–12):1044–1049
52. Yilmaz Y (2012) Review article: non-alcoholic fatty liver disease and osteoporosis—clinical and molecular crosstalk. Aliment Pharmacol Ther 36(4):345–352
53. Mensink RP et al (2003) Effects of dietary fatty acids and carbohydrates on the ratio of serum total to HDL cholesterol and on serum lipids and apolipoproteins: a meta-analysis of 60 controlled trials. Am J Clin Nutr 77(5):1146–1155
54. Saravanan N et al (2005) Differential effects of dietary saturated and trans-fatty acids on expression of genes associated with insulin sensitivity in rat adipose tissue. Eur J Endocrinol 153(1):159–165
55. Akinkuolie AO et al (2011) Omega-3 polyunsaturated fatty acid and insulin sensitivity: a meta-analysis of randomized controlled trials. Clin Nutr 30(6):702–707
56. Maury E, Ramsey KM, Bass J (2010) Circadian rhythms and metabolic syndrome: from experimental genetics to human disease. Circ Res 106(3):447–462
57. Duez H, Staels B (2010) Nuclear receptors linking circadian rhythms and cardiometabolic control. Arterioscler Thromb Vasc Biol 30(8):1529–1534
58. Sahar S, Sassone-Corsi P (2012) Regulation of metabolism: the circadian clock dictates the time. Trends Endocrinol Metab 23(1):1–8
59. Huang W et al (2011) Circadian rhythms, sleep, and metabolism. J Clin Invest 121(6):2133–2141
60. Antunes LC et al (2010) Obesity and shift work: chronobiological aspects. Nutr Res Rev 23(1):155–168
61. Semple RK et al (2011) Genetic syndromes of severe insulin resistance. Endocr Rev 32(4):498–514
62. Zhou D et al (2012) Common variant (rs9939609) in the FTO gene is associated with metabolic syndrome. Mol Biol Rep 39(6):6555–6561
63. Sookoian S, Pirola CJ (2011) Metabolic syndrome: from the genetics to the pathophysiology. Curr Hypertens Rep 13(2):149–157
64. Kraja AT et al (2011) A bivariate genome-wide approach to metabolic syndrome: STAMPEED consortium. Diabetes 60(4):1329–1339
65. Vattikuti S, Guo J, Chow CC (2012) Heritability and genetic correlations explained by common SNPs for metabolic syndrome traits. PLoS Genet 8(3):e1002637
66. Kristiansson K et al (2012) Genome-wide screen for metabolic syndrome susceptibility Loci reveals strong lipid gene contribution but no evidence for common genetic basis for clustering of metabolic syndrome traits. Circ Cardiovasc Genet 5(2):242–249

67. Zabaneh D, Balding DJ (2010) A genome-wide association study of the metabolic syndrome in Indian Asian men. PLoS One 5(8):e11961
68. Fraga MF et al (2005) Epigenetic differences arise during the lifetime of monozygotic twins. Proc Natl Acad Sci USA 102(30):10604–10609
69. Bruce KD, Hanson MA (2010) The developmental origins, mechanisms, and implications of metabolic syndrome. J Nutr 140(3):648–652
70. Rinaudo P, Wang E (2012) Fetal programming and metabolic syndrome. Annu Rev Physiol 74:107–130
71. Warner MJ, Ozanne SE (2010) Mechanisms involved in the developmental programming of adulthood disease. Biochem J 427(3):333–347
72. Barres R et al (2012) Acute exercise remodels promoter methylation in human skeletal muscle. Cell Metab 15(3):405–411
73. Pogribny IP et al (2006) Irreversible global DNA hypomethylation as a key step in hepatocarcinogenesis induced by dietary methyl deficiency. Mutat Res 593(1–2):80–87
74. Burcelin R et al (2011) Gut microbiota and diabetes: from pathogenesis to therapeutic perspective. Acta Diabetol 48(4):257–273
75. Reaven GM (1995) Pathophysiology of insulin resistance in human disease. Physiol Rev 75(3):473–486
76. Befroy DE et al (2007) Impaired mitochondrial substrate oxidation in muscle of insulin-resistant offspring of type 2 diabetic patients. Diabetes 56(5):1376–1381
77. Bonen A et al (2004) Triacylglycerol accumulation in human obesity and type 2 diabetes is associated with increased rates of skeletal muscle fatty acid transport and increased sarcolemmal FAT/CD36. FASEB J 18(10):1144–1146
78. Hancock CR et al (2008) High-fat diets cause insulin resistance despite an increase in muscle mitochondria. Proc Natl Acad Sci 105(22):7815
79. Chavez JA, Summers SA (2012) A ceramide-centric view of insulin resistance. Cell Metab 15(5):585–594
80. Adams JM 2nd et al (2004) Ceramide content is increased in skeletal muscle from obese insulin-resistant humans. Diabetes 53(1):25–31
81. Straczkowski M et al (2004) Relationship between insulin sensitivity and sphingomyelin signaling pathway in human skeletal muscle. Diabetes 53(5):1215–1221
82. Amati F et al (2011) Skeletal muscle triglycerides, diacylglycerols, and ceramides in insulin resistance: another paradox in endurance-trained athletes? Diabetes 60(10):2588–2597
83. Schmitz-Peiffer C (2010) Targeting ceramide synthesis to reverse insulin resistance. Diabetes 59(10):2351–2353
84. Boushel R et al (2007) Patients with type 2 diabetes have normal mitochondrial function in skeletal muscle. Diabetologia 50(4):790–796
85. Kelley DE et al (2002) Dysfunction of mitochondria in human skeletal muscle in type 2 diabetes. Diabetes 51(10):2944–2950
86. Menshikova EV et al (2005) Effects of weight loss and physical activity on skeletal muscle mitochondrial function in obesity. Am J Physiol Endocrinol Metab 288(4):E818–E825
87. Morino K et al (2005) Reduced mitochondrial density and increased IRS-1 serine phosphorylation in muscle of insulin-resistant offspring of type 2 diabetic parents. J Clin Invest 115(12):3587
88. Petersen KF et al (2004) Impaired mitochondrial activity in the insulin-resistant offspring of patients with type 2 diabetes. N Engl J Med 350(7):664–671
89. Petersen KF, Dufour S, Shulman GI (2005) Decreased insulin-stimulated ATP synthesis and phosphate transport in muscle of insulin-resistant offspring of type 2 diabetic parents. PLoS Med 2(9):e233
90. Ritov VB et al (2010) Deficiency of electron transport chain in human skeletal muscle mitochondria in type 2 diabetes mellitus and obesity. Am J Physiol Endocrinol Metab 298(1):E49–E58
91. Patti ME et al (2003) Coordinated reduction of genes of oxidative metabolism in humans with insulin resistance and diabetes: potential role of PGC1 and NRF1. Proc Natl Acad Sci 100(14):8466

92. Ortenblad N et al (2005) Reduced insulin-mediated citrate synthase activity in cultured skeletal muscle cells from patients with type 2 diabetes: evidence for an intrinsic oxidative enzyme defect. Biochim Biophys Acta 1741(1–2):206–214
93. Toledo FGS, Watkins S, Kelley DE (2006) Changes induced by physical activity and weight loss in the morphology of intermyofibrillar mitochondria in obese men and women. J Clin Endocrinol Metab 91(8):3224–3227
94. Mogensen M et al (2007) Mitochondrial respiration is decreased in skeletal muscle of patients with type 2 diabetes. Diabetes 56(6):1592–1599
95. Phielix E et al (2008) Lower intrinsic ADP-stimulated mitochondrial respiration underlies in vivo mitochondrial dysfunction in muscle of male type 2 diabetic patients. Diabetes 57(11):2943–2949
96. Mensink M et al (2007) Improved skeletal muscle oxidative enzyme activity and restoration of PGC-1α and PPARβ/δ gene expression upon rosiglitazone treatment in obese patients with type 2 diabetes mellitus. Int J Obes 31(8):1302–1310
97. Hwang H et al (2010) Proteomics analysis of human skeletal muscle reveals novel abnormalities in obesity and type 2 diabetes. Diabetes 59(1):33–42
98. Bach D et al (2005) Expression of Mfn2, the Charcot-Marie-Tooth Neuropathy Type 2A gene, in human skeletal muscle. Diabetes 54(9):2685–2693
99. Meex RCR et al (2010) Restoration of muscle mitochondrial function and metabolic flexibility in type 2 diabetes by exercise training is paralleled by increased myocellular fat storage and improved insulin sensitivity. Diabetes 59(3):572–579
100. Toledo FGS et al (2008) Mitochondrial capacity in skeletal muscle is not stimulated by weight loss despite increases in insulin action and decreases in intramyocellular lipid content. Diabetes 57(4):987–994
101. Rabol R et al (2010) Regional anatomic differences in skeletal muscle mitochondrial respiration in type 2 diabetes and obesity. J Clin Endocrinol Metab 95(2):857–863
102. Emanuela F et al (2012) Inflammation as a link between obesity and metabolic syndrome. J Nutr Metab 2012:476380
103. Elks CM, Francis J (2010) Central adiposity, systemic inflammation, and the metabolic syndrome. Curr Hypertens Rep 12(2):99–104
104. Glass CK, Olefsky JM (2012) Inflammation and lipid signaling in the etiology of insulin resistance. Cell Metab 15(5):635–645
105. Newsholme P et al (2007) Amino acid metabolism, insulin secretion and diabetes. Biochem Soc Trans 35(5):1180–1186
106. Wang TJ et al (2011) Metabolite profiles and the risk of developing diabetes. Nat Med 17(4):448–453
107. Gall WE et al (2010) α-Hydroxybutyrate is an early biomarker of insulin resistance and glucose intolerance in a nondiabetic population. PLoS One 5(5):e10883
108. Huffman KM et al (2009) Relationships between circulating metabolic intermediates and insulin action in overweight to obese, inactive men and women. Diabetes Care 32(9):1678–1683
109. Fiehn O et al (2010) Plasma metabolomic profiles reflective of glucose homeostasis in non-diabetic and type 2 diabetic obese African–American women. PLoS One 5(12):e15234
110. Hills S et al (2004) The EGIR-RISC study (The European group for the study of insulin resistance: relationship between insulin sensitivity and cardiovascular disease risk): I. Methodology and objectives. Diabetologia 47(3):566–570
111. Shah S et al (2011) Branched-chain amino acid levels are associated with improvement in insulin resistance with weight loss. Diabetologia 2011:1–10
112. Laferrère B et al (2011) Differential metabolic impact of gastric bypass surgery versus dietary intervention in obese diabetic subjects despite identical weight loss. Sci Transl Med 3(80):80re2

The Metabolic Syndrome and Cardiovascular Disease

4

Frank Pistrosch, Frank Schaper, and Markolf Hanefeld

4.1 Association Between Metabolic Syndrome and CVD in the Population

The global prevalence of the metabolic syndrome in the adult population varies between 15 and 50 %. The prevalence is affected by multiple factors such as age, sex, nutrition habits, lifestyle factors, socio-economic conditions and ethnicity as major determinants and not at least definitions and arbitrary cut-off limits of single components [1, 2].

Environmental factors, however, interact not only with the traits of the metabolic syndrome but also with traditional risk factors such as cholesterol and smoking. Thus, we are confronted with a very complex network of coronary risk factors, which makes it more difficult to evaluate metabolic syndrome as cardiovascular risk factor in its own right. Therefore, it is not surprising that metabolic syndrome as a cardiovascular risk factor is a matter of controversy. In two large prospective studies, Sattar et al. [3] found that the metabolic syndrome has only weak or no association with cardiovascular risk in elderly population representative for the United Kingdom. In these prospective trials, the metabolic syndrome was, however, a major risk factor for type 2 diabetes. Therefore, the authors concluded that there is no common soil for diabetes and CVD. The metabolic syndrome by NCEP III criteria could, however, be confirmed to be associated with CVD in Asian populations [4, 5]. Nevertheless, in all related studies we found a approximately twofold higher prevalence of the metabolic syndrome in comparable cohorts with major CVD (coronary heart disease, cerebrovascular disease, stroke) [6, 7]. Interestingly, in the United States, obesity, diabetes and coronary heart disease develop in parallel with some lag time for development of coronary heart disease (Table 4.1) [9]. The same

F. Pistrosch • F. Schaper • M. Hanefeld (✉)
Study Centre Professor Hanefeld, GWT-TUD GmbH, Fiedlerstrasse 34, 01307 Dresden, Germany
e-mail: Hanefeld@gwtonline-zks.de

H. Beck-Nielsen (ed.), *The Metabolic Syndrome*,
DOI 10.1007/978-3-7091-1331-8_4, © Springer-Verlag Wien 2013

Table 4.1 Prevalence of the metabolic syndrome by NCEP 1998 and WHO criteria 1999

Age	1998 WHO ($N = 35.8M$) (%)	1999 WHO ($N = 41.3M$) (%)	NCEP III ($N = 48.4M$) (%)	DM ($N = 14.0M$) (%)	CHD ($N = 12.2$) (%)
20–29 years (36M)	4.9	4.9	6.0	0.5	1.9
30–39 years (42M)	11.0	11.1	14.2	2.0	3.4
40–49 years (42M)	19.3	21.2	24.6	5.0	4.5
50–59 years (30M)	28.5	32.4	36.5	12.9	7.5
60–69 years (20M)	35.3	42.0	48.1	17.7	11.9
70–79 years (16M)	35.0	44.3	48.4	18.4	16.1
80+ years (9M)	22.4	27.7	43.3	15.5	17.9

Diabetes and CHD by age group among US population ≥20 years [9]
CHD coronary heart disease, *NCEP* National Cholesterol Education Program, *WHO* World Health Organization

phenomenon can be observed in the process of globalisation and westernisation in all other countries [10].

In a meta-analysis for patients with quantitative coronary angiography using intravascular ultrasound including a total population of 3,459 patients, 57.8 % met the criteria of the metabolic syndrome by NCEPIII definition [11]. Metabolic syndrome was associated greater likely of undergoing progression in plaque atheroma volume. Significant progression in plaque atheroma volume was defined as an increase of 5 % or greater. The main predicting factors for progression were hypertriglyceridaemia (odds ratio 1.26) and a body mass index >30 kg/m^2 (odds ratio 1.18). However, after adjusting of these two components metabolic syndrome itself disappeared as an independent predictor for plaque atheroma progression. This is in line with some studies from Wilson et al. [12] and Sundström et al. [13], who reported that metabolic syndrome did not predict cardiovascular mortality independently of its individual components. This illustrates that the components of the metabolic syndrome have partially overlapping mechanisms of pathogenic actions mediated through common effects. Therefore, their total combined effect could be less than the sum of individual effects.

In the Acute Coronary Syndrome (ACS) Israeli Survey, 1,060 consecutive patients with non-clinically diagnosed diabetes were admitted due to ACS. Three hundred and fifty nine patients with metabolic syndrome (modified NCEP III criteria) were compared with 701 subjects without metabolic syndrome. Patients with metabolic syndrome had higher 30-day mortality rates compared with patients with hyperglycaemia without metabolic syndrome (8.3 % vs. 2.5 %, $p < 0.05$). Multivariate analysis identified the metabolic syndrome as a strong independent predictor of 30-day and 1-year mortality with hazard ratios of 2.54 (95 % confidence interval (CI) 1.22–5.31) and 1.96 (95 % CI 1.18–3.24), respectively [14].

In a total of 633 unselected, consecutive patients hospitalised with acute myocardial infarction patients with ($n = 290$) and without ($n = 343$) metabolic syndrome were compared. Acute myocardial infarction characteristics and left ventricular (LV) ejection fraction at admission were similar for both groups. In-hospital case fatality was higher in patients with metabolic syndrome compared with those without, as was the incidence of severe heart failure (Killip class >II). In a multivariate analysis, metabolic syndrome was a strong and independent predictor of severe heart failure, but not in-hospital death. Analysis of the predictive value of each of the five metabolic syndrome components for severe heart failure showed that hyperglycaemia was the major determinant (odds ratio, 3.31; 95 % CI, 1.86–5.87) [15].

In the Strong Heart Study with American Indians, participants with metabolic syndrome had a greater LV dimension, mass, and relative wall thickness, and left atrial diameter (all $p <\neq 0.01$), and a higher prevalence of LV hypertrophy ($p < 0.001$), with lower ejection fraction ($p < 0.05$), midwall shortening ($p < 0.001$) and mitral *E*/*A* ratio ($p < 0.05$) than participants without metabolic syndrome [16].

A further study examined the association between left ventricular diastolic dysfunction (LVDD) and metabolic syndrome. The prevalence of LVDD was 68 % in subjects with metabolic syndrome vs. 19 % in patients without metabolic syndrome ($p < 0.001$). A severe form of LVDD was observed in 34 % and 15 % of patients with and without metabolic syndrome, respectively ($p = 0.001$). The prevalence of mild and severe diastolic dysfunction increased with the number of metabolic syndrome traits ($p = 0.001$). In the metabolic syndrome group, early diastolic tissue relaxation velocity (*E*) was significantly reduced (6.9 ± 1.8 cm/s vs. 7.7 ± 2.1 cm/s; $p = 0.009$) and the E/E' ratio was significantly higher (10.5 ± 3.9 vs. 9.1 ± 3.0 cm/s, $P = 0.015$) as compared with the group without metabolic syndrome ($n = 69$). In conclusion, metabolic syndrome was associated with a higher prevalence and severity of LVDD [17].

Recently published data from three large meta-analyses are in line with the 1999 statement of the AHA with metabolic syndrome to be associated with increased risk of cardiovascular events [9]. The largest of them included more than 900,000 patients. In this large population-based meta-analysis, the metabolic syndrome was associated with a twofold increase in cardiovascular events and a 1.5-fold increase in all-cause mortality rates. The cardiovascular risk was still high in patients with metabolic syndrome but without diabetes. The relative risk for coronary heart disease was higher in women than in men with metabolic syndrome [18]. These new data on the cardiovascular burden in association with the metabolic syndrome fits well into the overall estimation of the AHA published in 1999 using the NCEP III criteria [9].

There are less data available concerning metabolic syndrome and cerebrovascular disease.

In the Nijmegen Biomedical Study, several non-invasive measurements of atherosclerosis (NIMA) were carried out in 1,517 participants aged 50–70 years with and without metabolic syndrome [19]. Participants with metabolic syndrome by NCEP III criteria were characterised by increased subclinical atherosclerosis compared with participants without any trait of the metabolic syndrome, as reflected by lower ankle-brachial index at rest [percent change (95 % CI), men: −5.2 % (−9; −1), women: −3.1 % (−6; −1)] and after exercise [men: −7.7 % (−17; +2), F: −6.6 % (−11; −2)], higher augmentation index [men: +4.8 % (+3; +7), women: +1.9 % (+4; +18)], increased pulse wave velocity [men: +22.8 % (+15; +32), women: +20.5 % (+14; +28)], increased intima-media thickness (IMT) [men: +9.3 % (+5; +13), women: +6.9 % (+3; +11)], and thicker plaques [men: +17.6 % (−2; +41), women: +26.6 % (+5; +53)]. The number of traits was strongly associated with the severity of subclinical atherosclerosis. Interestingly, NIMA were already deteriorated when one or two traits were present and further deteriorated when four or five traits of the metabolic syndrome were diagnosed.

The carotid IMT and the plaque volume were examined by ultrasound in a total of 166 individuals (73 with metabolic syndrome vs. 93 without metabolic syndrome) [20]. Increased IMT was measured in patient with metabolic syndrome (0.818 mm) vs. (0.746 mm) in subjects without metabolic syndrome as well as total plaque volume (125 ± 26 vs. 77.3 ± 17.0 mm^3) ($p = 0.039$). The higher the number of risk factors that characterises the metabolic syndrome, the higher the increase in IMT.

In a cross-sectional study, metabolic syndrome ($n = 95$) resulted in an increased thickness of >16 % ($p = 0.002$) and increased stiffness of >32 % ($p = 0.012$) of the IMT of common carotid arteries compared with patients without metabolic syndrome ($n = 376$) [21].

A 14-year follow-up study in 1,131 men (114 with [only 9 %!] and 1,017 without metabolic syndrome) showed that metabolic syndrome was associated with all types of stroke (odds ratio 2.05)—65 strokes occurred during the monitoring, 47 of them were ischaemic [22].

After a 14-year follow-up in 2,097 individuals with initially high prevalence of the metabolic syndrome (men 30.3 %, women 24.7 %), 75 men and 55 women suffered the first stroke. The relative risk of stroke in individuals with diabetes and metabolic syndrome was high (odds ratio 3.28), higher than that of any other metabolic syndrome phenotype. In this study with high prevalence of metabolic syndrome, the metabolic syndrome was an independent risk factor for stroke also in individuals without diabetes [23].

4.2 CVD and Metabolic Syndrome in Patients with Abnormal Glucose Tolerance

It is a consistent finding that type 2 diabetes is associated in >70 % of subjects with metabolic syndrome [24, 25]. In the Diabetes in Germany (DIG) Study, a population-based observational study with more than 4,000 patients >74 % had

Table 4.2 Prevalence of metabolic syndrome (NCEPIII) and its traits in patients with type 2 diabetes: the Diabetes-In-Germany Study (DIG) [8]

	Prevalence (%)		
Traits	Total	Men	Women
Obesity*	49.8	44.4	55.9
Hypertension	91.3	91.3	91.4
HTG	55.4	56.5	54.1
Low HDL-C	9.3	10.0	8.4
Only diabetes	2.4	2.6	2.2
+1 trait	20.5	21.5	19.3
+2 traits	35.3	36.4	34.1
+3 traits	27.2	25.1	29.5
+4 traits	4.0	4.2	3.8
Overall metabolic syndrome	74.4	73.2	75.8

*Difference by gender $p \leq 0.001$ χ^2-test; obesity: body mass index ≥ 30 kg/m^2
NCEPIII National Cholesterol Education Program, *HTG* hypertriglyceridaemia, *HDL-C* high-density lipoprotein cholesterol

metabolic syndrome by NCEP III criteria [8]. In the majority, we observed triple traits and quartets (Table 4.2). Among individual phenotypes, triplets of hypertension plus obesity/hypertriglyceridaemia dominate.

Therefore, the WHO expert panel recommended excluding clinical type 2 diabetes as component of the metabolic syndrome [26]. This is in striking contrast to the first descriptions of the metabolic syndrome in the past century, which were based on the coincidence of diabetes with hypertension and hyperuricaemia [27, 28].

Already patients with impaired glucose tolerance (IGT) exhibit an increase in the prevalence of the metabolic syndrome compared with subjects with normal glucose tolerance in the same age range. About every second subject with IGT is diagnosed with metabolic syndrome [29–31].

Dysglycaemia as cardiovascular risk factor develops along a continuum up to the upper normal range for fasting and postprandial plasma glucose levels [32, 33]. Overwhelming evidence exists that cardiovascular events and progression of vascular lesions in diabetes strongly depend on the presence of comorbidities such as hypertension and dyslipidaemia, two major traits of the metabolic syndrome. As shown in Table 4.2, hypertension and hypertriglyceridaemia are the most frequent single traits in the DIG database [8].

With the dominance of hypertension and lipids as single risk factors it is not surprising that different phenotypes or combinations of the metabolic syndrome bear a different cardiovascular risk. In the DIG study the highest risk for all 11 combinations was for those with hypertension and its triplets with all other traits (Table 4.3). In all combinations with hypertension, women had a higher cardiovascular risk than men. However, quartets and quintets had no higher risk than triplets. This may be biased by small numbers of quartets and quintets. Overall, metabolic syndrome was associated with an odds ratio of 1.38 (CI 1.04–1.82) for men and 1.67 (CI 1.08–2.59) for women.

Table 4.3 Odds ratios (95 % confidence interval) for cardiovascular disease of different phenotypes of the metabolic syndrome in the Diabetes in Germany study (DIG) population by sex (NCEP III criteria) [8]

Phenotype	Total population	Men	Women
Triads			
DM + HBP + LHDL	5.67 (2.84–11.31)	4.25 (1.92–9.41)	10.90 (2.51–47.46)
DM + HBP + HTG	5.64 (2.29–13.87)	4.96 (1.80–13.71)	8.78 (1.21–63.91)
DM + HBP + Obes	6.17 (2.51–15.16)	6.11 (2.22–16.85)	9.19 (1.26–66.82)
DM + LHDL + HTG	1.14 (0.82–1.58)	0.85 (0.55–1.31)	1.78 (1.07–2.96)
DM + LHDL + Obes	0.90 (0.59–1.37)	0.54 (0.29–1.01)	1.76 (0.97–3.19)
DM + HTG + Obes	0.96 (0.79–1.17)	0.91 (0.71–1.17)	1.20 (0.86–1.68)
Quartets			
DM + HBP + LHDL + HTG	1.21 (0.87–1.69)	0.90 (0.58–1.39)	1.90 (1.13–3.20)
DM + HBP + LHDL + Obes	0.95 (0.62–1.46)	0.56 (0.30–1.04)	1.92 (1.05–3.50)
DM + HBP + HTG + Obes	1.01 (0.82–1.23)	0.93 (0.72–1.21)	1.29 (0.92–1.79)
DM + LHDL + HTG + Obes	0.86 (0.54–1.38)	0.47 (0.23–0.95)	1.85 (0.97–3.52)
Quintet			
DM + HBP + LHDL + HTG + Obes	0.92 (0.57–1.47)	0.49 (0.24–1.00)	2.03 (1.06–3.87)
Overall MetS	1.41 (1.12–1.78)	1.38 (1.04–1.82)	1.67 (1.08–2.59)

DM diabetes mellitus, *HBP* high blood pressure, *HTG* hypertriglyceridaemia, *Obes* obesity, *LHDL* low high density cholesterol, *NCEP* National Cholesterol Education Program

As demonstrated in Fig. 4.1, hypertension in the DIG study is the most important risk factor for CVD in type 2 diabetes with an odds ratio twice of that for overall metabolic syndrome. This is, however, not an argument against the concept of the metabolic syndrome in type 2 diabetes. In the DIG study, stepwise regression analysis to determine the significance of the metabolic syndrome together with major established risk factors confirms overall metabolic syndrome, age, men, sex, LDL-Cholesterol and smoking as independent risk factors [8]. The lesson from this and other studies is that a careful consideration of all traits of the metabolic syndrome in patients with type 2 diabetes is highly clinical relevant and can be used as guide for patient-centred treatment. For example triple combinations with obesity and hypertension will need weight neutral or weight-reducing antidiabetic drugs and should avoid ß-blockers to control hypertension in younger ages in patients with abnormal glucose tolerance if they are free of CVD.

4.3 Metabolic Syndrome and Related Cardiovascular Risk Factors

Metabolic syndrome is closely linked to insulin resistance together with visceral obesity. Thus, it includes other cardiovascular risk factors such as albuminuria [34, 35], non-alcoholic fatty liver [36, 37] and sleep apnoea [38, 39].

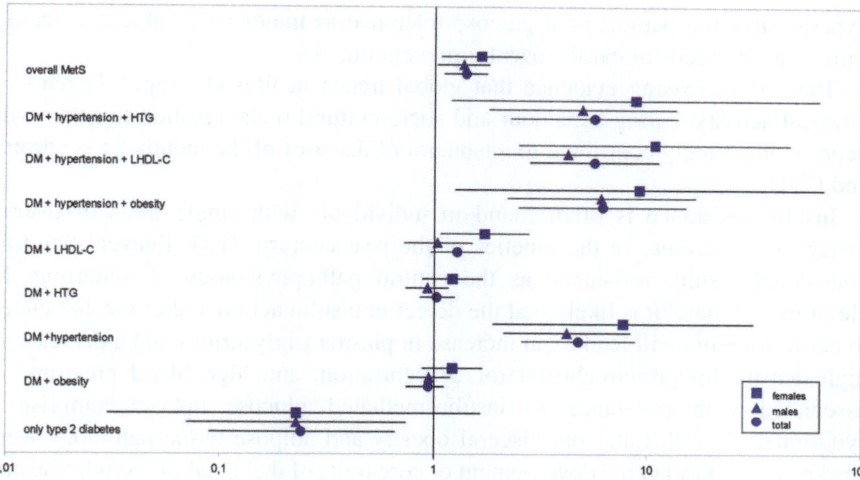

Fig. 4.1 Odds ratios for major cardiovascular diseases in patients with type 2 diabetes (DIG-study) in different traits of and overall metabolic syndrome [8]

Table 4.4 Diseases and emerging risk factors related to the metabolic syndrome

Non-alcoholic fatty liver
Sleep apnoea
Albuminuria
Minor sexual, nerval and psychological abnormalities
Social depression
Increased subclinical inflammation
Endothelial dysfunction
Increased intima-media thickness
Thrombophilia

Table 4.4 summarises typical clinical findings which may be associated with increased cardiovascular risk in patients with metabolic syndrome. Making the diagnosis of these diseases, therefore, indicates to look for all traits of the metabolic syndrome. Vice versa it should be good clinical practice in subjects with metabolic syndrome to look for these related diseases. We, however, find no specific complications related to the 'diagnosis' metabolic syndrome. All these diseases can be found in connection with single traits, particularly in visceral obesity, but this provides further support to the concept of this syndrome since lifestyle intervention with weight reduction and increased physical activity is the common basis of treatment for all diseases related to the metabolic syndrome.

4.4 Common Soil for the Metabolic Syndrome and CVD?

Metabolic syndrome became a mass phenomenon together with the worldwide epidemic of obesity and diabetes. When the statins allowed an effective and safe control of hypercholesterolaemia, traits of the metabolic syndrome such as hypertension and pathological glucose tolerance as major modifiable risk factors came into the focus of cardiovascular prevention.

There is increasing evidence that global trends in lifestyle, rapid decrease in physical activity, eating behaviour and socio-cultural maladaptation together with depression strongly contribute to a tsunami of diseases of the metabolic syndrome and CVD.

Insulin resistance is often found in individuals with single traits or overall metabolic syndrome. In the nineties of the past century, G.M. Reaven therefore considered insulin resistance as the central pathophysiology of syndrome X. He proposed that: "it is likely that the defect in insulin action and/or the associated hyperinsulinemia will lead to an increase in plasma triglycerides and a decrease in high density lipoprotein-cholesterol concentration, and high blood pressure … associated with resistance to insulin-mediated glucose uptake comprise a syndrome…" [40]. Later on, visceral obesity and adipose tissue pathology were worked out as keys to the development of core traits of the metabolic syndrome and related diseases based on the worldwide epidemic in obesity and the parallel increase in the global prevalence of the metabolic syndrome. Eventually traits of the metabolic syndrome entered the top league of cardiovascular risk factors [41–43]. Regional or visceral obesity is closely connected with another link of the metabolic syndrome to CVD: Low-grade inflammation. Adipocyte hypertrophy and visceral obesity are associated with an increase in secretion of biomarkers of low-grade inflammation such as interleukin (IL)-6, tumour necrosis factor α (TNFα) and resistin and a decrease in anti-inflammatory adipokine adiponectin [44, 45]. At the same time, we observe a massive immigration of activated macrophages into the adipose tissue [46, 47]. Furthermore, together with the fatty liver level of the C-reactive protein [44] and fetuin A [48, 49] is increased—both emerging new cardiovascular risk factors. By extrapolation, we see a very complex pathophysiology as soil for the metabolic syndrome and associated diseases, which are also relevant for cardiovascular risk. This overlapping of risk factors with a strong impact on lifestyle and environment applies for both the metabolic syndrome and CVD.

Therefore, if we consider a possible common soil for the metabolic syndrome and CVD, we have to focus not on a one-dimensional genetic or pathophysiology axis, but on lifestyle changes, rapid behavioural and cultural transitions and socio-economic stress in the process of globalisation and westernisation [10, 50]. As a prominent example, a close correlation between job stress and the metabolic syndrome was shown in the prospective Whitehall II study [51]. The age-adjusted odds ratio for metabolic syndrome, after adjustment for age, for the grade of stress exposure in the highest grade was >2 versus low and moderate exposure. Korenblum et al. [52] compared prevalence of type 2 diabetes and the metabolic syndrome between native Germans and different groups of immigrants in North Rhine Westphalia. Those with high social stress had about twice as high prevalence compared with well-integrated immigrants and with native Germans. A high social gradient for the metabolic syndrome, which could not be explained by behavioural factors, was reported from the Copenhagen City Heart study [53, 54]. In general, lower class people have higher risk of developing metabolic syndrome and CVD, as demonstrated for the transition time in Eastern bloc countries [55].

Thus, we find the common soil for the metabolic syndrome and CVD in times of globalisation in an unhealthy lifestyle and in changes of socio-economic conditions and environmental factors.

4.5 Metabolic Syndrome as Guide for Patient-Centred Treatment

As pointed out the metabolic syndrome is a simple term for a heterogenic cluster of interrelated diseases with complex interaction with CVD. However, there are core elements of a common soil such as nutrition, physical activity, social behaviour and stress as a basis for lifestyle intervention.

In the next step with individualised drug treatment or interventional measures such as bariatric surgery, the traits of metabolic disease and presence or absence of cardiovascular complications can be used as a guide for a patient-centred but integrated approach.

As we learned from the Steno 2 study [56], an integrated approach of major risk factors results in significant benefit compared with treatment only directed to control blood glucose. In the Study to Prevent Non-Insulin-Dependent Diabetes Mellitus (STOP-NIDDM) in patients with IGT, the number needed to treat to prevent one case of newly diagnosed diabetes in patients with metabolic syndrome was 5.8 vs. 16.5 in those without metabolic syndrome [31].

In the Antihypertensive and Lipid-Lowering Treatment to Prevent Heart Attach Trial (ALLHAT), a study to control hypertension with different blood pressure-lowering drugs to prevent cardiovascular complications treatment with ß-blockers and diuretics was associated with significantly higher risk of developing type 2 diabetes in the presence of the metabolic syndrome[57]. Thus, individual use of antidiabetic drugs or ß-blockers should be guided by presence or absence of traits of the metabolic syndrome and CVD. Pleiotropic effects of drugs for treatment of hypertension and dysglycaemia can be used for an integrated approach of this cluster of interrelated diseases.

The Steno 2 study, provides clear evidence, that an integrated approach to control major risk factors is most effective to prevent CVD and reduce all-cause mortality [56].

In conclusion, currently available data strongly support the evolving concept of the metabolic syndrome as an important cluster of cardiovascular risk factors and metabolic vascular diseases. The concept provides an integrated approach of diagnostics, prevention and treatment of diseases of the metabolic syndrome as major cardiovascular risk factors. Well-designed randomised controlled trials are needed to develop and evaluate patient-centred strategies. With a common soil of lifestyle factors and unhealthy environment, public health strategies are essential to stop the metabolic syndrome tsunami.

References

1. Cameron AJ et al (2004) The metabolic syndrome: prevalence in worldwide populations. Endocrinol Metab Clin North Am 33:351–375
2. Wilson PW, Meigs JB (2008) Cardiometabolic risk: a Framingham perspective. Int J Obes (Lond) 32(Suppl 2):17–20
3. Sattar N et al (2008) Can metabolic syndrome usefully predict cardiovascular disease and diabetes? Outcome data from two prospective studies. Lancet 371(9628):1927–1935
4. Jia W et al. (2004) A comparison of the application of two working definitions of metabolic syndrome in Chinese population. Zhonghua Yi Xue Za Zhi 84(7):534–538
5. Cameron AJ et al (2003) Comparison of WHO and NCEP metabolic syndrome definitions over 5 years in Mauritius. Diabetologia 46:A3068
6. Grundy SM (2008) Metabolic syndrome pandemic. Arterioscler Thromb Vasc Biol 28(4):629–636
7. Alberti KG et al (2006) Metabolic syndrome—a new world-wide definition. A Consensus Statement from the International Diabetes Federation. Diabet Med 23(5):469–480
8. Hanefeld M et al (2007) Impact of the individual components of the metabolic syndrome and their different combinations on the prevalence of atherosclerotic vascular disease in type 2 diabetes: the Diabetes in Germany (DIG) study. Cardiovasc Diabetol 6:13
9. Alexander CM et al (2003) NCEP-defined metabolic syndrome, diabetes, and prevalence of coronary heart disease among NHANES III participants age 50 years and older. Diabetes 52(5):1210–1214
10. Bornstein SR (2008) Is the worldwide epidemic of obesity a communicable feature of globalization? Exp Clin Endocrinol Diabetes 116(Suppl 1):S30–S32
11. Bayturan O et al (2010) The metabolic syndrome, its component risk factors, and progression of coronary atherosclerosis. Arch Intern Med 170(5):478–484
12. Wilson PW et al (2005) Metabolic syndrome as a precursor of cardiovascular disease and type 2 diabetes mellitus. Circulation 112(20):3066–3072
13. Sundström J et al (2008) Blood pressure-independent relations of left ventricular geometry to the metabolic syndrome and insulin resistance: a population-based study. Heart 94(7):874–878
14. Feinberg MS et al (2007) Impact of the metabolic syndrome on the clinical outcomes of non-clinically diagnosed diabetic patients with acute coronary syndrome. Am J Cardiol 99(5):667–672
15. Zeller M et al (2005) Prevalence and impact of metabolic syndrome on hospital outcomes in acute myocardial infarction. Arch Intern Med 165(10):1192–1198
16. Chinali M et al (2004) Comparison of cardiac structure and function in American Indians with and without the metabolic syndrome (the Strong Heart Study). Am J Cardiol 93(1):40–44
17. Dinh W et al (2011) Metabolic syndrome with or without diabetes contributes to left ventricular diastolic dysfunction. Acta Cardiol 66(2):167–174
18. Mottillo S et al (2010) The metabolic syndrome and cardiovascular risk a systematic review and meta-analysis. J Am Coll Cardiol 56(14):1113–1132
19. Holewijn S et al (2009) The metabolic syndrome and its traits as risk factors for subclinical atherosclerosis. J Clin Endocrinol Metab 94(8):2893–2899
20. Pollex RL et al (2006) Relationship of the metabolic syndrome to carotid ultrasound traits. Cardiovasc Ultrasound 4:28
21. Scuteri A et al (2004) Metabolic syndrome amplifies the age-associated increases in vascular thickness and stiffness. J Am Coll Cardiol 43(8):1388–1395
22. Kurl S et al (2006) Metabolic syndrome and the risk of stroke in middle-aged men. Stroke 37(3):806–811
23. Najarian RM et al (2006) Metabolic syndrome compared with type 2 diabetes mellitus as a risk factor for stroke: the Framingham Offspring Study. Arch Intern Med 166(1):106–111
24. Bruno G et al (2004) Casale Monferrato Study: metabolic syndrome as a predictor of all-cause and cardiovascular mortality in type 2 diabetes: the Casale Monferrato Study. Diabetes Care 27:2689–2694

25. Ilanne-Parikka P et al (2004) Prevalence of the metabolic syndrome and its components: findings from a Finnish general population sample and the Diabetes Prevention Study cohort. Diabetes Care 27:2135–2140
26. Simmons RK et al (2010) The metabolic syndrome: useful concept or clinical tool? Report of a WHO Expert Consultation. Diabetologia 53(4):600–605
27. Maranon G (1922) About hypertension and sugar disease. Z Inn Med 43:169–176
28. Kylin E et al (1923) Studien ueber das Hypertonie-Hyperglykaemie- Hyperurikaemiesyndrom. Zentralblatt fuer Innere Medizin 44:105–127
29. Hu G et al (2004) Prevalence of the metabolic syndrome and its relation to all-cause and cardiovascular mortality in nondiabetic European men and women. Arch Intern Med 164(10):1066–1076
30. Liu SJ et al (2008) Risks for type-2 diabetes associated with the metabolic syndrome and the interaction between impaired fasting glucose and other components of metabolic syndrome the study from Jiangsu, China of 5 years follow-up. Diabetes Res Clin Pract 81(1):117–123
31. Hanefeld M et al (2009) Metabolic syndrome and its single traits as risk factors for diabetes in people with impaired glucose tolerance: the STOP-NIDDM trial. Diab Vasc Dis Res 6(1):32–37
32. Gerstein HC (2009) Dysglycemia and cardiovascular risk in the general population. Circulation 119(6):773–775
33. Ning F et al (2012) Development of coronary heart disease and ischemic stroke in relation to fasting and 2-hour plasma glucose levels in the normal range. Cardiovasc Diabetol 11(1):76
34. van der Velde M et al (2012) Do albuminuria and hs-CRP add to the International Diabetes Federation definition of the metabolic syndrome in predicting outcome? Nephrol Dial Transplant 27(6):2275–2283
35. Sheen YJ, Sheu WH (2011) Metabolic syndrome and renal injury. Cardiol Res Pract 2011:567389
36. Sung KC (2012) Fatty liver, insulin resistance, and features of metabolic syndrome: relationships with coronary artery calcium in 10,153 people. Diabetes Care 35(11):2359–2364
37. Targher G et al (2010) Risk of cardiovascular disease in patients with nonalcoholic fatty liver disease. N Engl J Med 363(14):1341–1350
38. Ambrosetti M et al (2006) Metabolic syndrome in obstructive sleep apnea and related cardiovascular risk. J Cardiovasc Med (Hagerstown) 7(11):826–829
39. Kostapanos MS et al (2012) Obstructive sleep apnea and cardiovascular risk: is metabolic syndrome the link? Angiology 63(8):569–573
40. Reaven GM (1993) Role of insulin resistance in human disease (syndrome X): an expanded definition. Annu Rev Med 44:121–131
41. Cameron AJ et al (2009) Health and mortality consequences of abdominal obesity: evidence from the AusDiab study. Med J Aust 191(4):202–208
42. Lee CM (2008) The metabolic syndrome identifies a heterogeneous group of metabolic component combinations in the Asia-Pacific region. Diabetes Res Clin Pract 81(3):377–380
43. Eckel RH et al (2005) The metabolic syndrome. Lancet 365(9468):1415–1428
44. Ridker PM, Cook NR (2007) Biomarkers for prediction of cardiovascular events. N Engl J Med 356(14):1472–1473
45. Fernández-Real JM (2003) Insulin resistance and chronic cardiovascular inflammatory syndrome. Endocr Rev 24:278–301
46. Bouloumié A et al (2008) Adipose tissue lymphocytes and macrophages in obesity and insulin resistance: makers or markers, and which comes first? Arterioscler Thromb Vasc Biol 28(7):1211–1213
47. Heilbronn LK, Campbell LV (2008) Adipose tissue macrophages, low grade inflammation and insulin resistance in human obesity. Curr Pharm Des 14(12):1225–1230
48. Laughlin GA et al (2012) The association of fetuin-A with cardiovascular disease mortality in older community-dwelling adults: the Rancho Bernardo study. J Am Coll Cardiol 59(19):1688–1696

49. Weikert C et al (2008) Plasma fetuin-a levels and the risk of myocardial infarction and ischemic stroke. Circulation 118(24):2555–2562
50. Suchday S et al (2008) Subjective and objective measures of socioeconomic status: predictors of cardiovascular risk in college students in Mumbai, India. Ethn Dis 18(2 Supp 2):S2-235–S2-237
51. Stringhini S et al (2012) Socioeconomic status, structural and functional measures of social support, and mortality: the British Whitehall II Cohort Study, 1985–2009. Am J Epidemiol 175 (12):1275–1283
52. Korenblum W et al (2005) Elevated cortisol levels and increased rates of diabetes and mood symptoms in Soviet Union-born Jewish immigrants to Germany. Mol Psychiatry 10 (11):974–975
53. Rod NH et al (2011) Psychosocial risk factors and heart failure hospitalization: a prospective cohort study. Am J Epidemiol 174(6):672–680
54. Prescott E et al (2007) Social gradient in the metabolic syndrome not explained by psychosocial and behavioural factors: evidence from the Copenhagen City Heart Study. Eur J Cardiovasc Prev Rehabil 14(3):405–412
55. Stelmach W et al (2005) How education, income, control over life and life style contribute to risk factors for cardiovascular disease among adults in a post-communist country. Public Health 119(6):498–508
56. Gaede P et al (2003) Multifactorial intervention and cardiovascular disease in patients with type 2 diabetes. N Engl J Med 348(5):383–393
57. Black HR et al (2008) Metabolic and clinical outcomes in nondiabetic individuals with the metabolic syndrome assigned to chlorthalidone, amlodipine, or lisinopril as initial treatment for hypertension: a report from the Antihypertensive and Lipid-Lowering Treatment to Prevent Heart Attack Trial (ALLHAT). Diabetes Care 31(2):353–360

The Metabolic Syndrome and Cancer

5

Frank Pistrosch and Markolf Hanefeld

5.1 Epidemiology

Epidemiological studies have clearly demonstrated an association of many types of cancer with several traits of the metabolic syndrome [1–3]. The strongest associations were found between central obesity and cancers of the breast (in postmenopausal women), colorectum, endometrium, pancreas, liver, gallbladder, kidney and oesophagus [4] whereas type 2 diabetes was mainly associated with cancers of the pancreas, liver and endometrium [2]. The Women's Health Initiative Observational Study (WHI-OS) reported that patients with insulin resistance had a higher risk of developing postmenopausal breast cancer [5]. Data from case–control and cohort studies have determined hazard ratios between 1.1 and 2.3 for cancer incidence in obesity and type 2 diabetes. However, a coincidence of these two conditions or of other traits of the metabolic syndrome may further increase the risk [1, 2]. The metabolic syndrome is not only associated with an increased risk of cancer incidence but also mortality. About 10 % of the excess mortality in patients with type 2 diabetes may be attributable to death from cancer [6]. Comparable data have been reported from obese individuals [7]. After adjustment for age, sex, smoking status and body mass index, the hazard ratio for death from cancer among patients with type 2 diabetes was 1.25 (95 % confidence interval (CI), 1.19–1.31) compared with persons without diabetes. An increased risk of death from cancer was detectable even in persons with impaired glucose tolerance (hazard ratio 1.13; 95 % CI 1.06–1.20) [6].

F. Pistrosch • M. Hanefeld (✉)
Study Centre Professor Hanefeld, GWT-TUD GmbH, Fiedlerstrasse 34, 01307 Dresden, Germany
e-mail: Hanefeld@gwtonline-zks.de

H. Beck-Nielsen (ed.), *The Metabolic Syndrome*,
DOI 10.1007/978-3-7091-1331-8_5, © Springer-Verlag Wien 2013

5.2 Pathophysiology

Although the amount of epidemiological data supporting the association between traits of the metabolic syndrome and cancer is substantial, these data did not allow deriving a causal relationship. Therefore in vitro and in vivo studies were performed to identify common biological factors and to understand the connection between the two conditions.

The primary reason for the implementation of the term "metabolic syndrome" was to indicate a cluster of metabolic diseases and hypertension which occurred more frequently than by chance [8]. Later on, a common pathophysiological pathway for the development of the different traits of the syndrome has been suggested, which eventually contributes to the development of arteriosclerosis [9], and today the term metabolic syndrome describes not only a cluster of metabolic diseases but also a cluster of pathophysiologically linked cardiovascular risk factors.

Inflammation—the common soil for the development of different traits of the metabolic syndrome—was the most promising candidate for a causal relationship between cancer and metabolic syndrome, too. Carcinogenesis describes a process of malignant transformation, which involves initiation, promotion and progression of cancer. Whereas multiple genetic damages are a prerequisite for a complete neoplastic transformation of a cell, every step of carcinogenesis can be influenced by environmental factors.

Adipose tissue is the largest endocrine organ of the human body producing free fatty acids, different cytokines (interleukin 6, monocyte chemoattractant protein1, tumour necrosis factor-α) and hormones (leptin, aromatase, adiponectin, plasminogen activator inhibitor 1), which may be involved in cancer genesis and progression [10]. Interleukin 6 has been shown to enhance cancer cell growth and invasion via activation of signal transducer and activator of transcription protein pathway [11], whereas free fatty acids or cytokines like tumour necrosis factor-α cause insulin resistance and subsequently hyperinsulinaemia [12, 13]. The role of insulin resistance and hyperinsulinaemia in cancer development and progression has been extensively studied [14]. Insulin and insulin-like growth factor (IGF) receptors are expressed on most cancer cells, and its activation by insulin can stimulate cancer cell proliferation [15]. Furthermore, hyperinsulinaemia increases circulating IGF-1 levels by suppression of hepatic IGF-binding protein production [16]. Animal studies demonstrated a direct involvement of IGF-1 in cancer cell growth [17], and higher circulating IGF-1 levels in humans were associated with increased risk of cancer mortality [18]. Indirect effects of hyperinsulinaemia are mediated by the reduction of hepatic synthesis of sex hormone binding globulin, which resulted in increased levels of bioavailable sex hormones [1]. A stimulated aromatase activity of adipose tissue with an increased production of estradiol may additionally aggravate the risk of breast and endometrial cancer in postmenopausal women [4]. A direct pathophysiological role of hyperglycaemia in cancer cell proliferation remains to be proven and human studies assessing the effect of hyperglycaemia on cancer progression were inconclusive due to confounding effects of hyperinsulinaemia and comorbidities [1, 19]. In conclusion, there are convincing pathophysiological links between the metabolic syndrome and cancer development or progression which support the hypothesis of a causal association between these conditions.

5.3 Cancer Risk and Medical Treatment of the Metabolic Syndrome

The metabolic syndrome as a cluster of cardiovascular risk factors often requires pharmacological therapy. For most of its single traits therapeutic goals exist which cannot be achieved by lifestyle intervention alone in most cases. It has been demonstrated that the combination of improved glucose control, lipid-lowering therapy and blood pressure therapy can reduce death from any cause and from cardiovascular causes [20]. However, the extended use of meta-analyses and analyses of prescription databases have raised concerns about possible associations between the risk of cancer and often prescribed drugs in patients with metabolic syndrome. In 2010, a meta-analysis of nine randomised trials described an increased relative risk of cancer incidence in patients randomised to angiotensin receptor blocker compared with placebo (relative risk (RR) 1.07, 95 % CI 0.97–1.18) [21]. A second meta-analysis, which included 23 trials, did not confirm these results and reported an identical risk of cancer incidence between angiotensin receptor blocker and placebo (odds ratio 1.01, 95 % CI 0.93–1.09) [22]. These two examples illustrate the problem of pooled analyses of different prospective studies: Authors of meta-analyses did not have access to individual data, confirmation of cancer diagnosis was not uniformly regulated and trial duration was too short for evaluation of cancer outcomes since trials were primarily designed for other outcomes. Therefore, results of meta-analyses should be interpreted with caution since selection bias and poor quality of data may lead to erroneous conclusions [23]. To date there are no concerns that the benefits of angiotensin receptor use outweigh its possible risk and that an increased risk of cancer cannot be derived from currently available data.

Statins as most commonly prescribed lipid-lowering drugs in patients with metabolic syndrome did not affect the risk of cancer incidence or mortality [24, 25]. Data about ezetimibe, which inhibits dietary and biliary cholesterol absorption into enterocytes, demonstrated to increase cancer mortality in one prospective randomised trial (hazard ratio 1.67, 95 % CI 1.00–2.79) [26], but this finding has not been confirmed by other trials [27]. Since the number of patients in the above trials was rather small and the follow-up time too short for a reliable evaluation of cancer incidence or mortality, this issue remains to be clarified by further investigations.

Pharmacologic therapies for glucose control has undergone a critical evaluation during the recent years due to conflicting results of large trials, which did not demonstrate an improvement of cardiovascular outcomes by intensification of glucose-lowering therapy [28, 29]. In this context an updated guideline for the management of hyperglycaemia recommended an individualised approach including a risk benefit analysis of pharmacological therapy for each patient [30].

Since hyperinsulinaemia and stimulation of IGF-1 may be involved in the pathophysiology of cancer progression, recent studies focused on a possible risk of cancer from insulin secretagogues, incretin-based therapies and insulin/insulin analogues [1]. Few observational studies have described a possible increased risk of cancer mortality in patients treated with sulfonylurea [31]. However, the number of cancer cases was small and the study power limited [1].

A recent analysis of the United States Food and Drug Administration's database of reported adverse events for those associated with the dipeptidyl peptidase-4 (DPP-4) inhibitor sitagliptin and the glucagon-like peptide-1 mimetic exenatide revealed an increased risk of pancreatic cancer [32], whereas a recent meta-analysis of trials with DPP-4 inhibitors could not confirm this association [33]. However, due to the limited use of this new class of drugs, the possible risk of cancer cannot be finally evaluated.

Insulin, which is required for most patients with type 2 diabetes during the course of the disease, has been suspected to be associated with cancer in recent epidemiologic studies, especially if patients were treated with the long-acting insulin glargine [1, 34, 35]. In addition to insulin receptor-mediated effects, insulin glargine has a substantial affinity to the IGF-1 receptor and a higher mitogenic potency in vitro compared with human insulin [36]. This higher mitogenic potency has been suspected to result in a higher risk of cancer development in insulin glargine-treated patients. The poor quality of data from prescription registries, which were used in one of the epidemiologic analyses [35], may be the consequence of a selection bias. Insulin is usually prescribed late in the course of the disease after the failure of oral antidiabetic therapies, and patients using insulin have more comorbid conditions or traits of the metabolic syndrome, which may increase the risk of cancer. A large prospective open-label study with a 7-year follow-up with insulin glargine versus standard care—the Outcome Reduction with an Initial Glargine Intervention (ORIGIN) study—did not find an increased risk of cancer in insulin glargine-treated patients compared with the control group [37].

In conclusion, to date there is no convincing evidence that any specific treatment for single traits of the metabolic syndrome increases the risk of cancer morbidity or mortality. However, this lack of evidence for an increased cancer risk does not mean an exclusion of an increased risk. Further studies are necessary for a final statement.

5.4 Treatment of the Metabolic Syndrome and Cancer Risk Reduction

If the metabolic syndrome is associated with an increased cancer risk, one would expect a significant risk reduction by treatment of its traits. Lifestyle intervention is the most causal treatment of the metabolic syndrome. It has been demonstrated that physical activity is inversely associated with cancer incidence [38, 39].

The association of weight loss in central obesity and cancer risk in observational studies is less consistent and may be biased by accidentally weight loss due to undiagnosed cancer. However, there are clear evidence from animal studies that caloric restriction can reduce tumour growth [40]. In addition meta-analyses of patients who have undergone bariatric surgery demonstrated a decrease of cancer incidence together with weight loss and improved insulin sensitivity [41]. The cancer protective role of metabolic surgery was strongest for female obesity-related tumours, which may underline the contribution of both weight dependent and independent effects such as improvement of insulin resistance and beneficial modulation of sex hormones.

Metformin as recommended first-line treatment of type 2 diabetes may have advantages compared with other antidiabetic therapies regarding the risk of cancer. Several epidemiological studies demonstrated an association between metformin use and reduced cancer incidence [42, 43]. Metformin-induced activation of AMP activated protein kinase may play a crucial role in the inhibition of cancer cell proliferation [19, 44]. Additional observational studies suggest that metformin may improve cancer prognosis. Results of prospective trials, which are currently performed, might further clarify these possible drug-specific effects against cancer [19].

References

1. Giovannucci E, Harlan DM, Archer MC, Bergenstal RM, Gapstur SM, Habel LA, Pollak M, Regensteiner JG, Yee D (2010) Diabetes and cancer: a consensus report. Diabetes Care 33:1674–1685
2. Inoue M, Tsugane S (2012) Insulin resistance and cancer: epidemiological evidence. Endocr Relat Cancer 19(5):F1–F8
3. Stocks T, Van Hemelrijck M, Manjer J, Bjorge T, Ulmer H, Hallmans G, Lindkvist B, Selmer R, Nagel G, Tretli S, Concin H, Engeland A, Jonsson H, Stattin P (2012) Blood pressure and risk of cancer incidence and mortality in the Metabolic Syndrome and Cancer Project. Hypertension 59:802–810
4. Renehan AG, Tyson M, Egger M, Heller RF, Zwahlen M (2008) Body-mass index and incidence of cancer: a systematic review and meta-analysis of prospective observational studies. Lancet 371:569–578
5. Gunter MJ, Hoover DR, Yu H, Wassertheil-Smoller S, Rohan TE, Manson JE, Li J, Ho GY, Xue X, Anderson GL, Kaplan RC, Harris TG, Howard BV, Wylie-Rosett J, Burk RD, Strickler HD (2009) Insulin, insulin-like growth factor-I, and risk of breast cancer in postmenopausal women. J Natl Cancer Inst 101:48–60
6. Seshasai SR, Kaptoge S, Thompson A, Di Angelantonio E, Gao P, Sarwar N, Whincup PH, Mukamal KJ, Gillum RF, Holme I, Njolstad I, Fletcher A, Nilsson P, Lewington S, Collins R, Gudnason V, Thompson SG, Sattar N, Selvin E, Hu FB, Danesh J (2011) Diabetes mellitus, fasting glucose, and risk of cause-specific death. N Engl J Med 364:829–841
7. Calle EE, Rodriguez C, Walker-Thurmond K, Thun MJ (2003) Overweight, obesity, and mortality from cancer in a prospectively studied cohort of U.S. adults. N Engl J Med 348:1625–1638
8. Hanefeld M, Schaper F, Ceriello A (2007) History and definition(s) of metabolic syndrome. Internist (Berl) 48:117–125
9. Hotamisligil GS (2006) Inflammation and metabolic disorders. Nature 444:860–867

10. van Kruijsdijk RC, van der Wall E, Visseren FL (2009) Obesity and cancer: the role of dysfunctional adipose tissue. Cancer Epidemiol Biomarkers Prev 18:2569–2578
11. Yu H, Pardoll D, Jove R (2009) STATs in cancer inflammation and immunity: a leading role for STAT3. Nat Rev Cancer 9:798–809
12. Hotamisligil GS, Shargill NS, Spiegelman BM (1993) Adipose expression of tumor necrosis factor-alpha: direct role in obesity-linked insulin resistance. Science 259:87–91
13. Ozcan U, Cao Q, Yilmaz E, Lee AH, Iwakoshi NN, Ozdelen E, Tuncman G, Gorgun C, Glimcher LH, Hotamisligil GS (2004) Endoplasmic reticulum stress links obesity, insulin action, and type 2 diabetes. Science 306:457–461
14. Pollak M (2012) The insulin and insulin-like growth factor receptor family in neoplasia: an update. Nat Rev Cancer 12:159–169
15. Tran TT, Naigamwalla D, Oprescu AI, Lam L, McKeown-Eyssen G, Bruce WR, Giacca A (2006) Hyperinsulinemia, but not other factors associated with insulin resistance, acutely enhances colorectal epithelial proliferation in vivo. Endocrinology 147:1830–1837
16. Powell DR, Suwanichkul A, Cubbage ML, DePaolis LA, Snuggs MB, Lee PD (1991) Insulin inhibits transcription of the human gene for insulin-like growth factor-binding protein-1. J Biol Chem 266:18868–18876
17. Wu Y, Yakar S, Zhao L, Hennighausen L, LeRoith D (2002) Circulating insulin-like growth factor-I levels regulate colon cancer growth and metastasis. Cancer Res 62:1030–1035
18. Major JM, Laughlin GA, Kritz-Silverstein D, Wingard DL, Barrett-Connor E (2010) Insulin-like growth factor-I and cancer mortality in older men. J Clin Endocrinol Metab 95:1054–1059
19. Gallagher EJ, LeRoith D (2011) Diabetes, cancer, and metformin: connections of metabolism and cell proliferation. Ann N Y Acad Sci 1243:54–68
20. Gaede P, Lund-Andersen H, Parving HH, Pedersen O (2008) Effect of a multifactorial intervention on mortality in type 2 diabetes. N Engl J Med 358:580–591
21. Sipahi I, Debanne SM, Rowland DY, Simon DI, Fang JC (2010) Angiotensin-receptor blockade and risk of cancer: meta-analysis of randomised controlled trials. Lancet Oncol 11:627–636
22. Bangalore S, Kumar S, Kjeldsen SE, Makani H, Grossman E, Wetterslev J, Gupta AK, Sever PS, Gluud C, Messerli FH (2011) Antihypertensive drugs and risk of cancer: network meta-analyses and trial sequential analyses of 324,168 participants from randomised trials. Lancet Oncol 12:65–82
23. Bloch MJ, Basile JN (2010) Meta-analysis concludes angiotensin receptor blocker use increases the risk of developing cancer: concerns about the science and the message. J Clin Hypertens (Greenwich) 12:661–663
24. Baigent C, Blackwell L, Emberson J, Holland LE, Reith C, Bhala N, Peto R, Barnes EH, Keech A, Simes J, Collins R (2010) Efficacy and safety of more intensive lowering of LDL cholesterol: a meta-analysis of data from 170,000 participants in 26 randomised trials. Lancet 376:1670–1681
25. Strandberg TE, Pyorala K, Cook TJ, Wilhelmsen L, Faergeman O, Thorgeirsson G, Pedersen TR, Kjekshus J (2004) Mortality and incidence of cancer during 10-year follow-up of the Scandinavian Simvastatin Survival Study (4S). Lancet 364:771–777
26. Rossebo AB, Pedersen TR, Boman K, Brudi P, Chambers JB, Egstrup K, Gerdts E, Gohlke-Barwolf C, Holme I, Kesaniemi YA, Malbecq W, Nienaber CA, Ray S, Skjaerpe T, Wachtell K, Willenheimer R (2008) Intensive lipid lowering with simvastatin and ezetimibe in aortic stenosis. N Engl J Med 359:1343–1356
27. Baigent C, Landray MJ, Reith C, Emberson J, Wheeler DC, Tomson C, Wanner C, Krane V, Cass A, Craig J, Neal B, Jiang L, Hooi LS, Levin A, Agodoa L, Gaziano M, Kasiske B, Walker R, Massy ZA, Feldt-Rasmussen B, Krairittichai U, Ophascharoensuk V, Fellstrom B, Holdaas H, Tesar V, Wiecek A, Grobbee D, de Zeeuw D, Gronhagen-Riska C, Dasgupta T, Lewis D, Herrington W, Mafham M, Majoni W, Wallendszus K, Grimm R, Pedersen T, Tobert J, Armitage J, Baxter A, Bray C, Chen Y, Chen Z, Hill M, Knott C, Parish S, Simpson D, Sleight P, Young A, Collins R (2011) The effects of lowering LDL cholesterol with simvastatin plus ezetimibe in patients with chronic kidney disease (Study of Heart and Renal Protection): a randomised placebo-controlled trial. Lancet 377:2181–2192

28. Duckworth W, Abraira C, Moritz T, Reda D, Emanuele N, Reaven PD, Zieve FJ, Marks J, Davis SN, Hayward R, Warren SR, Goldman S, McCarren M, Vitek ME, Henderson WG, Huang GD (2009) Glucose control and vascular complications in veterans with type 2 diabetes. N Engl J Med 360:129–139
29. Gerstein HC, Miller ME, Byington RP, Goff DC Jr, Bigger JT, Buse JB, Cushman WC, Genuth S, Ismail-Beigi F, Grimm RH Jr, Probstfield JL, Simons-Morton DG, Friedewald WT (2008) Effects of intensive glucose lowering in type 2 diabetes. N Engl J Med 358:2545–2559
30. Inzucchi SE, Bergenstal RM, Buse JB, Diamant M, Ferrannini E, Nauck M, Peters AL, Tsapas A, Wender R, Matthews DR (2012) Management of hyperglycemia in type 2 diabetes: a patient-centered approach: position statement of the American Diabetes Association (ADA) and the European Association for the Study of Diabetes (EASD). Diabetes Care 35:1364–1379
31. Bowker SL, Majumdar SR, Veugelers P, Johnson JA (2006) Increased cancer-related mortality for patients with type 2 diabetes who use sulfonylureas or insulin. Diabetes Care 29:254–258
32. Elashoff M, Matveyenko AV, Gier B, Elashoff R, Butler PC (2011) Pancreatitis, pancreatic, and thyroid cancer with glucagon-like peptide-1-based therapies. Gastroenterology 141:150–156
33. Monami M, Dicembrini I, Martelli D, Mannucci E (2011) Safety of dipeptidyl peptidase-4 inhibitors: a meta-analysis of randomized clinical trials. Curr Med Res Opin 3(Suppl):57–64
34. Colhoun HM (2009) Use of insulin glargine and cancer incidence in Scotland: a study from the Scottish Diabetes Research Network Epidemiology Group. Diabetologia 52:1755–1765
35. Hemkens LG, Grouven U, Bender R, Gunster C, Gutschmidt S, Selke GW, Sawicki PT (2009) Risk of malignancies in patients with diabetes treated with human insulin or insulin analogues: a cohort study. Diabetologia 52:1732–1744
36. Kurtzhals P, Schaffer L, Sorensen A, Kristensen C, Jonassen I, Schmid C, Trub T (2000) Correlations of receptor binding and metabolic and mitogenic potencies of insulin analogs designed for clinical use. Diabetes 49:999–1005
37. The ORIGIN Trial Investigators (2012) Basal insulin and cardiovascular and other outcomes in dysglycemia. N Engl J Med 367(4):319–328
38. Tardon A, Lee WJ, Delgado-Rodriguez M, Dosemeci M, Albanes D, Hoover R, Blair A (2005) Leisure-time physical activity and lung cancer: a meta-analysis. Cancer Causes Control 16:389–397
39. Wolin KY, Yan Y, Colditz GA, Lee IM (2009) Physical activity and colon cancer prevention: a meta-analysis. Br J Cancer 100:611–616
40. Dunn SE, Kari FW, French J, Leininger JR, Travlos G, Wilson R, Barrett JC (1997) Dietary restriction reduces insulin-like growth factor I levels, which modulates apoptosis, cell proliferation, and tumor progression in p53-deficient mice. Cancer Res 57:4667–4672
41. Ashrafian H, Ahmed K, Rowland SP, Patel VM, Gooderham NJ, Holmes E, Darzi A, Athanasiou T (2011) Metabolic surgery and cancer: protective effects of bariatric procedures. Cancer 117:1788–1799
42. Evans JM, Donnelly LA, Emslie-Smith AM, Alessi DR, Morris AD (2005) Metformin and reduced risk of cancer in diabetic patients. Br Med J 330:1304–1305
43. Yang X, So WY, Ma RC, Kong AP, Lee HM, Yu LW, Chow CC, Ozaki R, Ko GT, Chan JC (2011) Low HDL cholesterol, metformin use, and cancer risk in type 2 diabetes: the Hong Kong Diabetes Registry. Diabetes Care 34:375–380
44. Luo Z, Zang M, Guo W (2010) AMPK as a metabolic tumor suppressor: control of metabolism and cell growth. Future Oncol 6:457–470

Lifestyle Intervention: Prevention of Complications to the Metabolic Syndrome

6

Pirjo Ilanne-Parikka and Jaakko Tuomilehto

6.1 The Metabolic Syndrome and the Risk of Type 2 Diabetes and Cardiovascular Disease

The metabolic syndrome is clinically important because of its association with the subsequent development of type 2 diabetes [1–7] and increased risk of cardiovascular disease (CVD) ([8–18]). In a systematic review and meta-analysis of longitudinal studies, Gami et al. [19] found 37 eligible studies including 43 cohorts with 172,573 individuals showing that individuals with the metabolic syndrome had a risk ratio of cardiovascular events of 1.78.

In recent years some controversy has emerged surrounding the clinical significance of the metabolic syndrome compared to other tools that identify individuals at elevated risk of cardiovascular diseases (CVD) [20, 21]. A review of prospective studies by Ford [22] concluded that the predictive value of the metabolic syndrome for all-cause mortality was unremarkable with an estimated summary relative risk of ~1.2 to ~1.4, and that the metabolic syndrome has a modest predictive value for CVD with an estimated summary relative risk of ~1.7 to ~1.9, depending on the definition of the metabolic syndrome [22].

A position statement of the American Association for Clinical Endocrinology pointed out that the metabolic syndrome should not be used as a disease unto itself [23]. A recent World Health Organization (WHO) report by Simmons et al. [24] came to a conclusion that the metabolic syndrome has a limited use as diagnostic or management tool. The metabolic syndrome is rather a concept that focuses attention on complex multifactorial health problems and should be

P. Ilanne-Parikka
Finnish Diabetes Association, Kirjoniementie 15, 33680 Tampere, Finland

J. Tuomilehto (✉)
Center for Vascular Prevention, Danube-University Krems, Dr-Karl-Dorrek-Strasse 30, 3500 Krems, Austria
e-mail: Jaakko.tuomilehto@donau-uni.ac.at

H. Beck-Nielsen (ed.), *The Metabolic Syndrome*,
DOI 10.1007/978-3-7091-1331-8_6, © Springer-Verlag Wien 2013

considered a pre-morbid condition excluding individuals with diagnosed diabetes or CVD [24].

In general, the metabolic syndrome has been most widely promoted for the identification of individuals at risk of CVD. The traditional risk scores may be more accurate for the prediction of future risk of CVD. However, the metabolic syndrome is an understandable and useful tool in clinical work. After recognition of a person at risk, awareness and lifestyle counselling and/or specific treatment for different features of the metabolic syndrome can be offered.

6.2 Management of the Metabolic Syndrome

Clinical management of the metabolic syndrome involves the modification of risk factors to prevent or delay the onset of CVD and delay of the onset of type 2 diabetes. The prevention and treatment of the metabolic syndrome is based on the management of its individual components. This by definition requires multiple targets and several management strategies to be applied simultaneously. Each of the components of the metabolic syndrome (Fig. 1.1, Chap. 1) can be improved by healthy lifestyle. Lifestyle modification should always be the primary intervention in people with the metabolic syndrome, but the residual risk of CVD that often remains usually requires pharmacotherapy [25]. Weight control, weight reduction and/or prevention of further weight gain, deserves first priority in individuals with abdominal obesity and the metabolic syndrome [26]. However, it must be kept in mind that weight reduction/control is only possible by the modification of diet and/or increased physical activity.

6.3 Dietary Considerations in the Prevention and Treatment of the Metabolic Syndrome

The optimal fat, protein, and carbohydrate composition for weight loss and for prevention and treatment of the metabolic syndrome and type 2 diabetes has been debated [27–30]. Excessive energy intake is the major driving force, but the quality of fats and carbohydrates also have important and independent effects. High glycaemic load is associated with increased diabetes risk, whereas high consumption of dietary fibre and poly/monounsaturated (PUFA/MUFA) fats is associated with decreased risk [31].

6.3.1 Dietary Fat Intake

In a review article on studies addressing the association between dietary fat intake and obesity, metabolic syndrome and diabetes, Melanson et al. [32] concluded that the data on the association between total fat intake and/or saturated fat intake and body weight remains inconclusive. However, the study further concluded that there are a sufficient number of studies suggesting that total fat and saturated fat intake increases the risk of having the components of metabolic syndrome, and that higher intake of MUFA and PUFA has a beneficial effect in reducing the risk [32].

On the role of reducing intake of saturated fat in the prevention of CVD, a panel of dietary experts [33] reached the following conclusions: "The evidence from epidemiological, clinical, and mechanistic studies is consistent in finding that the risk of coronary heart disease is reduced when saturated fatty acids (SAFA) are replaced with PUFA. No clear benefit of substituting carbohydrates for SAFA has been shown, although there might be a benefit if the carbohydrate is unrefined and has a low glycemic index".

6.3.2 Carbohydrate Intake

In obese individuals, low-carbohydrate diets result in greater initial weight loss and improvements in CVD risk factors for up to 1 year, as compared with conventional low-fat diets [34]. There have been only a few long-term trials, and none of them is primarily intended to treat the metabolic syndrome or prevent type 2 diabetes. After either 1 year (Foster et al. 2003) or 2 years [35] of treatment, no significant differences in weight loss were found between low carbohydrate and conventional low fat diets. However, Shai et al. [36] found that a dietary regimen lower in carbohydrates (~40 energy %) resulted in greater weight loss (4.7 kg) than a Mediterranean diet (4.4 kg) or calorie-restricted low-fat diet (2.9 kg), after a 2-year period.

The effects of low-carbohydrate diet on CVD risk factors and the metabolic syndrome have been inconclusive. There are studies showing more improvements with a low-carbohydrate diet (Foster et al. 2003; [36, 37]), while others do not show any significant associations [30, 38], especially when weight loss was taken into account. Sacks et al. [30] reported similar reduction in the prevalence of the metabolic syndrome in all dietary groups, from 32 % to 18–22 % among 811 overweight adults randomised to four different diet modalities.

Dietary glycaemic load is estimated from glycaemic index by multiplying it by the amount of carbohydrates. A high glycaemic load diet, which increases insulin demand and may lead to pancreatic beta-cell exhaustion in the long run, has been implicated in increased risk of type 2 diabetes and CVD [39]. In a meta-analysis of 37 prospective studies, Barclay et al. [40] found that diets with high glycaemic index and/or glycaemic load increased the risk of type 2 diabetes and heart disease.

6.3.3 Dietary Patterns

The role of a single nutrient, food item or lifestyle factor does not seem to be as important as dietary patterns or the combined effects of lifestyle change and dietary factors in the prevention and treatment of the metabolic syndrome and type 2 diabetes. Hu et al. [41] followed 84,941 women from 1980 to 1996 in the Nurses

Health Study. They defined a low-risk group for type 2 diabetes according to five variables: (1) body mass index (BMI) <25 kg/m^2; (2) a diet high in cereal fibre and PUFA and low in trans fat; (3) moderate-to-vigorous physical activity for at least half an hour/day; (4) no current smoking; and (5) an average intake of a half-serving of an alcoholic beverage/day.

With regard to CVD risk factors, several epidemiological and intervention studies support the benefits of Mediterranean diet low in SAFA and high in MUFA [33, 42]. A meta-analysis by Kastorini et al. [43] of prospective epidemiological studies and clinical trials assessing the effect of Mediterranean diet on the metabolic syndrome and its components showed that adherence to diet was associated with a reduced risk of the metabolic syndrome, and the results from clinical studies revealed a protective effect against the components of the metabolic syndrome.

Several diet-quality scores have been developed [44] to provide healthy dietary guidelines targeting major chronic diseases [45]. De Koning et al. [44] compared associations of different scores with incidence of type 2 diabetes among men from the Health Professionals Follow-up study. They concluded that several diet-quality scores, especially Alternative Healthy Eating Index (AHEI) and Dietary Approaches to Stop Hypertension (DASH), were associated with a lower risk of type 2 diabetes. These scores reflect a dietary pattern characterised by high intakes of plant-based foods such as whole grains; moderate alcohol; low intakes of red and processed meat, sodium, sugar-sweetened beverages and trans fat [44]. High scores of AHEI have earlier been shown to associate with decreased risk of CVD [46] and type 2 diabetes [45] and higher odds of the metabolic syndrome resolution [47]. A recent population-based cross-sectional study among elderly Finns showed that a healthy diet (vegetables $\geq$ 400 g/day, fish $\geq$ 2 servings/week, fibre $\geq$ 14 g/1,000 kcal, saturated fat $<$ 10 energy %/day) is associated with a reduced risk of having the metabolic syndrome [48].

6.3.4 Dietary Recommendations for the Treatment of the Metabolic Syndrome

For an overall healthy diet, the 2010 USA dietary guidelines emphasise three major goals: (1) balance calories with physical activity to manage weight; (2) consume more fruits, vegetables, whole grains, fat-free and low-fat dairy products and seafood; and (3) consume fewer foods with sodium, saturated fats, trans fats, cholesterol, added sugars and refined grains [49]. New dietary recommendations for the Nordic countries are under revision.

Current care guidelines for adult obesity in Finland emphasise individualised approach, but support regular meals with avoidance of "empty" calories. Energy deficit of ~600 kcal/day can be achieved by reducing (saturated) fats, sugar, sweets, pastry, white cereal and alcohol as well as portion sizes of pasta, rice and potatoes and increasing consumption of vegetables, berries and fruits [50].

6.4 Physical Activity and the Metabolic Syndrome

Increased time spent engaging in sedentary behaviours and decreased time spent engaging in moderate-to-vigorous physical activity have been reported to independently correlate with the risk of the metabolic syndrome and its components in cross-sectional studies [22, 51–56].

In a meta-analysis of ten prospective cohort studies, Jeon et al. [57] found a substantial inverse correlation between physical activity of moderate intensity and risk of type 2 diabetes. Those who were regularly engaged in physical activity of moderate intensity had ~30 % lower risk of type 2 diabetes as compared with sedentary individuals. A similar decrease in diabetes risk was observed when they specifically examined regular walking. After adjustment for BMI, the reduction in diabetes risk remained substantial for both regular moderately intense activity and walking.

6.4.1 Leisure Time Physical Activity

Data on the role of leisure time physical activity (LTPA) in the treatment of the metabolic syndrome is limited. More is known about the effect of exercise on insulin resistance and the metabolic syndrome components, especially obesity, in cross-sectional and prospective cohorts.

Borodulin et al. [58] found in the FINRISK 2002 cross-sectional survey that higher levels of LTPA were associated with lower 2-h plasma glucose and fasting insulin levels and reduced risk of having impaired glucose tolerance (IGT) and type 2 diabetes, independent of the level of abdominal obesity. A 16-year follow-up of 18,414 women in the Nurses Health Study II showed that bicycling, when of an intensity similar to that of brisk walking, was associated with less weight gain with an inverse dose–response relationship, especially among overweight and obese women [59]. Ekelund et al. [60] followed 84,511 men and 203,097 women in a prospective cohort study for 5 years and found that a higher level of physical activity reduced abdominal adiposity, independent of body weight and weight changes. Ekelund et al. [61] also found that an increase in physical activity energy expenditure lowered plasma triglycerides, fasting insulin, and 2-h glucose even in the absence of improved aerobic fitness and weight loss among 393 individuals followed for 5.6 years. On the other hand, cardiorespiratory fitness, even without weight loss, has been shown to prevent the metabolic syndrome [62]. Hassinen et al. [63] found that higher cardiorespiratory fitness at baseline, measured by maximum VO_2 uptake, was associated with a reduced metabolic syndrome development and a higher metabolic syndrome resolution rate in a 2-year follow-up.

There are some intervention trials that examine the role of LTPA on insulin resistance, abdominal obesity and the metabolic syndrome. Boule et al. [64] studied the effect of a 20-week endurance training programme in 596 healthy but sedentary individuals. They found that insulin sensitivity, measured by an intravenous glucose tolerance test, increased by 10 % following the intervention, although the variability was high. In this study, improvements in fasting insulin were transitory and disappeared within 72 h after the last bout of exercise. They concluded that in the absence of substantial weight loss, regular exercise is required for sustained improvement in glucose homeostasis. Lee et al. [65] found that regular exercise for 60 min five times per week was associated with reduction in total and visceral fat and muscle lipids among 24 men participating in 13 weeks of supervised aerobic exercise. Johnson et al. [66] used a metabolic syndrome score and found that, compared with the inactive controls, moderate intensity exercise—at an amount calorically equivalent to walking approximately 17 km over an average of 170 min per week—resulted in a significant improvement in calculated metabolic syndrome scores.

6.4.2 Resistance Training

Physical inactivity and ageing reduce muscle mass and contribute to obesity, insulin resistance, type 2 diabetes, dyslipidaemia and hypertension [67]. Increase in muscle mass may reduce multiple CVD risk factors [68]. Cross-sectional studies have demonstrated that muscular strength is inversely associated with the prevalence of the metabolic syndrome [69], and resistance training improves the components of the metabolic syndrome [70].

6.4.3 Sedentary Lifestyle

In the Nurses Health Study, independent of exercise levels, sedentary behaviours were found to be correlated with elevated risk of obesity and type 2 diabetes, whereas even light to moderate activity was associated with substantially lower risk [71]. In a cross-sectional cohort of 4,864 subjects in the Australian Diabetes Obesity and Lifestyle (AusDiab) study, sitting time, independent of central adiposity, and TV viewing time were deleteriously associated with CVD risk markers [72].

Healy et al. [73] examined the associations of objectively measured sedentary time, light-intensity physical activity and moderate-to-vigorous intensity activity with fasting and 2-h plasma glucose in a cross-sectional cohort. Physical activity was measured by accelerometers worn by participants during waking hours for seven consecutive days. Light-intensity physical activity was shown to be beneficially associated and sedentary time unfavourably associated with plasma glucose levels. They also found that independent of time spent in moderate-to-vigorous physical activity, there were significant associations of sedentary time, light-intensity time and mean activity intensity with waist circumference and clustered metabolic risk. Independent of waist circumference, moderate-to-vigorous physical activity time was significantly associated with triglycerides [74]. In a cross-sectional analysis with 4,757 participants from the National Health and Nutrition Examination Survey (NHANES), Healy et al. [75] found associations between prolonged sedentary time and CVD and inflammatory biomarkers such as waist circumference, high-density lipoprotein (HDL) cholesterol, C-reactive protein, triglycerides and insulin.

6.4.4 Exercise Recommendation for the Prevention of Type 2 Diabetes and for the Treatment of the Metabolic Syndrome

The American College of Sport Medicine and the American Diabetes Association published a joint statement on exercise and type 2 diabetes in 2010 [76]. It recommends at least 2.5 h/week of moderate-to-vigorous physical activity as part of lifestyle changes to prevent the onset of type 2 diabetes in high-risk adults. The current care guidelines for health-related physical activity recommend at least 30 min of any moderate-intensity physical activity, consisting of one or several shorter bouts at least 5 days a week, or vigorous exercise for 1 h 15 min once per week for the treatment of the metabolic syndrome. Additionally, muscle-strengthening activity like push-ups, sit-ups and lifting weight at least twice weekly, and a personal exercise programme is recommended.

6.5 Lifestyle Trials in Type 2 Diabetes Prevention

The best evidence for the benefit of lifestyle intervention to reduce weight and insulin resistance comes from intervention studies that were designed to investigate the possibility of preventing or delaying type 2 diabetes in high-risk groups via intensive lifestyle intervention. These studies have recruited overweight or obese individuals with abnormal glucose tolerance, mainly IGT. They have mostly aimed at achieving weight loss through a combination of dietary changes and physical activity. The DPP has reported the prevalence of the metabolic syndrome among the participants or the effects of the intervention on metabolic syndrome development or resolution [77]. It is, however, not clear how the results of these trials apply to a non-IGT population with the metabolic syndrome.

6.5.1 Finnish Diabetes Prevention Study

The DPS in Finland is a multicentre, randomised, prospective and controlled lifestyle intervention trial with the main aim of assessing prevention of type 2 diabetes in subjects with IGT [78, 79]. Overweight (BMI $\geq$ 25 kg/m^2) and middle-aged (40–64 years) individuals without previous diagnosis of diabetes other than gestational diabetes were eligible for DPS. Persons who were already participating in regular vigorous exercise programmes or had a chronic disease that would make a 6-year survival unlikely were excluded from the study. After the first screening oral glucose tolerance test (OGTT), a repeated OGTT was done in those within the IGT range, i.e. 2-h plasma glucose 7.8–11.0 mmol/l and fasting plasma glucose less than 7.8 mmol/l at the first visit. The mean of the 2-h glucose concentrations was used as the criterion for inclusion. The primary endpoint of DPS was the diagnosis of type 2 diabetes by WHO 1985 criteria [80] with a repeated plasma glucose value in the diabetes range, i.e. a fasting plasma glucose $\geq$ 7.8 mmol/l or 2-h value $\geq$ 11.1 mmol/l during OGTT (75 g).

The participants were randomised to an intensive and individually tailored diet and exercise counselling group and to a usual care control group. In addition, the effects of the intervention on insulin sensitivity and CVD risk factors were assessed [81, 82]. The main goals of the intensive intervention in DPS were: (1) weight reduction of $\geq$5 %; (2) $<$30 % of the daily energy intake from fat; (3) $<$10 % of the daily energy intake from saturated fat; (4) fibre intake $\geq$15 g per 1,000 kcal; and (5) moderately intense physical activity $\geq$30 min per day. The study participants were categorised according to their success in achieving these five predefined intervention goals (0 = not achieved, 1 = achieved) by the third year visit (mean LTPA and nutrient intake during the years 1, 2 and 3). A success score from 0 to 5 was calculated as the sum of the achieved goals.

The primary results of DPS showed that lifestyle changes can prevent the progression from IGT to type 2 diabetes with a relative risk reduction of 58 % [78]. Significantly greater improvements were seen at year 3 in waist circumference, serum total cholesterol to HDL cholesterol ratio and serum triglycerides in the intervention group compared with the control group [82].

6.5.2 Diabetes Prevention Program in the USA

Men and women with BMI > 24 kg/m^2, age > 25 years and both IGT and elevated fasting plasma glucose that participated in the DPP in the United States. During the average intervention and follow-up of 2.8 years, lifestyle intervention reduced the incidence of diabetes by 58 % and metformin by 31 %, as compared with placebo [83]. The DPP researchers also reported that the intensive lifestyle intervention improved CVD risk factor status [including hypertension, high triglyceride levels, low HDL levels and small dense low-density lipoprotein (LDL)] compared with placebo and metformin therapy [84].

The DPP researchers conducted post hoc analyses to evaluate changes in the resolution and incidence of the metabolic syndrome. By the third year the prevalence of the metabolic syndrome increased from 55 to 61 % in the placebo group, from 54 to 55 % in the metformin group, and decreased from 51 to 43 % in the lifestyle group [77]. Of those having the metabolic syndrome at baseline, 18 % of the placebo group, 23 % of the metformin group and 38 % of the lifestyle group, had recovered from the metabolic syndrome by the third study year. Among those without the metabolic syndrome at baseline, 53 % of the placebo group, 47 % of the metformin group and 38 % of the lifestyle group, had developed metabolic syndrome by the third year. The incidence of the metabolic syndrome was reduced by 41 % in the lifestyle group and by 17 % in the metformin group compared with placebo. Lifestyle intervention reduced the incidence of all components of the metabolic syndrome except HDL-cholesterol level, while metformin was effective only in reducing the incidence of elevated waist circumference and fasting glucose.

The study participants were categorised according to their success in achieving these five predefined intervention goals (0 = not achieved, 1 = achieved) by the third year visit (mean LTPA and nutrient intake during the years 1, 2 and 3). A success score from 0 to 5 was calculated as the sum of the achieved goals.

6.5.3 Intensive Lifestyle Counselling in the Intervention and Control Group

The methods used for the implementation of the programme have been published and described in detail elsewhere [82, 85]. The participants were advised to increase their overall level of physical activity, and endurance exercise was recommended in order to increase aerobic capacity and cardiorespiratory fitness. This was promoted by the study nurses and the nutritionist during the counselling sessions and highlighted by the study physicians. Sessions for supervised, individually tailored and progressive circuit-type resistance training with moderate intensity were recommended twice a week. Sessions were offered free of charge in three of the study centres with the aim to improve functional capacity and strength of large muscle groups of the upper and lower body.

The participants in the standard care control group were given general verbal and written health behaviour information about food choices, physical activity and weight loss at baseline, but no individualised counselling was offered. Control group participants filled out the same annual questionnaires and food diaries. The participants visited the study centre once a year for measurements and met the study nurse, nutritionist and physician.

6.5.4 Blood pressure and lipid management in the DPS

Drug treatment of hypertension blood pressure and/or dyslipidaemia was initiated according to guidelines if necessary. The use of blood pressure-lowering medications increased during the study in both groups: 34.5 % vs. 35.4 % ($p = 0.822$ between the groups) used antihypertensive medication at baseline and 40.7 % vs. 42.9 % ($p = 0.521$ between the groups) used antihypertensive medication at the end of the study in the intervention group and in the control group, respectively. The same trend was seen for the lipid-lowering medication: 4.6 % vs. 5.8 % ($p = 0.623$ between the groups) used lipid-lowering medication at baseline, whereas the corresponding figures were 14,4 % vs. 13.8 % ($p = 0.382$ between the groups) for the intervention and control groups at the end of the study.

Table 6.1 Prevalence of the metabolic syndrome and its components in the DPS at baseline by gender

	Men	Women	*p*
MetS	**78.4**	**72.2**	0.082
Obesity	**96.5**	**86.3**	<0.001
BMI ≥ 30 kg/m^2	45.3	59.1	0.004
Waist-to-hip ratio >0.90 men, >0.85 women	96.5	75.3	<0.001
Hypertension	**62.9**	**60.9**	0.647
Systolic blood pressure ≥140 mmHg	38.2	44.0	0.181
Diastolic blood pressure ≥90 mmHg	39.4	33.1	0.161
Use of blood pressure medication	29.1	29.2	0.745
Dyslipidaemia	**51.2**	**48.6**	0.599
Triglycerides ≥1.7 mmol/l	44.8	39.0	0.205
HDL-cholesterol <0.9 in men and <1.0 mmol/l in women	22.7	17.8	0.183
Use of lipid medication	5.8	5.4	0.857

Data are percentages. Obesity: BMI ≥ 30 kg/m^2 or waist-to-hip ratio >0.90 in men and >0.85 in women. Hypertension: Systolic blood pressure ≥140 mmHg or diastolic blood pressure ≥90 mmHg or use of oral antihypertensive medication. Dyslipidaemia: HDL-cholesterol <0.9 mmol/l in men and <1.0 mmol/l in women or triglycerides ≥1.7 mmol/l or use of lipid lowering medication.

MetS metabolic syndrome, *BMI* body mass index, *HDL* high-density lipoprotein

6.5.5 Effects of the Lifestyle Intervention on the Metabolic Syndrome in the DPS

Altogether 78.4 % of the men and 72.2 % of the women in the DPS fulfilled the modified WHO 1998 criteria for the metabolic syndrome [86]. The prevalence of obesity, hypertension and dyslipidaemia in men and women is shown in Table 6.1.

The metabolic syndrome status of the DPS participants was reassessed by the National Cholesterol Education Program (NCEP) 2005 definition [87]. There were no significant differences in these variables between the intervention group and control group, except for slightly lower saturated fat intake in the intervention group. Reported dietary intakes did not differ between those with the metabolic syndrome and those without at baseline. On the other hand, those with the metabolic syndrome exercised significantly less than those without the metabolic syndrome at baseline.

Body weight, dietary intakes and physical activity of the participants at baseline, year 1 and year 3 are shown in Table 6.2. Weight and intake of total fat and saturated fat were lower, while intake of carbohydrates and fibres and the proportion of physical activity were higher in the intervention group than in the control group during the intervention.

Table 6.2 Mean weight, mean dietary intakes and proportion (%) of physical active at baseline, at year 1 and at year 3 in the DPS intervention and control group

	Control group	Control group	*p*
Weight			
Baseline	86.7 ± 14.0	85.5 ± 14.4	0.327
Year 1	82.2 ± 13.6	84.8 ± 14.6	<0.001
Year 3[a]	83.4 ± 14.1	85.1 ± 15.5	<0.001
Fat (E%)			
Baseline	36.0 ± 6.7	37.1 ± 6.5	0.067
Year 1	32.6 ± 6.7	35.0 ± 6.2	<0.001
Year 3[a]	31.6 ± 6.2	34.4 ± 6.1	<0.001
Saturated fat (E%)			
Baseline	16.2 ± 4.0	17.0 ± 4.3	0.019
Year 1	13.5 ± 3.8	15.8 ± 4.1	<0.001
Year 3[a]	13.0 ± 3.8	15.4 ± 4.1	<0.001
Carbohydrate (E%)			
Baseline	43.6 ± 7.5	43.2 ± 6.7	0.506
Year 1	47.0 ± 7.5	44.9 ± 7.0	0.002
Year 3[a]	47.2 ± 7.4	45.0 ± 7.1	0.001
Fiber (g/1 000 kcal)			
Baseline	11.7 ± 4.0	11.7 ± 3.9	0.943
Year 1	14.2 ± 4.6	12.5 ± 3.7	<0.001
Year 3[a]	14.0 ± 4.7	12.6 ± 4.1	<0.001
Proportion of physically active (%)			
Baseline	64	67	0.519
Year 1	86	69	<0.001
Year 3[a]	82	71	<0.001

[a]Last observation carried forward for individuals who dropped out or developed diabetes during the study
[b]*p* for test of equality between groups adjusted for baseline level. *N* varied between 252 and 265 in the intervention group and between 245 and 257 in the control group

All five of the predefined goals were met by year 3 more often in the intervention group than in the control group. Three or more goals were fulfilled by 30.3 % of the participants in the intervention group and by 13.1 % in control group. The percentage of those with dietary fat intake ≤30 energy % was 38.2 % vs. 23.6 % ($p < 0.001$), the percentage of those with saturated fat intake ≤10 energy % was 21.3 % vs. 10.6 % ($p = 0.001$) and the percentage of those with fibre intake ≥15 g/1,000 kcal was 32.6 % vs. 26.0 % ($p = 0.014$) in the intervention group and in the control group, respectively. Weight reduction of ≥5 % was achieved by 39.1 % in the intervention group and in 18.7 % in the control group ($p < 0.001$), and 51.0 % in the intervention group exercised at least 2.5 h per week with moderate-to-vigorous intensity compared with 41.3 % in the control group ($p = 0.030$). In a logistic regression analysis adjusted for age, sex and baseline metabolic syndrome, lower BMI and BMI change were shown to be associated with the metabolic syndrome prevalence. No goals other than achieving weight loss of

≥5 % were associated alone with metabolic syndrome prevalence. However, the number of the predefined goals (0–5) that were met at year 3, analysed as a continuous variable, was associated with the metabolic syndrome prevalence ($p = 0.047$ adjusted for sex, age and baseline metabolic syndrome).

6.5.6 Changes in the Prevalence of the Metabolic Syndrome

The prevalence of the metabolic syndrome decreased during the first year with the most intensive dietary intervention—from 74.0 to 58.0 % and from 73.9 to 67.7 % ($p = 0.018$) in the intervention group and control group, respectively. At the end of the study, with a mean intervention time of 3.9 years, 62.6 % of the subjects in the intervention group and 71.2 % of the subjects in the control group ($p = 0.025$) had the metabolic syndrome (Fig. 6.1), which corresponds to 38 % relative risk reduction (odds ratio 0.62 with 95 % confidence interval (CI) 0.40–95; adjusted for age, sex and baseline value) in the intervention group.

The prevalence of the different components of the metabolic syndrome at year 1 and at the end of the DPS intervention is shown in Fig. 6.1. During the study, there were significant improvements in all of the components except fasting glucose in the intervention group, but there were only improvements in HDL cholesterol in the control group. Significant differences between the groups were seen in abdominal obesity and fasting glucose after the first year. By the end of the study only abdominal obesity and the overall prevalence of the metabolic syndrome were significantly different between the groups. The risk reduction for abdominal obesity was 52 % (odds ratio 0.48; 95 % CI 0.2–0.81 adjusted for age, sex and baseline value) in the intervention group from baseline to the end of the study.

6.5.7 Effects of Lifestyle Changes in Those with the Metabolic Syndrome at Baseline

Among those 386 participants with the metabolic syndrome at baseline the mean weight loss was 4.8 ± 5.1 kg vs. 0.9 ± 3.4 kg ($p < 0.001$) after the first year and 2.4 ± 5.3 kg vs. 0.4 ± 5.1 kg ($p < 0.001$) at the end of the intervention period in the intervention group and control group, respectively [88].

Comparisons within the groups showed that indicators for obesity or insulin resistance, i.e. fasting and 2-h plasma insulin, homeostasis assessment model for insulin resistance (HOMA-IR) index, dyslipidaemia and hypertension, improved significantly in the intervention group during the study, whereas only HDL cholesterol, triglycerides and diastolic blood pressure improved in the control group. Fasting plasma glucose and 2-h plasma glucose were significantly lower within the intervention group after the first year compared with baseline, but the glucose values increased significantly within both of the groups during the study (Table 6.3).

Comparison between the groups at the first annual visit showed significantly more improvements in all parameters studied in the intervention group. At the end of the

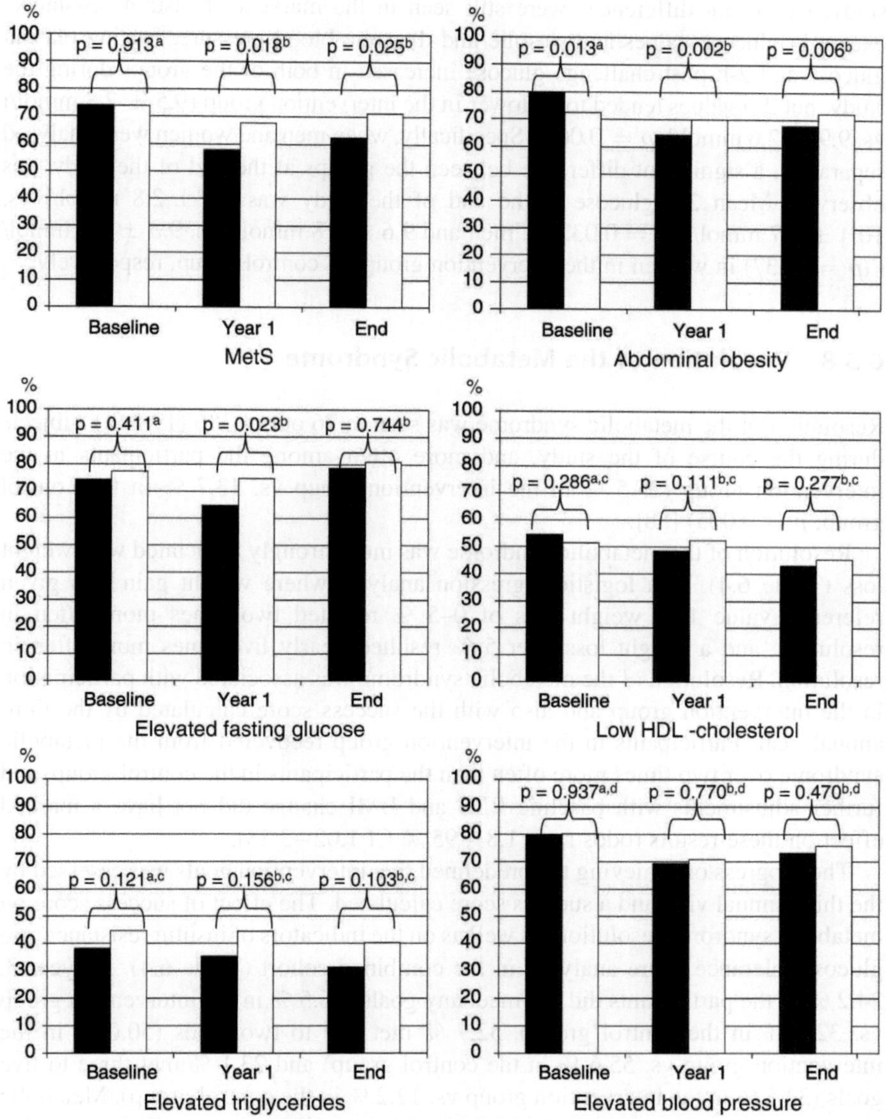

p = difference between intervention group and control group; a, adjusted for age and sex; b, adjusted for age, sex and baseline value; c, adjusted for lipid medication at baseline and end; d, adjusted for blood pressure medication at baseline and at end.

Abdominal obesity: waist circumference ≥ 102 cm in men and ≥ 88 cm in women;

Elevated fasting glucose: fasting plasma glucose ≥ 5.6 mmol/l; Elevated blood pressure: systolic blood pressure ≥ 130 mmHg and/or diastolic blood pressure ≥ 85 mmHg and/or blood pressure lowering medication; Low HDL-cholesterol: HDL cholesterol < 1.03 mmol/l in men and < 1.3 mmol/l in women; Elevated triglycerides: serum fasting triglycerides ≥ 1.7 mmol/l

Fig. 6.1 Prevalence of the metabolic syndrome and its components in the intervention group *filled bar* and in the control group *open bar* at baseline, at year 1 and at the end of the DPS

study, significant differences were still seen in the markers of insulin resistance, except in glucose values and systolic and diastolic blood pressure. Fasting plasma glucose and 2-h post challenge glucose increased in both of the groups during the study, but 2-h values tended to be lower in the intervention group (9.5 ± 2.8 mmol/l vs. 9.9 ± 2.6 mmol/l; $p = 0.064$). Specifically, when men and women were analysed separately, a significant difference between the groups at the end of the study was observed. Mean 2-h glucose at the end of the study was 9.2 ± 2.8 mmol/l vs. 10.4 ± 2.7 mmol/l ($p = 0.032$) in men and 9.6 ± 2.8 mmol/l vs. 9.8 ± 2.6 mmol/l ($p = 0.437$) in women in the intervention group vs. control group, respectively.

6.5.8 Resolution of the Metabolic Syndrome

Resolution of the metabolic syndrome was seen in 76 out of 386 (19.7 %) subjects during the course of the study, and more often among the participants in the intervention group (25.5 % in the intervention group vs. 13.7 % in the control group; $p = 0.005$) [88].

Resolution of the metabolic syndrome was most strongly associated with weight loss (Table 6.4). In a logistic regression analysis where weight gain was given reference value 1, a weight loss of 0–5 % resulted two times more often in resolution, and a weight loss over 5 % resulted nearly five times more often in resolution. Resolution of the metabolic syndrome was associated with participation in the intervention group and also with the success score calculated by the third annual visit. Participants in the intervention group recovered from the metabolic syndrome over two times more often than the participants in the control group, and further adjustments with baseline BMI and BMI change did not have a marked effect on these results (odds ratio 1.81; 95 % CI 1.02−3.23).

The progress of achieving the predefined five intervention goals was assessed by the third annual visit and a success score calculated. The effect of success score on metabolic syndrome resolution, as well as on the indicators of insulin resistance and glucose tolerance, were analysed in the combined cohort (Table 6.4). By year 3, 24.2 % of the participants did not meet any goals (16.5 % in the intervention group vs. 32.2 % in the control group), 52.7 % met one to two goals (50.0 % in the intervention group vs. 55.6 % in the control group) and 23.1 % met three to five goals (33.5 % in the intervention group vs. 12.2 % in the control group). Metabolic syndrome resolution was seen in 30.7 % of the participants who met three to five goals and in 12.0 % of those who did no meet any of the goals.

6.5.9 Weight Change and the Metabolic Syndrome

Weight loss is the most important target in the treatment of the metabolic syndrome. Some weight regain occurred after the first year, but a difference between the groups remained throughout the study. Mean BMI was 32.1 ± 4.6 kg/m^2 vs. 32.1 ± 4.5 kg/m^2 ($p = 0.839$, adjusted for age and sex) at baseline, 30.3 ± 4.5

Table 6.3 Biochemical parameters of those with metabolic syndrome at baseline, taken at baseline, at year 1 and at the end of the DPS

	Intervention group	Control group	p^e
Fasting plasma glucose (mmol/l)			
Baseline	6.3 ± 0.7	6.3 ± 0.7	0.739[a]
Year 1	6.0 ± 0.7	6.3 ± 0.8	<0.001[b]
End	6.5 ± 1.0	6.6 ± 0.9	0.155[b]
p^d for change within group	0.001	<0.001	
2-h plasma glucose (mmol/l)			
Baseline	9.0 ± 1.6	9.0 ± 1.4	0.706[a]
Year 1	8.2 ± 1.9	8.9 ± 2.1	<0.001[b]
End	9.5 ± 2.8	9.9 ± 2.6	0.064[b]
p^d for change within group	0.030	<0.001	
Fasting insulin (mU/l)			
Baseline	14 (11–19)	15 (11–20)	0.185[a]
Year 1	12 (9–15)	14 (11–19)	<0.001[b]
End	12 (9–17)	15 (11–21)	<0.001[b]
p^d for change within group	<0.001	0.488	
2-h insulin (mU/l)			
Baseline	90 (61–134)	88 (65–135)	0.665[a]
Year 1	58 (37–108)	78 (50–123)	<0.001[b]
End	61 (43–108)	90 (56–128)	<0.001[b]
p^d for change within group	<0.001	0.370	
HOMA-IR			
Baseline	4.1 (2.9–5.4)	4.0 (3.1–5.6)	0.264[a]
Year 1	3.2 (2.3–4.1)	4.0 (2.8–5.4)	<0.001[b]
End	3.5 (2.4–5.0)	4.4 (3.1–6.4)	<0.001[b]
p^d for change within group	0.001	0.268	
HDL-cholesterol (mmol/l)			
Baseline	1.14 ± 0.3	1.16 ± 0.26	0.527[a,c]
Year 1	1.19 ± 0.27	1.17 ± 0.29	0.015[b,c]
End	1.25 ± 0.33	1.23 ± 0.33	0.007[b,c]
p^d for change within group	<0.001	<0.001	
Triglycerides			
Baseline	1.68 (1.29–2.26)	1.79 (1.40–2.35)	0.108[a,c]
Year 1	1.50 (1.10–1.95)	1.75 (1.33–2.39)	<0.001[b,c]
End	1.47 (1.13–2.02)	1.65 (1.21–2.30)	0.075[b,c]
p^d for change within group	<0.001	0.013	

Data are mean ± SD or median (with 0.2–0.75 interquartile range)
[a]Adjusted for age and sex
[b]Adjusted for age, sex and baseline value
[c]Adjusted for lipid lowering medication
[d]p for change within group from baseline to end
[e]p for difference between groups; general linear model

Table 6.4 Odds ratios for metabolic syndrome resolution by randomisation group, weight change group and lifestyle success score by year 3 during the DPS

Variable	*n* (%)	Odds ratio[a]	95 % CI
Group			
Control group		1	
Intervention group		2.11	(1.25–3.59)
Weight change by year 3			
Weight gain		1	
Weight loss 0–5 %		2.10	(1.02–4.37)
Weight loss >5 %		4.89	(2.44–9.79)
Success score by year 3			
0 goal achieved	89 (24.2)	1	
1 goal achieved	121 (32.9)	2.46	(1.09–5.55)
2 goals achieved	73 (19.8)	2.31	(0.95–5.63)
≥3 goals achieved	85 (23.1)	3.10	(1.33–7.21)

[a]Adjusted for age and sex

kg/m^2 vs. 31.8 ± 4.7 kg/m^2 ($p < 0.001$ additionally adjusted for baseline value) at year 1, and 30.7 ± 4.7 kg/m^2 vs. 31.9 ± 5.0 kg/m^2 ($p < 0.001$) at the end in the intervention group vs. in the control group participants, respectively. Those in the intervention group showed ≥5 % weight loss over three times more often than those in the control group after the first year and nearly twice as often at the end of the study. A weight loss of ≥5 % was seen in 47.9 % in the intervention group and in 14.0 % in the control group at year 1 and in 35.2 % in the intervention group and 18.4 % in the control group at the end. Weight gain was observed in 14.2 % in the intervention group and 43.5 % in the control group at year 1 and in 31.6 % in the intervention group and 49.5 % in the control group at the end of the study [88].

The effects of weight change on indicators of insulin resistance and glucose tolerance were analysed in the combined cohort. Both fasting and 2-h plasma glucose, as well as insulin and HOMA-IR index, improved significantly in those with a weight loss. Significant improvements were also seen in blood pressure and lipid values.

Resolution of the metabolic syndrome was observed in 39.4 % of those with weight loss of ≥5 % and in 7.1 % of those with weight gain. In a logistic regression model for the resolution of the metabolic syndrome (age, sex, group, baseline weight and percentage of weight change by the year 3 as explanatory variables), the odds ratio for weight change was 0.89 (95 % CI 0.84−0.93), conferring to 10 % relative odds for the metabolic syndrome resolution for one percentage of weight loss.

6.5.10 LTPA Changes and Metabolic Syndrome Resolution and Development

The averaged total, low and moderate-to-vigorous intensity LTPA changes during the study years were categorised into thirds and the association with the metabolic

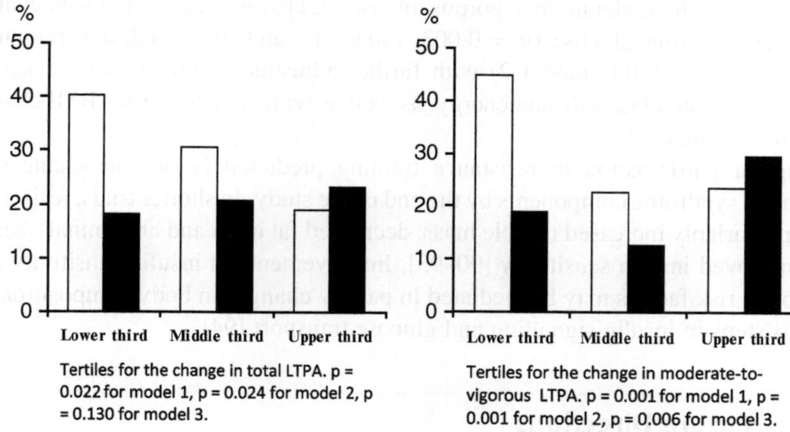

Fig. 6.2 Incidences (%) of the development *open bar* and the resolution *filled bar* of the metabolic syndrome according to tertiles for total (*left panel*) and for moderate-to-vigorous intensity leisure time physical activity (LTPA) (*right panel*) change. Model 1: Adjustments for age, sex, group and DPS study years. The change in moderate-to-vigorous intensity LTPA was also adjusted for change in low intensity LTPA. Model 2: Model 1 and adjustments for change in dietary intakes of total fat, saturated fat, fibre and energy. Model 3: Model 2 and change in body mass index (BMI)

syndrome status change (metabolic syndrome resolution, metabolic syndrome development and unchanged status) during the study was examined. Change in total LTPA was associated with change in the metabolic syndrome status after adjustments for age, sex, intervention group, DPS study years (model 1) and dietary intakes (model 2), but the association was no more significant after adjustments for BMI change (model 3; Fig. 6.2, left panel). However, the association of moderate-to-vigorous LTPA change with the metabolic syndrome status change was significant even after adjustments for dietary intakes and weight change (Fig. 6.2, right panel). The resolution of the metabolic syndrome was seen in 29.7 % vs. 19.1 % ($p = 0.004$) of those with the metabolic syndrome at baseline and the development of the metabolic syndrome was seen in 23.5 % vs. 44.7 % ($p = 0.041$) of those without metabolic syndrome at baseline in the upper vs. lower third of change in moderate-to-vigorous LTPA. The change in low-intensity LTPA did not associate with the metabolic syndrome status change [89].

6.5.11 LTPA Changes and Components of the Metabolic Syndrome

There was a significant association between the total LTPA change (adjusted for age, intervention group and DPS study years; model 1) and elevated fasting plasma glucose ($p = 0.003$), low HDL cholesterol ($p = 0.018$) and elevated triglycerides ($p = 0.002$). However, the association remained significant only for elevated triglycerides ($p = 0.003$) when the analysis was adjusted for dietary changes (model 2) and further for BMI change (model 3).

The change in moderate-to-vigorous intensity LTPA was correlated with change in elevated fasting glucose ($p = 0.003$; model 1), and the correlation remained significant ($p = 0.011$; model 2) with further adjustments for dietary intakes of total fat, saturated fat, fibre and energy, as well as with adjustment for BMI change ($p = 0.018$; model 3).

Regular participation in resistance training predicted favourable changes in metabolic syndrome components by the end of the study. In shorter trials, resistance training variably increased muscle mass, decreased fat mass and abdominal obesity and improved insulin sensitivity [90–93]. Improvements in insulin sensitivity and metabolic risk factors may be mediated in part by changes in body composition, as well as steps in insulin signalling and glucose transport [94].

6.6 Future Directions

The increase in the number of people with the metabolic syndrome and type 2 diabetes will progress while urbanisation continues with more sedentary lifestyles, "obesogenic" environments and the constant availability of energy-rich foods. People also live longer and the number of senior citizens is set to increase, while childhood mortality declines at the same time. In addition, the management targeted to the individual components of the metabolic syndrome has become more successful, and therefore the survival of people with metabolic syndrome, even in those who have developed type 2 diabetes and/or CVD, is improving. Thus, this will further increase the number of people (survivors) with the metabolic syndrome. More community-based preventive actions especially targeted to young people are clearly needed. However, this will only help the future situation. Meanwhile, we must find out better solutions to the already existing epidemic of the metabolic syndrome and assist the large number of people who suffer from one or several components of the metabolic syndrome.

The most significant modifiable risk factors for the metabolic syndrome and type 2 diabetes are overweight, abdominal obesity, physical inactivity and dietary factors. Lifestyle changes are the first choice of therapy both in the primary and secondary prevention of the metabolic syndrome. The potential to prevent type 2 diabetes in high-risk individuals, like those having the metabolic syndrome, through reinforced lifestyle intervention has been established in several clinical trials (Table 6.5), and the long-term follow-up in present studies shows that the effect is maintained for many years after discontinuation of active intervention [102].

In addition to high-risk approaches, population-based strategies and community awareness are needed. Programmes approaching families and children are important. Everyday living environments that have low barriers for commuting and leisure time physical activities are of benefit. While socioeconomic differences show associations with chronic diseases and the use of healthcare services, more information about optimal and attainable implementation programmes is needed.

Table 6.5 Major lifestyle intervention studies to prevent type 2 diabetes

Authors(s), year Name of the study [reference]	Area	Study population N	 Age (years)	 Glucose tolerance	Duration (years)	RRR (%)
Eriksson and Lindgärde 1991 Malmö Feasibility Study [94]	Sweden	181	47–49	IGT	6	63
Pan et al. 1997 DaQing Study [95]	China	577	~45	IGT	6	31/46/42[a]
Tuomilehto et al. 2001 DPS [77]	Finland	522	40–64	IGT	3.2	58
Knowler et al. 2002 DPP [82]	USA	3234	≥25	IGT+ IFG	2.8	58
Kosaka et al. 2005 Toranomon Study [96]	Japan	458	~55	IGT	4	67
Ramachandran et al. 2006 Indian DPP [97]	India	531	35–55	IGT	3	28
Roumen et al. 2008 SLIM Study [98]	Netherlands	147	>40	IGT	3	58
Penn et al. 2009 Newcastle Study [99]	UK	102	>40	IGT	3.1	55
Saito et al. Zensharen Study [100]	Japan	641	30–60	IFG	3	44

DPS diabetes prevention study, *DPP* diabetes prevention program, *SLIM* study on lifestyle intervention and impaired glucose tolerance Maastricht, *IGT* impaired glucose tolerance, *IFG* impaired fasting glucose, *RR* relative risk reduction
[a]DaQing had three intervention groups: diet/exercise/diet+exercise

References

1. Laaksonen DE et al (2002) Metabolic syndrome and development of diabetes mellitus: application and validation of recently suggested definitions of the metabolic syndrome in a prospective cohort study. Am J Epidemiol 156:1070–1077
2. Ford ES et al (2008) Metabolic syndrome and incident diabetes. Diabetes Care 31:1898–1904
3. Ford ES et al (2008) Metabolic syndrome and risk of incident diabetes: findings from the European Prospective Investigation into Cancer and Nutrition-Potsdam Study. Cardiovasc Diabetol 7:35
4. Lorenzo C et al (2003) The metabolic syndrome as predictor of type 2 diabetes: the San Antonio Heart Study. Diabetes Care 26:3153–3159
5. Wang J et al (2004) The metabolic syndrome and incident diabetes: assessment of four suggested definitions of the metabolic syndrome in a Chinese population with high post-prandial glucose. Horm Metab Res 36:708–715
6. Wang J et al (2007) How well does the metabolic syndrome defined by five definitions predict incident diabetes and incident coronary heart disease in a Chinese population? Atherosclerosis 192:161–168
7. Gupta AK et al (2008) Determinants of new-onset diabetes among 19 257 hypertensive patients randomized in the Anglo-Scandinavian Cardiac Outcomes Trial - Blood pressure lowering arm and the relative influence of antihypertensive medication. Diabetes Care 31:982–988
8. Mente A et al (2010) Metabolic syndrome and risk of acute myocardial infarction: a case-control study of 26,903 subjects from 52 countries. J Am Coll Cardiol 55:2390–2398

9. Lakka H-M et al (2002) The metabolic syndrome and total and cardiovascular disease mortality in middle-aged men. JAMA 288:2709–2716
10. Ärnlöv J et al (2010) Impact of BMI and the metabolic syndrome on the risk of diabetes in middle-aged men. Diabetes Care 34:61–65
11. Jeppesen J et al (2007) Insulin resistance, the metabolic syndrome, and risk of incident cardiovascular disease: a population-based study. J Am Coll Cardiol 49:2112–2119
12. Malik S et al (2004) Impact of the metabolic syndrome on mortality from coronary heart disease, cardiovascular disease, and all causes in United States adults. Circulation 110:1245–1250
13. Wilson PW et al (2005) Metabolic syndrome as a precursor of cardiovascular disease and type 2 diabetes mellitus. Circulation 112:3066–3072
14. Broekhuizen LN et al (2011) Physical activity, metabolic syndrome, and coronary risk: the EPIC-Norfolk prospective population study. Eur J Cardiovasc Prev Rehabil 18:209–217
15. Hu G et al (2004) Prevalence of the metabolic syndrome and its relation to all-cause and cardiovascular mortality in nondiabetic European men and women. Arch Intern Med 164:1066–1076
16. Hunt KJ et al (2004) National Cholesterol Education Program versus World Health Organization metabolic syndrome in relation to all-cause and cardiovascular mortality in the San Antonio Heart Study. Circulation 110:1251–1257
17. Isomaa B et al (2001) The metabolic syndrome influences the risk of chronic complications in patients with Type II diabetes. Diabetologia 44:1148–1154
18. Sattar N et al (2003) Metabolic syndrome with and without C-reactive protein as a predictor of coronary heart disease and diabetes in the West of Scotland Coronary Prevention Study. Circulation 108:414–419
19. Gami AS et al (2007) Metabolic syndrome and risk of incident cardiovascular events and death: a systematic review and meta-analysis of longitudinal studies. J Am Coll Cardiol 49:403–414
20. Kahn R et al (2005) The metabolic syndrome: time for a critical appraisal: joint statement from the American Diabetes Association and the European Association for the Study of Diabetes. Diabetes Care 28:2289–2304
21. Reaven GM (2006) The metabolic syndrome: is this diagnosis necessary? Am J Clin Nutr 83:1237–1247
22. Ford ES et al (2005) Sedentary behavior, physical activity, and the metabolic syndrome among U.S. adults. Obesity 13:608–614
23. Mechanick JI et al (2005) American College of Endocrinology/American Association for Clinical Endocrinologists: Reaffirmation of the 2003 ACE Insulin Resistance Syndrome Position Statement. Retrieved 1.5.2011 from http://www.aace.org
24. Simmons R et al (2010) The metabolic syndrome: useful concept or clinical tool? Report of a WHO Expert Consultation. Diabetologia 53:600–605
25. Eckel RH et al (2010) The metabolic syndrome. Lancet 375:181
26. Grundy SM et al (2005) Diagnosis and management of the metabolic syndrome: an American Heart Association/National Heart, Lung, and Blood Institute Scientific Statement. Circulation 112:2735–2752
27. Accurso A et al (2008) Dietary carbohydrate restriction in type 2 diabetes mellitus and metabolic syndrome: time for a critical appraisal. Nutr Metab 5:9
28. Feinglos MN, Totten SE (2008) Are you what you eat, or how much you eat? The case of type 2 diabetes mellitus. Arch Intern Med 168:1485–1486
29. Nordmann AJ et al (2006) Effects of low-carbohydrate vs. low-fat diets on weight loss and cardiovascular risk factors: a meta-analysis of randomized controlled trials. Arch Intern Med 166:285–293
30. Sacks FM et al (2009) Comparison of weight-loss diets with different compositions of fat, protein, and carbohydrates. N Engl J Med 360:859–873
31. Hu FB (2011) Globalization of diabetes. Diabetes Care 34:1249–1257

32. Melanson EL et al (2009) The relationship between dietary fat and fatty acid intake and body weight, diabetes and the metabolic syndrome. Ann Nutr Metab 55:229–243
33. Astrup A et al (2011) The role of reducing intakes of saturated fat in the prevention of cardiovascular disease: where does the evidence stand in 2010? Am J Clin Nutr 93:684–688
34. Hession M et al (2009) Systematic review of randomized controlled trials of low-carbohydrate vs. low-fat/low-calorie diets in the management of obesity and its comorbidities. Obes Rev 10:36–50
35. Foster GD et al (2010) Weight and metabolic outcomes after 2 years on a low-carbohydrate versus low-fat diet. Ann Intern Med 153:147–157
36. Shai I et al (2008) Weight loss with a low-carbohydrate, mediterranean, or low-fat diet. N Engl J Med 359:229–241
37. Frisch S et al (2009) A randomized controlled trial on the efficacy of carbohydrate-reduced or fat-reduced diets in patients attending a telemedically guided weight loss program. Cardiovasc Diabetol 8:36
38. Goldstein T et al (2011) The effect of a low carbohydrate energy-unrestricted diet on weight loss in obese type 2 diabetes patients - a randomized controlled trial. Eur E J Clin Nutr Metab: e121–e125
39. Hu FB, Willett WC (2002) Optimal diets for prevention of coronary heart disease. JAMA 288:2569–2578
40. Barclay AW et al (2008) Glycemic index, glycemic load, and chronic disease risk: a meta-analysis of observational studies. Am J Clin Nutr 87:627–637
41. Hu FB et al (2001) Diet, lifestyle, and the risk of type 2 diabetes mellitus in women. N Engl J Med 345:790–797
42. Sofi F et al (2010) Accruing evidence on benefits of adherence to the Mediterranean diet on health: an updated systematic review and meta-analysis. Am J Clin Nutr 92:1189–1196
43. Kastorini C-M et al (2011) The effect of Mediterranean diet on metabolic syndrome and its components: a meta-analysis of 50 studies and 534 906 individuals. J Am Coll Cardiol 57:1299–1313
44. de Koning L et al (2011) Diet–quality scores and the risk of type 2 diabetes in men. Diabetes Care 34:1150–1156
45. McCullough ML et al (2002) Diet quality and major chronic disease risk in men and women: moving toward improved dietary guidance. Am J Clin Nutr 76:1261–1271
46. Fung TT et al (2007) A prospective study of overall diet quality and risk of type 2 diabetes in women. Diabetes Care 30:1753–1757
47. Akbaraly TN et al (2010) Overall diet history and reversibility of the metabolic syndrome over 5 years. Diabetes Care 33:2339–2341
48. Kouki R et al (2011) Food consumption, nutrient intake and the risk of having metabolic syndrome: the DR's EXTRA Study. Eur J Clin Nutr 65:368–377
49. U.S. Department of Agriculture and U.S. Department of Health and Human Services (2010) Dietary guidelines for Americans. Retrieved 25.3.2011 from http://www.dietaryguidelines.org
50. Adult Obesity (2011) Current care guideline. Working group by the Finnish Association for the Study of Obesity. Finnish Medical Society Duodecim, Helsinki. Available at: http://www.kaypahoito.fi/
51. Balkau B et al (2008) Physical activity and insulin sensitivity: the RISC study. Diabetes 57:2613–2618
52. Bertrais S et al (2005) Sedentary behaviors, physical activity, and metabolic syndrome in middle-aged French subjects. Obesity 13:936–944
53. Dunstan D et al (2005) Associations of TV viewing and physical activity with the metabolic syndrome in Australian adults. Diabetologia 48:2254–2261
54. Dunstan DW et al (2007) Association of television viewing with fasting and 2-hour post-challenge plasma glucose levels in adults without diagnosed diabetes. Diabetes Care 30:516–522
55. Healy GN et al (2006) Beneficial associations of physical activity with 2-hour but not fasting blood glucose in Australian adults: the AusDiab Study. Diabetes Care 29:2598–2604

56. Li C-L et al (2007) Associations between the metabolic syndrome and its components, watching television and physical activity. Public Health 121:83–91
57. Jeon CY et al (2007) Physical activity of moderate intensity and risk of type 2 diabetes: a systematic review. Diabetes Care 30:744–752
58. Borodulin K et al (2006) Association of leisure time physical activity and abdominal obesity with fasting serum insulin and 2-h post challenge plasma glucose levels. Diabet Med 23:1025–1028
59. Lusk AC et al (2010) Bicycle riding, walking, and weight gain in premenopausal women. Arch Intern Med 170:1050–1056
60. Ekelund U et al (2011) Physical activity and gain in abdominal adiposity and body weight: prospective cohort study in 288 498 men and women. Am J Clin Nutr 93:826–835
61. Ekelund U et al (2005) Physical activity energy expenditure predicts progression toward the metabolic syndrome independently of aerobic fitness in middle-aged healthy Caucasians: the medical research council Ely study. Diabetes Care 28:1195–1200
62. LaMonte MJ et al (2005) Cardiorespiratory fitness is inversely associated with the incidence of metabolic syndrome: a prospective study of men and women. Circulation 112:505–512
63. Hassinen M et al (2010) Cardiorespiratory fitness and metabolic syndrome in older men and women. Diabetes Care 33:1655–1657
64. Boule NG et al (2005) Effects of exercise training on glucose homeostasis: the HERITAGE family study. Diabetes Care 28:108–114
65. Lee S et al (2005) Exercise without weight loss is an effective strategy for obesity reduction in obese individuals with and without type 2 diabetes. J Appl Physiol 99:1220–1225
66. Johnson JL et al (2007) Exercise training amount and intensity effects on metabolic syndrome (from studies of a Targeted Risk Reduction Intervention through Defined Exercise). Am J Cardiol 100:1759–1766
67. Williams MA et al (2007) Resistance exercise in individuals with and without cardiovascular disease: 2007 update: a scientific statement from the American Heart Association Council on Clinical Cardiology and Council on Nutrition, Physical Activity, and Metabolism. Circulation 116:572–584
68. Braith RW, Stewart KJ (2006) Resistance exercise training: its role in the prevention of cardiovascular disease. Circulation 113:2642–2650
69. Jurca R et al (2005) Association of muscular strength with incidence of metabolic syndrome in men. Med Sci Sports Exerc 37:1849–1855
70. Strasser B et al (2010) Resistance training in the treatment of the metabolic syndrome: a systematic review and meta-analysis of the effect of resistance training on metabolic clustering in patients with abnormal glucose metabolism. Sports Med 40:397–415
71. Hu FB et al (2003) Television watching and other sedentary behaviors in relation to risk of obesity and type 2 diabetes mellitus in women. JAMA 289:1785–1791
72. Thorp AA et al (2010) Deleterious associations of sitting time and television viewing time with cardiometabolic risk biomarkers. Diabetes Care 33:327–334
73. Healy GN et al (2007) Objectively measured light-intensity physical activity is independently associated with 2-hour plasma glucose. Diabetes Care 30:1344–1389
74. Healy GN et al (2008) Objectively measured sedentary time, physical activity, and metabolic risk. Diabetes Care 31:369–371
75. Healy GN et al (2011) Sedentary time and cardio–metabolic biomarkers in US adults: NHANES 2003–2006. Eur Heart J 32:590–597
76. Colberg SR et al (2010) Exercise and type 2 diabetes. Diabetes Care 33:e147–e167
77. Orchard TJ et al (2005) The effect of metformin and intensive lifestyle intervention on the metabolic syndrome: the Diabetes Prevention Program randomized trial. Ann Intern Med 142:611–619
78. Tuomilehto J et al (2001) Prevention of type 2 diabetes mellitus by changes in lifestyle among subjects with impaired glucose tolerance. N Engl J Med 344:1343–1350
79. Uusitupa M et al (2000) The Finnish Diabetes Prevention Study. Br J Nutr 83:S137–S142

80. World Health Organization (1985) Diabetes mellitus: Report of WHO Study Group. Tech. Rep. Ser. No. 727. WHO, Geneva
81. Eriksson J et al (1999) Prevention of Type II diabetes in subjects with impaired glucose tolerance: the Diabetes Prevention Study (DPS) in Finland. Diabetologia 42:793–801
82. Lindström J et al (2003) Lifestyle intervention and 3-year results on diet and physical activity. Diabetes Care 26:3230–3236
83. Knowler WC et al (2002) Reduction in the incidence of type 2 diabetes with lifestyle intervention or metformin. N Engl J Med 346:393–403
84. The Diabetes Prevention Program Research Group (2005) Impact of intensive lifestyle and metformin therapy on cardiovascular disease risk factors in the Diabetes Prevention Program. Diabetes Care 28:888–894
85. Lindström J et al (2005) Lifestyle strategies for weight control: experience form the Finnish Diabetes Prevention Study. Proc Nutr Soc 64:81–88
86. Ilanne-Parikka P et al (2004) Prevalence of the metabolic syndrome and its components findings from a Finnish general population sample and the Diabetes Prevention Study (DPS) cohort. Diabetes Care 27:2135–2140
87. Alberti KGM et al (2005) The metabolic syndrome—a new worldwide definition. Lancet 366:1059–1062
88. Ilanne-Parikka P et al (2008) Effect of lifestyle intervention on the occurrence of metabolic syndrome and its components in the Finnish Diabetes Prevention Study. Diabetes Care 31:805–807
89. Ilanne-Parikka P et al (2010) Leisure-time physical activity and the metabolic syndrome in the Finnish Diabetes Prevention Study. Diabetes Care 33:1610–1617
90. Cuff DJ et al (2003) Effective exercise modality to reduce insulin resistance in women with type 2 diabetes. Diabetes Care 26:2977–2982
91. Lakka TA, Laaksonen DE (2007) Physical activity in prevention and treatment of the metabolic syndrome. Appl Physiol Nutr Metab 32:76–88
92. Miller JP et al (1994) Strength training increases insulin action in healthy 50- to 65-yr-old men. J Appl Phys 77:1122–1127
93. Sigal RJ et al (2007) Effects of aerobic training, resistance training, or both on glycemic control in type 2 diabetes: a randomized trial. Ann Intern Med 147:357–369
94. Holten MK et al (2004) Strength training increases insulin-mediated glucose uptake, GLUT4 content, and insulin signalling in skeletal muscle in patients with type 2 diabetes. Diabetes 53:294–305
95. Eriksson KF, Lingärde Fl (1991) Prevention of type 2 (non-insulin-dependent) diabetes mellitus by diet and physical exercise. The 6-year Malmö feasibility study. Diabetologia 34:891–898
96. Pan XR et al (1997) Effects of diet and exercise in preventing NIDDM in people with impaired glucose tolerance. The Da Qing IGT and Diabetes Study. Diabetes Care 20: 537–544
97. Kosaka K, Noda M, Kuzuya T (2005) Prevention of type 2 diabetes by lifestyle intervention: a Japanese trial in IGT males. Diabetes Res Clin Pract 67:152–162
98. Ramachandran A et al (2006) The Indian Diabetes Prevention Programme shows that lifestyle modification and metformin prevent type 2 diabetes in Asian Indian subjects with impaired glucose tolerance (IDPP-1). Diabetologia 49:289–297
99. Roumen C et al (2008) Impact of 3-year lifestyle intervention on postprandial glucose metabolism: the SLIM study. Diabetic Medicine 25:597–605
100. Penn L et al (2009) Prevention of type 2 diabetes in adults with impaired glucose tolerance: the European Diabetes Prevention RCT in Newcastle upon Tyne, UK. BMC Public Health. 9:342
101. Saito T et al (2011) Lifestyle modification and prevention of type 2 diabetes in overweight Japanese with impaired fasting glucose levels. A randomized controlled trial. Arch Intern Med 171:1352–1360
102. Lindström J et al (2013) Improved lifestyle and decreased diabetes risk over 13 years: long-term follow-up of the randomised Finnish Diabetes Prevention Study (DPS). Diabetologia 56:284–293

Low-Carbohydrate Diets in the Treatment of the Metabolic Syndrome

7

Marc-Andre Cornier and Boris Draznin

7.1 Introduction

Definitions, epidemiology, pathophysiology and various aspects of treatment of the metabolic syndrome are described thoroughly elsewhere in this book. The goal of this chapter is to outline the role of low-carbohydrate diets in the overall therapeutic approach to this important entity.

The metabolic syndrome by definition is a constellation of medical disorders related to excess adiposity, including dyslipidaemia, cardiovascular abnormalities, insulin resistance and inadequate utilisation of glucose [1, 2]. It remains unresolved whether all components of the metabolic syndrome are united by a single pathophysiological mechanism or simply co-exist in the various symbiotic relations based on genetic background and lifestyle choices [3].

Even though lifestyle modifications remain the keystone of therapy [4–6], other aspects of therapeutic interventions are critical for normalisation of many individual components of the metabolic syndrome in these patients, such as blood pressure, dyslipidaemia, glucose tolerance, etc. It is highly likely that treatment of the metabolic syndrome will remain multifaceted requiring a combination of therapeutic modalities.

In addition to physical activity, diet is a crucial component of lifestyle management [4]; however, consensus as to which dietary approach is most efficacious remains elusive [7]. Overall, energy restriction has been shown to consistently result in weight loss and to benefit adiposity-associated comorbidities, such as, dyslipidaemia, hypertension and insulin resistance. Most individuals are, however, unable to sustain long-term weight loss induced by chronic energy restriction because of hunger, dietary monotony, lack of variability of food items and

M.-A. Cornier • B. Draznin (✉)
Division of Endocrinology, Diabetes and Metabolism, University of Colorado School of Medicine, Anschutz Medical Campus, Mail Stop 8106, 12801 E 17th Ave, Aurora, CO, USA
e-mail: boris.draznin@ucdenver.edu

H. Beck-Nielsen (ed.), *The Metabolic Syndrome*,
DOI 10.1007/978-3-7091-1331-8_7, © Springer-Verlag Wien 2013

adaptations in energy expenditure [8, 9]. Recently, nutritional intervention studies have been focusing on decreasing hunger and promoting satiety in attempt to improve adherence to dietary interventions, the strongest predictor of ultimate weight loss success [10–12].

In experimental animals, metabolic syndrome can be induced by a combination of high-fat and high-fructose (carbohydrate) diet [13]. Even though both of these dietary interventions can induce certain cardiometabolic changes compatible with the metabolic syndrome, the combination of the two appears to rapidly and consistently induce a constellation of findings comparable to human metabolic syndrome [14]. Because high-fat and high-carbohydrate diets have been implicated in the pathogenesis of the metabolic syndrome [15], many investigators have used either low-fat or low-carbohydrate diet in an attempt to reverse the metabolic syndrome either in its entirety or at least some of its components.

7.2 Diets for the Metabolic Syndrome

It is well established that weight loss is beneficial for treating all of the components of the metabolic syndrome, including improving excessive adiposity, dyslipidaemia, hypertension, insulin resistance and hyperglycaemia [16]. The magnitude of weight loss needs not be drastic. The Finnish Diabetes Prevention Study showed that lifestyle intervention with modest weight loss significantly reduced the prevalence of the metabolic syndrome (OR of 0.62; 95 % CI 0.40–0.95) as compared with the control group [17]. A 41 % reduction in the incidence of the metabolic syndrome was also seen with the intensive lifestyle intervention of the Diabetes Prevention Program [18]. In addition, a weight loss of as small as 5–10 % of body weight can significantly reduce triglycerides and increase high-density lipoprotein (HDL) cholesterol [19]. Furthermore, both hypertensive individuals and individuals at risk of developing hypertension can see a significant reduction in blood pressure with a modest weight loss [20–22]. Fasting blood glucose, insulin and HbA1c can also be decreased with modest weight loss [23]; interestingly, a 7-day negative energy balance without measurable weight loss has also been shown to improve insulin sensitivity [24]. Notably, the Diabetes Prevention Program demonstrated that weight loss was the number one predictor of reduction in the incidence of diabetes [25]. In fact, for every kilogram of weight loss, the risk of diabetes development was decreased by 16 %. A decrease in caloric intake is an avenue by which to promote a chronic negative energy balance resulting in weight loss. Although the macronutrient classification of the eliminated calories is of lesser importance when addressing overall energy balance, the type of macronutrients habitually consumed can influence the health of the individual with metabolic syndrome.

This remainder of this chapter will concentrate on the utility of low-carbohydrate diets in treatment and management of the metabolic syndrome.

7.3 Why a Low-Carbohydrate Diet?

7.3.1 Low-Carbohydrate Diets and Insulin Secretion

The concept of lowering carbohydrate intake in individuals who have insulin resistance is not a new idea. Lower carbohydrate intake results in relatively less insulin secretion to maintain normal glycaemia, which may be especially beneficial in someone who is resistant to insulin and/or has some insulin secretion abnormalities as is seen in the metabolic syndrome [26]. This in theory would result in reduced glucose variability, which may be favourable. Furthermore, as insulin is an anabolic hormone, reduced insulin secretion may be beneficial from a fuel storage and oxidation perspective.

7.3.2 Low-Carbohydrate Diets and Energy Intake

It has been proposed that hyperinsulinaemia promotes hunger and food cravings and, therefore, a lower carbohydrate diet that lowers insulin levels would reduce hunger, cravings and thus food intake. While this concept has not been supported by research, carbohydrate restriction to the point of ketosis has been shown to be associated with reduced energy intake and may be a primary mechanism for the weight loss success of low-carbohydrate diets [27]. Any change in diet pattern, however, has also been shown to result in at least short-term weight loss, and thus simply changing one's diet from a relatively high to a low-carbohydrate diet may account for some of the short-term success of these diets. The macronutrient that is replaced during carbohydrate restriction may also be important. Studies have suggested that dietary protein may be the most important macronutrient regulating satiety [12, 28]. For example, a diet with moderate protein increase (30 %) at the expense of carbohydrates (40 %) has been shown to achieve a higher satiating effect than conventional energy-restricted diets.

7.3.3 Low-Carbohydrate Diets and Weight Loss

While weight loss has been shown to be greater with lower carbohydrate diets in the short term, up to 1 year [27, 29, 30], the effects on long-term weight loss have been mixed [31–34]. A large randomised 2-year study of four diets of differing levels of carbohydrate, fat and protein did not show significantly greater weight loss with lower carbohydrate intake although prescribed macronutrient intakes did not reach target levels [35]. Adherence, though, was the strongest predictor of weight loss as has been shown in other studies. Both a low-carbohydrate diet and a "Mediterranean Diet" were shown to be more effective at 2-year weight loss than a low-fat diet. The Mediterranean Diet, while not necessarily a low-carbohydrate diet, promotes mono- and poly-unsaturated fats and has also been associated with reduced mortality and cardiovascular disease (CVD) [36]. Higher protein diets can improve weight loss without reductions in the lean body mass [12, 28].

Interestingly, there is some evidence that the baseline degree of insulin sensitivity predicts the weight loss response to diets of varying macronutrient content. Specifically, it appears that insulin-resistant individuals may lose more weight on lower carbohydrate diets than those who are more insulin sensitive [37].

7.3.4 Metabolic Effects of Low-Carbohydrate Diets

Due in part to the recent rise in the popularity of low-carbohydrate diets, there has been interest in the effect of carbohydrate intake on metabolic factors. Investigations into this question have consistently reported that carbohydrate intake is positively associated with total cholesterol, low-density lipoprotein (LDL) cholesterol and triglycerides and negatively associated with HDL cholesterol [38, 39], and low-carbohydrate diets have been consistently associated with reductions in triglycerides and higher HDL cholesterol levels. Grundy et al. [40], for example, found that a diet high in monounsaturated fat reduced cholesterol and triglycerides while maintaining HDL cholesterol levels as compared with diets low in fat or high in saturated fats. Furthermore, lower carbohydrate diets have been associated with improved carbohydrate metabolism especially in those with insulin resistance and/or type 2 diabetes mellitus [41]. As with weight loss, individuals with greater degrees of insulin resistance may have greater benefits on metabolic parameters on lower carbohydrate diets than those who are more insulin sensitive [37, 42, 43].

7.4 Low-Carbohydrate Diets in the Metabolic Syndrome: Outcomes

Unfortunately, there is a relative paucity of data examining the effects of diet and macronutrient intake on clinical outcomes in individuals with metabolic syndrome, per se. Muzio et al. [7] compared a low-carbohydrate, high-protein and monosaturated fat diet with a high-carbohydrate diet in their ability to impact cardiometabolic risk factors over 5 months in 100 obese individuals with metabolic syndrome. Even though all components of the metabolic syndrome except HDL cholesterol improved significantly in both groups, each of the diets impacted facets of the metabolic syndrome uniquely. The low-carbohydrate diet resulted in better reduction in systolic blood pressure and heart rate as well as triglycerides, whereas the high-carbohydrate diet resulted in greater reduction in LDL cholesterol. Other studies found similar results in abdominally obese [44] and insulin-resistant, obese [26] persons. In contrast, McAuley et al. [45] found that both high-fat and high-protein diets not only improved triglycerides but also resulted in greater reductions in body weight and waist circumference than a high-carbohydrate diet in insulin-resistant, obese women but only over 8 weeks. The data in patients with diabetes are also not clear again primarily due to the paucity of studies. Small studies of relatively short duration suggest that diets lower in carbohydrate and higher in monounsaturated fat are generally not associated with greater weight loss but are associated with greater improvements in lipids and glycaemic control [46–52].

7.5 The "Type" of Macronutrient Is also Important

7.5.1 Carbohydrates

Currently, the United States Department of Agriculture (USDA) and the Institute of Medicine (IOM) recommend a carbohydrate intake of 45–65 % of total caloric intake [100]. This recommendation is appropriate for most populations, as total carbohydrate consumption has not been shown to be associated with the development of type 2 diabetes or the metabolic syndrome [53–55]. It must also be stressed, though, that dietary carbohydrate can be placed into two categories: simple and complex. It is the latter which should comprise the bulk of the carbohydrate intake, while simple carbohydrates, especially in the form of added sugars, should be limited [100]. Common sources of added sugars in the diet include soft drinks, cakes, cookies, pies, fruit drinks, dairy desserts and candy [56]. Although added sugars are chemically identical to naturally occurring simple sugars (e.g. sugars found in fruit), concern is warranted regarding the lack of nutrients found in foods laden with added sugars. It has been shown that individuals who consume a greater percentage of calories as added sugars consume significantly less vitamins and minerals [57].

Because various carbohydrates elicit distinct metabolic responses in terms of insulin release and glucose utilisation, a concept of glycaemic index (GI) of food items gained significant interest among researchers and clinicians [58–62]. GI is a well-recognised marker of how a given carbohydrate is processed postprandially [58]. The reader is referred to excellent reviews written on this topic [62, 63]. Studies in animal models have shown that diets based on high-GI food items promote weight gain and visceral adiposity [64–66]. In contrast, diets based on low-GI food items enhance weight loss, minimise postprandial insulin release and promote satiety [67–69]. In humans, low-GI diets, containing high amounts of fruit, vegetables, legumes and whole grains, have been shown to induce greater weight loss than conventional diets [70, 71].

The GI has received considerable attention in terms of classifying which carbohydrates are "good" or "bad" for disease risk. Low-GI foods (i.e. those that are minimally processed) have been shown to improve components of the metabolic syndrome including dyslipidaemia and hyperglycaemia [72], whereas a higher GI has been shown to be positively associated with insulin resistance and metabolic syndrome prevalence [55]. Therefore, a diet high in complex, unrefined carbohydrates with an emphasis on fibre (14 g/1,000 cal consumed daily) and low in added sugars (<25 % of caloric intake) has been recommended for individuals with or at risk of metabolic syndrome. This type of diet was recommended for participants in the lifestyle intervention group of the Diabetes Prevention Program (i.e. high carbohydrate, low fat); participants decreased their percent fat intake by an average of 6.6 % over a 1-year period [25]. This dietary change contributed to weight loss, which, as previously noted, was the primary predictor of the decrease in diabetes incidence in the study. Moreover, a lower glycaemic load was associated with a reduced risk of CVD in the Nurses' Health Study [73]. Interestingly, though, diet soda but not "regular" soda was found to be a predictor of the metabolic syndrome in the Atherosclerosis Risk in Communities (ARIC) Study [74]. Overall, controversy remains about the wide use of low-GI diets since evidence from some interventional studies have produced inconsistent results in terms of weight loss, especially in the long-term studies.

Even when one assumes that diets aimed at reductions in the postprandial glucose responses are the best for individuals with metabolic syndrome, the debate whether carbohydrate restriction vs. consumption of foods with low-GI values would result in more favourable outcomes is not settled. Future studies comparing head to head the effectiveness of a low-GI diet with a carbohydrate-restricted diet in patients with metabolic syndrome must be conducted.

7.5.2 Fat

Since the National Health and Nutritional Examination Survey (NHANES) 1971, the average % fat intake in the United States has decreased from 36.9 % to 32.8 % in men and from 36.1 % to 32.8 % in women [75], thus bringing fat intake within the recommended range of intake (i.e. 20–35 %; [100]). Despite these reductions, there has been a marked increase in obesity and the metabolic syndrome over the same time period [76]. Like carbohydrate, it may be the type of fats that are consumed, rather than the total amount, which has a greater effect on components of the metabolic syndrome. Several studies have shown no effect of increased fat intake (20–40 % of caloric intake) on insulin sensitivity [77–80], although some conflicting results have been reported [81]. Interestingly, it has been shown that obese insulin-resistant women lost more weight on a 16-week high-fat (40 %) low-carbohydrate (40 %) diet, while obese insulin-sensitive women lost more weight on a low-fat (20 %) high-carbohydrate diet (60 %) [37]. Therefore, the degree of insulin resistance may determine what macronutrient composition is most appropriate to promote weight loss.

Evidence points toward the type of fat that is consumed having an effect on insulin sensitivity. Saturated fat has consistently been shown to be positively associated with fasting insulin levels [81–83]. The substitution of unsaturated fats for saturated fats in the diet has been shown to either have no effect on [84–88] or improve [89–92] insulin sensitivity. Given the observed association between saturated fat intake and insulin levels, it is prudent to recommend a reduction in saturated fat intake (<7 % of caloric intake) and an increase in the unsaturated fatty acids, specifically linoleic (5–10 % of caloric intake) and α-linolenic (0.7–1.6 % of caloric intake), as is promoted by the 2010 USDA Dietary Guidelines [100]. These guidelines are also applicable in the case of CVD, as investigators have been researching this relationship as early as the 1960s. Both serum cholesterol and overall CVD risk have been shown to be improved by type of dietary fat, i.e. a reduction in saturated fat and an increase in unsaturated fat, more so than total fat intake [93–96]. The Nurses' Health Study investigators reported that a 5 % increase in saturated fat intake was associated with a 17 % increase in coronary risk, while monounsaturated and polyunsaturated fat intakes were inversely related to coronary disease [97].

7.6 Conclusions

Dietary intake clearly has an impact on all of the components of the metabolic syndrome. Even though energy deficit is the most important element of weight loss programmes, macronutrient composition of the diet may influence dietary effectiveness and long-term compliance. Although each case should be treated individually, it is prudent to recommend a diet low in saturated fat, higher in unsaturated fats, high in complex carbohydrates and low in sodium.

The treatment of the metabolic syndrome should correct and/or prevent metabolic and cardiovascular abnormalities in the affected individuals. Weight reduction is a powerful tool to prevent and treat the metabolic syndrome. Because hypocaloric low-carbohydrate diets combined with a reduction in saturated fat can improve insulin sensitivity, glucose tolerance, reduce triglyceridaemia, increase circulating HDL cholesterol and result in substantial weight loss, it should be recommended as a part of lifestyle modifications in patients with metabolic syndrome.

While definition of "an optimal diet" is still elusive, a lifestyle that includes a reasonable restriction of carbohydrates or a consumption of low-GI food items can improve metabolic risk profiles in men and women [98, 99]. Prospective studies examining glycaemic load, GI and carbohydrate restriction on the outcomes of the metabolic syndrome are urgently needed.

References

1. Reaven GM (1988) Banting lecture (1988). Role of insulin resistance in human disease. Diabetes 37(12):1595–1607
2. Grundy SM, Cleeman JI et al (2005) Diagnosis and management of the metabolic syndrome. An American heart association/national heart, lung, and blood institute scientific statement. Executive summary. Cardiol Rev 13(6):322–327
3. Sullivan VK (2006) Prevention and treatment of the metabolic syndrome with lifestyle intervention: where do we start? J Am Diet Assoc 106(5):668–671
4. American Heart Association Nutrition, Lichtenstein CAH et al (2006) Diet and lifestyle recommendations revision 2006: a scientific statement from the American Heart Association Nutrition Committee. Circulation 114(1):82–96
5. Minich DM, Bland JS (2008) Dietary management of the metabolic syndrome beyond macronutrients. Nutr Rev 66(8):429–444

6. Abete I, Astrup A et al (2010) Obesity and the metabolic syndrome: role of different dietary macronutrient distribution patterns and specific nutritional components on weight loss and maintenance. Nutr Rev 68(4):214–231
7. Muzio F, Mondazzi L et al (2007) Effects of moderate variations in the macronutrient content of the diet on cardiovascular disease risk factors in obese patients with the metabolic syndrome. Am J Clin Nutr 86(4):946–951
8. Anton SD, Han H et al (2009) Effect of calorie restriction on subjective ratings of appetite. J Hum Nutr Diet 22(2):141–147
9. Redman LM, Heilbronn LK et al (2009) Metabolic and behavioral compensations in response to caloric restriction: implications for the maintenance of weight loss. PLoS One 4(2):e4377
10. Paddon-Jones D, Westman E et al (2008) Protein, weight management, and satiety. Am J Clin Nutr 87(5):1558S–1561S
11. Parra D, Ramel A et al (2008) A diet rich in long chain omega-3 fatty acids modulates satiety in overweight and obese volunteers during weight loss. Appetite 51(3):676–680
12. Soenen S, Westerterp-Plantenga MS (2008) Proteins and satiety: implications for weight management. Curr Opin Clin Nutr Metab Care 11(6):747–751
13. Rutledge AC, Adeli K (2007) Fructose and the metabolic syndrome: pathophysiology and molecular mechanisms. Nutr Rev 65(6 Pt 2):S13–S23
14. Lee J, Xu Y et al (2010) Multiple abnormalities of myocardial insulin signaling in a porcine model of diet-induced obesity. Am J Physiol Heart Circ Physiol 298(2):H310–H319
15. Poudyal H, Panchal SK et al (2012) Chronic high-carbohydrate, high-fat feeding in rats induces reversible metabolic, cardiovascular, and liver changes. Am J Physiol Endocrinol Metab 302(12):E1472–E1482
16. Pasanisi F, Contaldo F et al (2001) Benefits of sustained moderate weight loss in obesity. Nutr Metab Cardiovasc Dis 11(6):401–406
17. Ilanne-Parikka P, Eriksson JG et al (2008) Effect of lifestyle intervention on the occurrence of metabolic syndrome and its components in the Finnish Diabetes Prevention Study. Diabetes Care 31(4):805–807
18. Orchard TJ, Temprosa M et al (2005) The effect of metformin and intensive lifestyle intervention on the metabolic syndrome: the Diabetes Prevention Program randomized trial. Ann Intern Med 142(8):611–619
19. Van Gaal LF, Wauters MA et al (1997) The beneficial effects of modest weight loss on cardiovascular risk factors. Int J Obes Relat Metab Disord 21(Suppl 1):S5–S9
20. Langford HG, Blaufox MD et al (1985) Dietary therapy slows the return of hypertension after stopping prolonged medication. JAMA 253(5):657–664
21. Stamler R, Stamler J et al (1987) Nutritional therapy for high blood pressure. Final report of a four-year randomized controlled trial–the Hypertension Control Program. JAMA 257 (11):1484–1491
22. Whelton PK, Appel LJ et al (1998) Sodium reduction and weight loss in the treatment of hypertension in older persons: a randomized controlled trial of nonpharmacologic interventions in the elderly (TONE). TONE Collaborative Research Group. JAMA 279(11):839–846
23. Wing RR, Koeske R et al (1987) Long-term effects of modest weight loss in type II diabetic patients. Arch Intern Med 147(10):1749–1753
24. Kelley DE, Wing R et al (1993) Relative effects of calorie restriction and weight loss in noninsulin-dependent diabetes mellitus. J Clin Endocrinol Metab 77(5):1287–1293
25. Hamman RF, Wing RR et al (2006) Effect of weight loss with lifestyle intervention on risk of diabetes. Diabetes Care 29(9):2102–2107
26. McLaughlin T, Carter S et al (2006) Effects of moderate variations in macronutrient composition on weight loss and reduction in cardiovascular disease risk in obese, insulin-resistant adults. Am J Clin Nutr 84(4):813–821
27. Brehm BJ, Seeley RJ et al (2003) A randomized trial comparing a very low carbohydrate diet and a calorie-restricted low fat diet on body weight and cardiovascular risk factors in healthy women. J Clin Endocrinol Metab 88(4):1617–1623

28. Latner JD, Schwartz M (1999) The effects of a high-carbohydrate, high-protein or balanced lunch upon later food intake and hunger ratings. Appetite 33(1):119–128
29. Samaha FF, Iqbal N et al (2003) A low-carbohydrate as compared with a low-fat diet in severe obesity. N Engl J Med 348(21):2074–2081
30. Yancy WS Jr, Olsen MK et al (2004) A low-carbohydrate, ketogenic diet versus a low-fat diet to treat obesity and hyperlipidemia: a randomized, controlled trial. Ann Intern Med 140(10):769–777
31. Foster GD, Wyatt HR et al (2003) A randomized trial of a low-carbohydrate diet for obesity. N Engl J Med 348(21):2082–2090
32. Stern L, Iqbal N et al (2004) The effects of low-carbohydrate versus conventional weight loss diets in severely obese adults: one-year follow-up of a randomized trial. Ann Intern Med 140(10):778–785
33. Dansinger ML, Gleason JA et al (2005) Comparison of the Atkins, Ornish, Weight Watchers, and Zone diets for weight loss and heart disease risk reduction: a randomized trial. JAMA 293(1):43–53
34. Gardner CD, Kiazand A et al (2007) Comparison of the Atkins, Zone, Ornish, and LEARN diets for change in weight and related risk factors among overweight premenopausal women: the A TO Z Weight Loss Study: a randomized trial. JAMA 297(9):969–977
35. Sacks FM, Bray GA et al (2009) Comparison of weight-loss diets with different compositions of fat, protein, and carbohydrates. N Engl J Med 360(9):859–873
36. de Lorgeril M, Renaud S et al (1994) Mediterranean alpha-linolenic acid-rich diet in secondary prevention of coronary heart disease. Lancet 343(8911):1454–1459
37. Cornier MA, Donahoo WT et al (2005) Insulin sensitivity determines the effectiveness of dietary macronutrient composition on weight loss in obese women. Obes Res 13(4):703–709
38. Ma Y, Li Y et al (2006) Association between carbohydrate intake and serum lipids. J Am Coll Nutr 25(2):155–163
39. Liese AD, Gilliard T et al (2007) Carbohydrate nutrition, glycaemic load, and plasma lipids: the Insulin Resistance Atherosclerosis Study. Eur Heart J 28(1):80–87
40. Grundy SM (1986) Comparison of monounsaturated fatty acids and carbohydrates for lowering plasma cholesterol. N Engl J Med 314(12):745–748
41. Harber MP, Schenk S et al (2005) Alterations in carbohydrate metabolism in response to short-term dietary carbohydrate restriction. Am J Physiol Endocrinol Metab 289(2): E306–E312
42. Pittas AG, Das SK et al (2005) A low-glycemic load diet facilitates greater weight loss in overweight adults with high insulin secretion but not in overweight adults with low insulin secretion in the CALERIE trial. Diabetes Care 28(12):2939–2941
43. Ebbeling CB, Leidig MM et al (2007) Effects of a low-glycemic load vs low-fat diet in obese young adults: a randomized trial. JAMA 297(19):2092–2102
44. Tay J, Brinkworth GD et al (2008) Metabolic effects of weight loss on a very-low-carbohydrate diet compared with an isocaloric high-carbohydrate diet in abdominally obese subjects. J Am Coll Cardiol 51(1):59–67
45. McAuley K, Hopkins C et al (2005) Comparison of high-fat and high-protein diets with a high-carbohydrate diet in insulin-resistant obese women. Diabetologia 48(1):8–16
46. Low CC, Grossman EB et al (1996) Potentiation of effects of weight loss by monounsaturated fatty acids in obese NIDDM patients. Diabetes 45(5):569–575
47. Gumbiner B, Low CC et al (1998) Effects of a monounsaturated fatty acid-enriched hypocaloric diet on cardiovascular risk factors in obese patients with type 2 diabetes. Diabetes Care 21(1):9–15
48. Heilbronn LK, Noakes M et al (1999) Effect of energy restriction, weight loss, and diet composition on plasma lipids and glucose in patients with type 2 diabetes. Diabetes Care 22(6):889–895
49. Parker B, Noakes M et al (2002) Effect of a high-protein, high-monounsaturated fat weight loss diet on glycemic control and lipid levels in type 2 diabetes. Diabetes Care 25(3):425–430

50. Brinkworth GD, Noakes M et al (2004) Long-term effects of advice to consume a high-protein, low-fat diet, rather than a conventional weight-loss diet, in obese adults with type 2 diabetes: one-year follow-up of a randomised trial. Diabetologia 47(10):1677–1686
51. Rizkalla SW, Taghrid L et al (2004) Improved plasma glucose control, whole-body glucose utilization, and lipid profile on a low-glycemic index diet in type 2 diabetic men: a randomized controlled trial. Diabetes Care 27(8):1866–1872
52. Sheard NF, Clark NG et al (2004) Dietary carbohydrate (amount and type) in the prevention and management of diabetes: a statement by the American Diabetes Association. Diabetes Care 27(9):2266–2271
53. Lundgren H, Bengtsson C et al (1989) Dietary habits and incidence of noninsulin-dependent diabetes mellitus in a population study of women in Gothenburg, Sweden. Am J Clin Nutr 49(4):708–712
54. Marshall JA, Hamman RF et al (1991) High-fat, low-carbohydrate diet and the etiology of non-insulin-dependent diabetes mellitus: the San Luis Valley Diabetes Study. Am J Epidemiol 134(6):590–603
55. McKeown NM, Meigs JB et al (2004) Carbohydrate nutrition, insulin resistance, and the prevalence of the metabolic syndrome in the Framingham Offspring Cohort. Diabetes Care 27(2):538–546
56. Guthrie JF, Morton JF (2000) Food sources of added sweeteners in the diets of Americans. J Am Diet Assoc 100(1):43–51, quiz 49–50
57. Lewis CJ, Park YK et al (1992) Nutrient intakes and body weights of persons consuming high and moderate levels of added sugars. J Am Diet Assoc 92(6):708–713
58. Jenkins DJ, Wolever TM et al (1981) Glycemic index of foods: a physiological basis for carbohydrate exchange. Am J Clin Nutr 34(3):362–366
59. Ford ES, Liu S (2001) Glycemic index and serum high-density lipoprotein cholesterol concentration among us adults. Arch Intern Med 161(4):572–576
60. Brand-Miller JC (2004) Postprandial glycemia, glycemic index, and the prevention of type 2 diabetes. Am J Clin Nutr 80(2):243–244
61. Levitan EB, Cook NR et al (2008) Dietary glycemic index, dietary glycemic load, blood lipids, and C-reactive protein. Metabolism 57(3):437–443
62. Radulian G, Rusu E et al (2009) Metabolic effects of low glycaemic index diets. Nutr J 8:5
63. Wood RJ, Fernandez ML (2009) Carbohydrate-restricted versus low-glycemic-index diets for the treatment of insulin resistance and metabolic syndrome. Nutr Rev 67(3):179–183
64. Kabir M, Rizkalla SW et al (1998) A high glycemic index starch diet affects lipid storage-related enzymes in normal and to a lesser extent in diabetic rats. J Nutr 128(11):1878–1883
65. Scribner KB, Pawlak DB et al (2007) Hepatic steatosis and increased adiposity in mice consuming rapidly vs. slowly absorbed carbohydrate. Obesity (Silver Spring) 15(9):2190–2199
66. Scribner KB, Pawlak DB et al (2008) Long-term effects of dietary glycemic index on adiposity, energy metabolism, and physical activity in mice. Am J Physiol Endocrinol Metab 295(5):E1126–E1131
67. Flint A, Moller BK et al (2006) Glycemic and insulinemic responses as determinants of appetite in humans. Am J Clin Nutr 84(6):1365–1373
68. de Rougemont A, Normand S et al (2007) Beneficial effects of a 5-week low-glycaemic index regimen on weight control and cardiovascular risk factors in overweight non-diabetic subjects. Br J Nutr 98(6):1288–1298
69. Brand-Miller J, McMillan-Price J et al (2008) Carbohydrates–the good, the bad and the whole grain. Asia Pac J Clin Nutr 17(Suppl 1):16–19
70. Agus MS, Swain JF et al (2000) Dietary composition and physiologic adaptations to energy restriction. Am J Clin Nutr 71(4):901–907
71. Roberts SB (2000) High-glycemic index foods, hunger, and obesity: is there a connection? Nutr Rev 58(6):163–169
72. Jenkins DJ, Kendall CW et al (2002) Glycemic index: overview of implications in health and disease. Am J Clin Nutr 76(1):266S–273S

73. Halton TL, Willett WC et al (2006) Low-carbohydrate-diet score and the risk of coronary heart disease in women. N Engl J Med 355(19):1991–2002
74. Lutsey PL, Steffen LM et al (2008) Dietary intake and the development of the metabolic syndrome: the Atherosclerosis Risk in Communities study. Circulation 117(6):754–761
75. Hedley AA, Ogden CL et al (2004) Prevalence of overweight and obesity among US children, adolescents, and adults, 1999–2002. JAMA 291(23):2847–2850
76. Ford ES, Giles WH et al (2004) Increasing prevalence of the metabolic syndrome among u.s. Adults. Diabetes Care 27(10):2444–2449
77. Borkman M, Campbell LV et al (1991) Comparison of the effects on insulin sensitivity of high carbohydrate and high fat diets in normal subjects. J Clin Endocrinol Metab 72 (2):432–437
78. Garg A, Grundy SM et al (1992) Comparison of effects of high and low carbohydrate diets on plasma lipoproteins and insulin sensitivity in patients with mild NIDDM. Diabetes 41(10):1278–1285
79. Sarkkinen E, Schwab U et al (1996) The effects of monounsaturated-fat enriched diet and polyunsaturated-fat enriched diet on lipid and glucose metabolism in subjects with impaired glucose tolerance. Eur J Clin Nutr 50(9):592–598
80. Bisschop PH, de Metz J et al (2001) Dietary fat content alters insulin-mediated glucose metabolism in healthy men. Am J Clin Nutr 73(3):554–559
81. Mayer EJ, Newman B et al (1993) Usual dietary fat intake and insulin concentrations in healthy women twins. Diabetes Care 16(11):1459–1469
82. Maron DJ, Fair JM et al (1991) Saturated fat intake and insulin resistance in men with coronary artery disease. The Stanford coronary risk intervention project investigators and staff. Circulation 84(5):2020–2027
83. Parker DR, Weiss ST et al (1993) Relationship of dietary saturated fatty acids and body habitus to serum insulin concentrations: the Normative Aging Study. Am J Clin Nutr 58 (2):129–136
84. Heine RJ (1993) Dietary fish oil and insulin action in humans. Ann N Y Acad Sci 683:110–121
85. Schwab U, Uusitupa M et al (1993) Effects of two fat-modified diets on glucose and lipid metabolism in healthy subjects. Ann N Y Acad Sci 683:279–280
86. Uusitupa M, Schwab U et al (1994) Effects of two high-fat diets with different fatty acid compositions on glucose and lipid metabolism in healthy young women. Am J Clin Nutr 59(6):1310–1316
87. Fasching P, Ratheiser K et al (1996) No effect of short-term dietary supplementation of saturated and poly- and monounsaturated fatty acids on insulin secretion and sensitivity in healthy men. Ann Nutr Metab 40(2):116–122
88. Lovejoy JC, Smith SR et al (2002) Effects of diets enriched in saturated (palmitic), monounsaturated (oleic), or trans (elaidic) fatty acids on insulin sensitivity and substrate oxidation in healthy adults. Diabetes Care 25(8):1283–1288
89. Budohoski L, Panczenko-Kresowska B et al (1993) Effects of saturated and polyunsaturated fat enriched diet on the skeletal muscle insulin sensitivity in young rats. J Physiol Pharmacol 44(4):391–398
90. Vessby B, Unsitupa M et al (2001) Substituting dietary saturated for monounsaturated fat impairs insulin sensitivity in healthy men and women: the KANWU Study. Diabetologia 44(3):312–319
91. Summers LK, Fielding BA et al (2002) Substituting dietary saturated fat with polyunsaturated fat changes abdominal fat distribution and improves insulin sensitivity. Diabetologia 45(3):369–377
92. Xiao C, Giacca A et al (2006) Differential effects of monounsaturated, polyunsaturated and saturated fat ingestion on glucose-stimulated insulin secretion, sensitivity and clearance in overweight and obese, non-diabetic humans. Diabetologia 49(6):1371–1379

93. Keys A, Parlin RW (1966) Serum cholesterol response to changes in dietary lipids. Am J Clin Nutr 19(3):175–181
94. Dayton S, Pearce ML (1969) Diet high in unsaturated fat. A controlled clinical trial. Minn Med 52(8):1237–1242
95. Turpeinen O, Karvonen MJ et al (1979) Dietary prevention of coronary heart disease: the Finnish Mental Hospital Study. Int J Epidemiol 8(2):99–118
96. de Lorgeril M, Salen P et al (1999) Mediterranean diet, traditional risk factors, and the rate of cardiovascular complications after myocardial infarction: final report of the Lyon Diet Heart Study. Circulation 99(6):779–785
97. Hu FB, Stampfer MJ et al (1997) Dietary fat intake and the risk of coronary heart disease in women. N Engl J Med 337(21):1491–1499
98. Finley CE, Barlow CE et al (2010) Glycemic index, glycemic load, and prevalence of the metabolic syndrome in the cooper center longitudinal study. J Am Diet Assoc 110 (12):1820–1829
99. Jones JL, Fernandez ML et al (2011) A Mediterranean-style low-glycemic-load diet improves variables of metabolic syndrome in women, and addition of a phytochemical-rich medical food enhances benefits on lipoprotein metabolism. J Clin Lipidol 5(3):188–196
100. US Department of Agriculture and US Department of Health and Human Services (2010) Dietary guidelines for Americans 2010, 7th edn. US Government Printing Office, Washington, DC

Treatment with Metformin

8

Clifford J. Bailey

8.1 General Overview

Metformin (dimethylbiguanide) is a biguanide agent now used widely in the treatment of type 2 diabetes. As a guanidine derivative (Fig. 8.1), its history can be traced from the use of *Galega officinalis* (goat's rue or French lilac) in mediaeval Europe as a treatment for symptoms of diabetes [1]. *Galega officinalis* is rich in guanidine, and the glucose-lowering properties of guanidine were noted early in the twentieth century, giving rise to the use of synthalin (decamethylene diguanidine) and galegine (isoamylene guanidine) as diabetes therapies [2, 3]. Although the synthesis and glucose-lowering effect of dimethylbiguanide was recorded in the late 1920s [4], the use of guanidine derivatives all but disappeared with increasing availability of insulin in the 1930s. It was not until the 1950s that Jean Sterne and Denise Duval, unaware of the previous studies, noted that guanidine derivatives used to treat malaria or influenza also lowered blood glucose. After extensive animal research they identified dimethylbiguanide as a low toxicity antihyperglycaemic agent [5]. Other more potent biguanides, notably phenformin and buformin, that were introduced as antidiabetic agents at or around this time were initially more popular, but were subsequently withdrawn due to associated lactic acidosis [3]. It was not until the introduction of metformin into the United States (1995) and the results of the United Kingdom Prospective Diabetes Study (UKPDS) (1998) that this agent became recognised as an important glucose-lowering therapy for type 2 diabetes [6, 7].

Metformin does not have an approved indication for use to treat metabolic syndrome, but it has been used "off-label" in many studies to determine its effect on the emergence, progression and treatment of features of the metabolic syndrome. We will first consider its approved indication for use in the treatment of type

C.J. Bailey (✉)
School of Life and Health Sciences, Aston University, Birmingham B4 7ET, UK
e-mail: c.j.bailey@aston.ac.uk

H. Beck-Nielsen (ed.), *The Metabolic Syndrome*,
DOI 10.1007/978-3-7091-1331-8_8, © Springer-Verlag Wien 2013

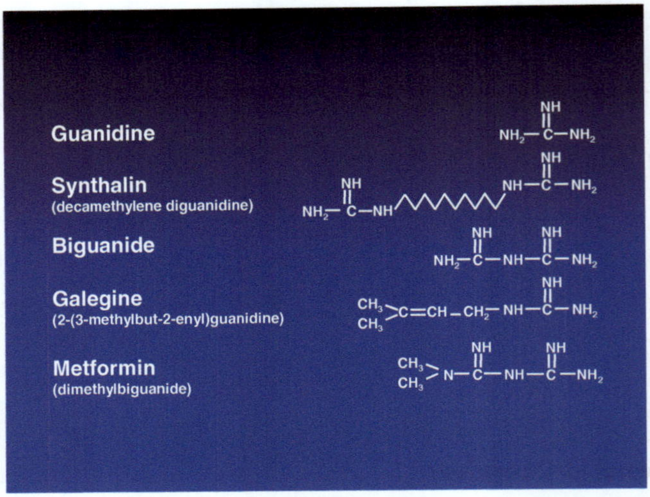

Fig. 8.1 Structures of guanidine, synthalin, biguanide, galegine and metformin

2 diabetes and then return to its "off-label" use against other features of the metabolic syndrome. A substantial proportion of type 2 diabetes patients exhibit sufficient of these other features of metabolic syndrome to qualify for a diagnosis of metabolic syndrome by current criteria [8]. However, it is not possible from most of the published literature on type 2 diabetes patients to tease out data that specifically apply or refer to those patients with metabolic syndrome. Nevertheless, the studies in type 2 diabetes patients provide the bulk of evidence for the effects of metformin on individual components of the metabolic syndrome (Table 8.1).

8.2 Glucose-Lowering Effect of Metformin in Type 2 Diabetes

Lifestyle measures, especially diet and exercise, are key elements at all stages of the management of type 2 diabetes. When these measures alone are unable to achieve or maintain adequate glycaemic control, most guidelines suggest metformin as a preferred first line pharmacological therapy, provided there are no contraindications and the drug is well tolerated [9, 10].

Metformin acts mainly to counter insulin resistance and its blood glucose-lowering effect in type 2 diabetes is attributed mainly to decreased hepatic glucose production through insulin-dependent and insulin-independent mechanisms elaborated in subsequent sections [11]. The extent of the glucose lowering is considerably influenced by the baseline level of hyperglycaemia and the patient's pathophysiological status of beta-cell function and insulin resistance. Most patients with mild to moderately severe fasting hyperglycaemia [e.g. 110–275 mg/dL (6.1–15.5 mmol/L) or HbA1C 7–12 % (53–108 mmol/mol)] exhibit a glucose-lowering effect. On average patients within this range of baseline, hyperglycaemia

Table 8.1 Effects of metformin that are relevant to "metabolic syndrome" and counter cardiometabolic risk

Clinical feature	Effect of metformin
Insulin resistance	Counters insulin resistance leading to improved insulin sensitivity in liver, muscle and possibly other (vascular) tissues
Hyperinsulinaemia	Reduces fasting hyperinsulinaemia
Abdominal obesity	Usually stabilises body weight; can facilitate reduction of excess adiposity
Hyperglycaemia	Improves glycaemic control in type 2 diabetes; reduces progression of impaired glucose tolerance (IGT) to type 2 diabetes
Dyslipidaemia	Modest improvements of lipid profile in some hypertriglyceridaemic and hypercholesterolaemic individuals.
Raised blood pressure	No significant effect on blood pressure in most studies but may be improved in overweight individuals achieving weight loss.
Pro-inflammatory state	Reduced C-reactive protein and some adipo-cytokines
Pro-coagulant state	Some anti-thrombotic activity e.g. decreases in plasminogen activator inhibitor 1, fibrinogen and platelet aggregation
Atherosclerosis	Reduced myocardial infarctions and increased survival in type 2 diabetes: reduced carotid intima-media thickness and reduced adhesion molecules; other evidence for anti-atherogenic activity, mostly from animal studies

respond to metformin with a lowering of fasting plasma glucose by about 25–75 mg/dL (1.5–4.2 mmol/L) and HbA1C by 1–2 % (11–22 mmol/mol) [12–14]. The reduction in glycaemia is usually greater at higher baseline glycaemia and earlier in the duration of the disease. Although the effect is mostly on fasting hyperglycaemia, reductions in the prandial increment in plasma glucose are also evident.

Glucose lowering with metformin in type 2 diabetes does not cause blood glucose to drop into frank hypoglycaemia, and even high doses of metformin have little effect on glycaemia in non-diabetic normoglycaemic subjects [3, 7, 11]. This is probably due in part to the lack of stimulation of basal insulin concentrations and to the counter-regulatory mechanisms remaining unimpeded by metformin [11, 15]. Many studies have confirmed the improvement in whole body insulin sensitivity using hyperinsulinaemic euglycaemic clamps and applying models based on glucose–insulin ratios such as homeostasis model assessment for insulin resistance (HOMA-IR) and the Matsuda index, suggesting that metformin enhances insulin-mediated effects to suppress hepatic glucose production and promotes peripheral glucose utilisation [3, 11, 16–18]. Basal insulin levels are typically slightly decreased as insulin sensitivity improves in type 2 diabetes patients receiving metformin [6, 11–13]. However, prandial insulin responses are often maintained relative to the glycaemic excursion, possibly aided by slightly raised prandial concentrations of the glucose-dependent incretin glucagon-like peptide-1, but consistent changes in glucagon concentrations have not emerged [7, 11, 19].

8.3 Non-Glycaemic Effects of Metformin in Type 2 Diabetes

8.3.1 Weight Control

In addition to its glucose-lowering effects, metformin exerts a variety of effects that are independent of glycaemic control and potentially beneficial to cardiovascular risk management [11, 13]. Most of these risk factors are components of the metabolic syndrome (Table 8.1). Thus, metformin does not induce weight gain and is generally regarded as weight neutral, although a small reduction in body weight (mean loss of 0.5–2 kg) is often observed in overweight and obese patients [20]. This has been ascribed to the reduction in basal insulinaemia, and possibly due to initial nausea or other initial adverse gastrointestinal effects, or to a possibly mild appetite suppression. However, animal studies suggest an increase in glucose turnover, which may also contribute [21].

8.3.2 Lipid Profile

Depending on the extent of dyslipidaemia, metformin therapy is often accompanied by a small decrease in plasma total cholesterol, low-density lipoprotein (LDL) cholesterol and triglycerides (of ~5 %), although there is little or no effect when these parameters are already within the normal range [3, 11, 22]. High-density lipoprotein (HDL) cholesterol is usually unaffected or very marginally raised, and it is generally considered that any improvement in the lipid profile would not be sufficient to explain the beneficial vascular outcomes observed in large prospective trials and retrospective database analyses [3, 7, 11, 22].

8.3.3 Vascular Effects

Several large studies have reported potentially anti-atherogenic and anti-thrombotic effects of metformin in type 2 diabetes (Fig. 8.2) [23]. The UKPDS noted that early and intensive anti-hyperglycaemic intervention with metformin in overweight and obese type 2 diabetes was associated with a long-term (10–15 years) reduction in the incidence of myocardial infarction and an increase in survival (Fig. 8.3) [6]. This was apparently independent of the glucose-lowering efficacy of metformin because other glucose-lowering medications that achieved similar glycaemic control were not associated with this cardiovascular protection. A decrease in cardiovascular events with metformin therapy has been supported by subsequent large retrospective analyses [24–28] and by observational studies [29, 30]. Additionally, there is prospective evidence that metformin reduced restenosis after percutaneous coronary angioplasty [31] and reduced carotid intima-media thickness [32, 33].

Anti-thrombotic effects attributed to metformin include increased fibrinolytic activity associated with decreased production of plasminogen activator inhibitor-1, decreased sensitivity to platelet-aggregating agents and possibly a reduced amount

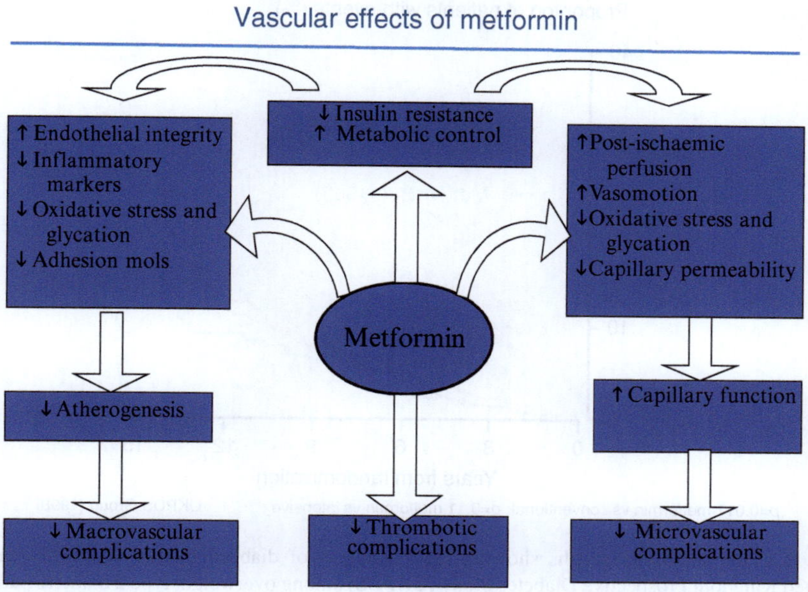

Fig. 8.2 Reduced macrovascular and microvascular complications in type 2 diabetic patients receiving metformin are mediated by direct effects on the vasculature as well as reduced insulin resistance and improved metabolic control. ↑ increase; ↓ decrease. Redrawn from [23]

of fibrinogen [34–38]. Metformin may also reduce circulating concentrations of coagulation factors VII and XIII, reducing the cross-linking of fibrin [39–41].

Most studies have failed to identify any consistent effect of metformin on blood pressure, although small reductions in blood pressure may accompany weight loss [23]. However, improved vascular reactivity consonant with improved endothelial function has been noted in several studies. For example, metformin has improved arterial flow during plethysmography studies in diabetic and non-diabetic individuals independently of glycaemic control, including subjects with metabolic syndrome [42–45]. Several studies indicate that metformin improves an endothelium-dependent vasodilatatory mechanism, but it is possible that non-endothelium-dependent mechanisms may also be involved [46–49].

With regard to the endothelium and athero-thrombotic activity, there is evidence that metformin can reduce monocyte adhesion to endothelial cells [50]. This appears to be due to reduced production of several vascular cell adhesion molecules, notably vascular cell adhesion module 1 (VCAM-1), intracellular cell adhesion module 1 (ICAM-1) and E-selectin, independently of glycaemic control [50, 51]. Metformin has also been reported to reduce markers of low grade inflammation such as C-reactive protein (CRP) and pro-inflammatory adipocytokines in diabetic and non-diabetic subjects, but this has not been consistently confirmed [51–56].

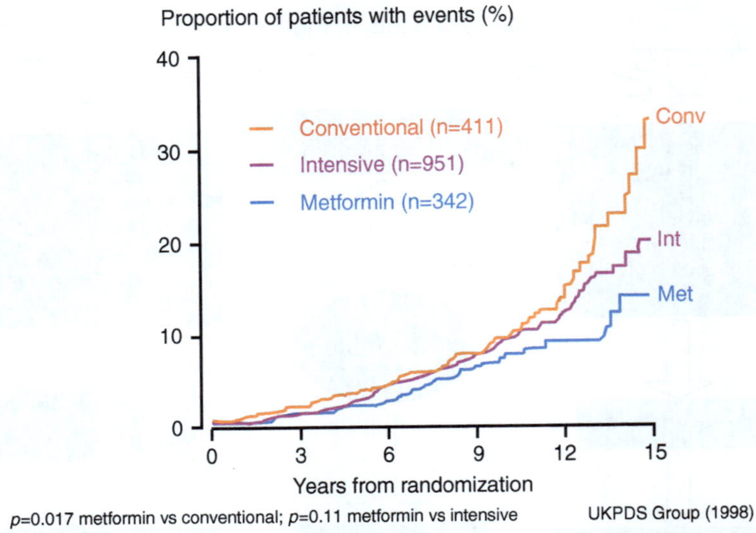

Fig. 8.3 Kaplan–Meier graphs showing the proportion of diabetes-related end points in the United Kingdom Prospective Diabetes Study (UKPDS) among overweight type 2 diabetes patients initially assigned to diet only (conventional therapy) or to intensive therapy with metformin or a sulphonylurea or insulin. Data for the sulphonylurea and insulin groups were similar, and these data have been pooled for this figure. Re-drawn from data [6]

8.3.4 Glycation and Oxidative Stress

Metformin would be expected to reduce non-enzymatic glycation of proteins through its anti-hyperglycaemic activity, and several studies have demonstrated reductions in advanced glycation end products [57, 58]. Increased antioxidant activity has been reported during metformin therapy [52, 53], and in vitro experiments suggest reduced production of reactive oxygen species [59–61].

8.4 Clinical Use of Metformin

Metformin (proprietary name Glucophage) is available in two tablet formulations: standard (immediate-release) and extended-release formulation. There are also now liquid and chewable formulations. Pharmacokinetic aspects of metformin are summarised in Table 8.2 and the clinical use in type 2 diabetes are summarised in Table 8.3.

When lifestyle measures are inadequate to achieve or maintain glycaemic control in type 2 diabetes, metformin is usually the preferred pharmacological

Table 8.2 Pharmacokinetic features of metformin

Feature	Comment
Bioavailability	50–60 %; absorbed mainly from the small intestine
T_{max}	0.9–2.6 h for standard (IR) formulation 4–8 h for extended-release formulation
C_{max}	1–2 μg/mL (Approximately 10^{-5} mol/L) 1–2 h after single oral dose of 500–1,000 mg for standard (IR) formulation; maximal concentration is ~20 % lower with extended-release formulation, but similar area under the curve
Plasma protein binding	Negligible
Plasma elimination half-life	~6 h
Metabolism	Not measurably metabolised
Elimination	About 90 % of absorbed drug is eliminated in urine in 24 h; multi-exponential renal elimination involving glomerular filtration and tubular secretion
Tissue distribution	Distributed in most tissues at concentrations similar to peripheral plasma; higher concentrations in liver and kidney; highest concentration in salivary glands and intestinal wall

T_{max} is time to maximum plasma concentration after single oral dose
C_{max} is maximum plasma concentration

Table 8.3 Clinical use of metformin in the treatment of type 2 diabetes

Feature	Comment
Indications	Monotherapy or in combination with other oral antidiabetic agents or insulin in type 2 diabetes patients inadequately controlled by diet, exercise and health education
Dose	500-, 850- and 1,000-mg Standard (IR) tablets: taken with meals 500-, 750- and 1,000-mg XR tablet: take with evening meal 500 mg/5 mL Liquid formulation
Titration	Increase dose slowly; monitor glycaemic control; maximal dose 2,550 or 3,000 mg/day depending on country (2,000 mg/day in children)
Contraindications	Renal and hepatic disease; cardiac or respiratory insufficiency; any hypoxic condition; severe infection; alcohol abuse; history of lactic acidosis; temporarily discontinue during use of intravenous radiographic contrast agents; pregnancy (although safe use demonstrated in several studies)
Side-effects	Gastrointestinal symptoms and metallic taste, likely to improve with dose reduction and re-titration; may impair absorption of vitamin B12 and folic acid
Adverse reactions	Risk of lactic acidosis in patients with a contraindication; hypoglycaemia can occur when taken in combination with another antidiabetic drug or during alcohol abuse
Monitoring	Check for contraindications; check plasma creatinine and haemoglobin periodically; possible interaction with cimetidine therapy

therapy: its efficacy is as good as other oral therapies, it does not cause weight gain or frank hypoglycaemia, and it offers various potentially cardio-protective actions that are independent of its glucose-lowering effect [9, 10]. Before initiating metformin therapy an important precaution is to check that renal function is adequate. This is usually based on a measure of serum creatinine (typically <1.5 mg/dL in men or <1.4 mg/dL in women, but <1.7 mg/dL in some guidelines) or creatinine clearance (>60 mL/min/1.73 m^2 or estimated glomerular filtration rate by modification of diet in renal disease (MDRD) of >45 mL/min/1.73 m^2 in some guidelines) [62]. Metformin taken with meals and the dose is titrated slowly to minimise initial gastrointestinal side-effects, which may be reduced with the extended-release formulation. About 5–10 % of patients do not tolerate a full therapeutic dose of metformin (2,000 mg/day). The most serious recognised adverse event associated with excess accumulation of metformin is lactic acidosis. This is rare (incidence ~0.03 cases/1,000 patient-years of treatment), but with a mortality of ~50 %. Since metformin is eliminated unchanged in the urine, periodic monitoring of renal function is therefore obligatory. Long-term therapy with metformin may cause a small decrease in the absorption of vitamin B12 and occasionally folate; however, development of anaemia from this cause is rare and is usually reversed by improved diet or vitamin B12 supplementation [7, 11].

Beyond its approved indication for type 2 diabetes, metformin has been used "off-label "in the treatment of polycystic ovary syndrome (PCOS) where several (but not all) studies have reported that, given in conjunction with clomiphene, it yields a greater improvement in rates of ovulation and pregnancy and fewer miscarriages [63]. Although not indicated for use in pregnancy, metformin has been found to improve maternal and foetal outcomes in patients with gestational diabetes [64]. Although thiazolidinedione insulin sensitizers have been reported to improve hepatic function in non-alcoholic fatty liver disease, similar benefits have not been confirmed with metformin [65]. In recent years evidence has emerged to suggest that metformin may have anti-neoplastic properties, and trials are now underway to assess the potential of metformin as a preventative or therapeutic agent against several types of cancers [66].

8.5 Pharmacological Mechanism of Action of Metformin

Many experimental studies have reported on the cellular mode of action of metformin. Many have failed to take account of the concentrations of the drug to which different tissues are exposed [67]. For example, most peripheral tissues see concentrations approximating circulating concentrations up to about $1\text{–}5 \times 10^{-5}$ mol/L. Liver can be exposed to up to fivefold to tenfold higher concentrations, and there are much higher concentrations still in the walls of the intestinal tract. Consequently different cellular mechanisms may operate to different extents in different tissues.

Metformin gains rapid entry into many cell types via the organic cation transporter-1 (OCT1) [68] and its effects are typically evident too quickly for a genomic mode of action alone [21]. At high concentrations, metformin will suppress the activity of the respiratory chain at complex I and reduce the adenosine triphosphate (ATP):adenosine monophosphate (AMP) ratio [69]. At low concentrations, metformin has been shown to modestly enhance insulin receptor tyrosine kinase activity, possibly by reducing receptor dephosphorylation through reduced phosphotyrosine phosphatase activity [70], providing a basis for improved insulin action. At intermediate concentrations, metformin demonstrably activates AMP-activated protein kinase (AMPK) with dependency on the presence of liver kinase B1 (LKB1) [71, 72]. Whether this is a direct effect of metformin or subsequent to a subtle change in cellular energy status is unclear [73]. However, activation of AMPK has diverse intracellular effects that could account for many of the low potency effects on nutrient metabolism. These include a suppression of gluconeogenesis by down regulation of phosphoenolpyruvate carboxykinase and glucose-6-phosphatase, reduced lipogenesis and increased fatty acid oxidation via phosphorylation and deactivation of acetyl-CoA carboxylase. Additionally, the AMPK route could mediate increased mitochondrial biogenesis via peroxisome proliferator-activated receptor-γ co-activator-1α (PGC-1α), with possible mechanisms for increased plasma membrane insertion and activation of the insulin-sensitive glucose transporter Glut4 [74–76].

Although the antidiabetic efficacy of metformin requires the presence of at least some circulating insulin, metformin does not appear to promote the genomically mediated proliferative and cell differentiation effects of insulin. The insulin-dependent and -independent AMPK-mediated effects of metformin contribute to a re-balancing of the glucose-fatty acid (Randle) cycle to favour glucose utilisation. Also, high concentrations of metformin in the walls of the intestine promote anaerobic glucose metabolism in this tissue, increasing glucose lactate turnover, which may enhance futile cycling and increased energy dissipation that help to prevent weight gain [21]. Potential anti-cancer mechanisms for metformin include AMPK-dependent and -independent decreases of mammalian target of rapamycin (mTOR) signalling and protein synthesis, respiratory chain suppression and a lowering of basal insulinaemia, possibly targeting cancer stem cells [77].

8.6 Metformin and Metabolic Syndrome in Non-Diabetic Subjects

Many studies have now affirmed that intensive lifestyle management and pharmacological intervention with metformin, thiazolidinediones, acarbose or orlistat can prevent or delay progression of impaired glucose tolerance (IGT) and impaired fasting glucose (IFG) to new onset type 2 diabetes [78, 79]. Preceding sections have examined the effects of metformin in type 2 diabetes: in this section we focus on the effects of metformin on features of the metabolic syndrome in non-diabetic subjects.

The idea that metformin might confer primary protection against a collective of cardiovascular risk factors in non-diabetic individuals was tested in the Biguanides and the Prevention of the Risk of Obesity (BIGPRO) 1 study started in 1991. This multicentre double-blind trial recruited 324 non-diabetic, middle-aged (35–65 years) subjects without cardiovascular disease but with abdominal adiposity (waist-to-hip ratio >0.95 in men and <0.80 in women) as an indicator of insulin resistance [80]. Participants were randomised to placebo or metformin (850 mg/day) with standard lifestyle advice to all. At 1 year metformin was associated with greater mean weight loss (by 1.2 kg), slightly lower fasting plasma glucose (by 0.2 mmol/L), slightly lower total cholesterol and LDL cholesterol (by 0.16 and 0.12 mmol/L, respectively) and lower fasting insulin (by 9 pmol/L). Blood pressure was not affected and there were no significant cardiovascular events, but five subjects in the placebo group and none in the metformin group were diagnosed with type 2 diabetes during the study. BIGPRO2 recruited subjects with raised triglyceride levels and raised blood pressure but revealed little more [81], reaffirming the need for larger and longer trials to investigate the potential prophylactic effect of metformin.

8.6.1 Diabetes Prevention Program

The Diabetes Prevention Program (DPP) was the first large prospective trial (started 1966) to assess whether metformin could reduce the progression of IGT (2 h post–75 g oral glucose tolerance test (OGTT) 7.8–11.0 mmol/L) with or without IFG (5.6–7.7 mmol/L) into type 2 diabetes [82]. The trial randomised 3,234 subjects to intensive lifestyle management or standard lifestyle advice with metformin (2 × 850 mg/day) or placebo: the metformin or placebo was given in a double-blinded manner. Most subjects were obese (mean weight 94 kg and body mass index (BMI) 34 kg/m^2) and hyperinsulinaemic (mean fasting insulin 185 pmol/L), 30 % were hypertensive (≥140/90 mmHg or receiving antihypertensive medication), 29 % were hypertriglyceridaemic (>2.3 mmol/L) and 44 % had raised LDL cholesterol values (≥3.4 mmol/L) or were on lipid-lowering medications [83]. Participants had to be healthy enough to cope with the intensive exercise and without a cardiovascular event for >6 months.

Over a mean study period of 2.8 years, with some patients followed for 5 years, the incidence of new diabetes was reduced by metformin (by 31 % vs. placebo), but not as much as intensive lifestyle (by 58 %) (Table 8.4 and Fig. 8.4). The incidence per 100 person years was 7.8, 11.0 and 4.8 for the metformin, placebo and intensive lifestyle, respectively [82]. Metformin was more effective in younger, more obese subjects and in those with higher fasting plasma glucose values near to the diagnostic threshold for diabetes [83]. Metformin was also associated with a reduction in insulin and proinsulin concentrations, and there was greater weight loss with metformin (−2.1 kg) than placebo (−0.1 kg), but not as much as intensive lifestyle (−5.6 kg), which came close to achieving the target objective of the study to achieve a weight loss of 7 %.

Metformin did not exert any clinically notable effects on the prevalence of dyslipidaemia (by the National Cholesterol Education Program Adult Treatment Panel (NCEP ATP) III criteria), which increased during the trial from 12 % at randomisation to 21 % with metformin, 19 % with placebo and 16 % with intensive lifestyle. A rise in the prevalence of hypertension during the trial (30 % at

Table 8.4 Key prospective randomised trials investigating the effect of metformin on the incidence of new diabetes in subjects with impaired glucose tolerance (IGT)

Trial	Number of subjects	Mean duration (years)	Treatment arms	Change in body weight (kg or BMI)	Change in risk of diabetes versus placebo or control
Diabetes Prevention Program (DPP)	3,324	2.8	Standard lifestyle + placebo	−0–1 kg	–
			Standard lifestyle + metformin	−2.1 kg	−31 %
			Intensive lifestyle	−5.6 kg	−58 %
Indian Diabetes Prevention Program (IDPP)	531	2.5	Standard lifestyle (control)	+0.8 kg	–
			Standard lifestyle + metformin	+0.4 kg	−26.4 %
			Intensive lifestyle	+0.5 kg	−28.5 %
			Intensive lifestyle + metformin	+0.5 kg	−28.2 %
Chinese diabetes prevention study	321	3	Standard lifestyle	+0.2 BMI	–
			Standard lifestyle + metformin	−0.3 BMI	−77 %
			Standard lifestyle + acarbose	−0.7 BMI	−88 %
			Intensive lifestyle	−0.4 BMI	−43 %

BMI Body mass index (kg/m^2)

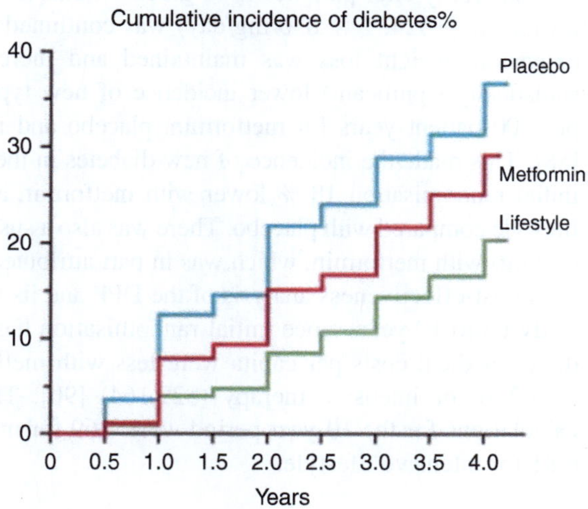

Fig. 8.4 Cumulative incidence of new diabetes during the Diabetes Prevention Program. The diagnosis of diabetes was based on the criteria of the American Diabetes Association. The incidence of diabetes differed significantly among the three groups ($P < 0.001$ for each comparison). Re-drawn from [82]

randomisation) was not affected by metformin (40 %) compared with placebo (39 %), whereas intensive lifestyle (29 %) prevented this rise. The incidence of cardiovascular events was numerically too small to derive any statistical variation although metformin was associated with least cardiovascular deaths (1, 4, 2 with metformin, placebo and intensive, respectively) and fewer non-fatal cardiovascular events (5.2, 7.3 and 9.7 per 1,000 person years with metformin, placebo and intensive, respectively) [84]. Analysis of data at 1 year noted a small reduction of

CRP with metformin (−7 % in men and −14 % in women) compared with placebo, but this was much less than the 30 % reduction seen with intensive lifestyle [85].

At randomisation, 53 % ($n = 1{,}711$) of subjects in the DPP trial were characterised as having metabolic syndrome according to the NCEP ATP III criteria (three or more of waist circumference >102 cm for men and >84 cm for women, blood pressure >130/85 mmHg, triglyceride >1.7 mmol/L, HDL cholesterol <1.03 mmol/L for men and <1.3 mmol/L for women and fasting plasma glucose >6.2 mmol/L) [86]. By 3 years the metformin group showed a smaller proportion with metabolic syndrome (45 %) than placebo (51 %), although a smaller proportion was seen with intensive lifestyle (34 %). Over the 3 years, metabolic syndrome resolved (or at least subjects no longer triggered three or more of the above criteria) in 23 % with metformin compared with 18 % on placebo and 38 % on intensive lifestyle. Amongst those without metabolic syndrome at randomisation, metformin also reduced the onset of metabolic syndrome, but not as effectively as intensive lifestyle. Thus after 3 years, the new occurrence of metabolic syndrome was 50, 61 and 38 per 100 person years for the metformin, placebo and intensive groups, respectively. The reduced onset of metabolic syndrome with metformin was more evident amongst men than women.

When the DPP trial concluded, withdrawal from metformin for 1–2 weeks did not materially alter parameters of glucose homeostasis [87]. However, when metformin ($n = 924$, 2×850 mg/day) was continued for 5.7 years as an open-label extension, weight loss was maintained and there was a numerically (but not statistically significant) lower incidence of new type 2 diabetes (4.9, 5.6 and 5.9 per 100 patient years for metformin, placebo and intensive therapy, respectively) [88]. This made the incidence of new diabetes in the 10 years of the DPP since the initial randomisation 18 % lower with metformin and 34 % lower with intensive lifestyle compared with placebo. There was also a sustained reduction in body weight (−2 kg) with metformin, which was in part attributed to good adherence [89].

A cost-effectiveness analysis of the DPP and its follow-up open-label outcomes study up to 10 years since initial randomisation has indicated that the cumulative direct medical costs per capita were less with metformin ($27,915) than placebo ($28,236) or intensive therapy ($29,164) [90]. The quality adjusted life years calculations for the 10-year period were 6.69 for metformin, 6.67 for placebo and 6.81 for intensive lifestyle.

8.6.2 Other Diabetes Prevention Programmes

Several studies in addition to the DPP have reported the effectiveness of metformin in reducing weight gain and preventing progression of IGT/IFG to diabetes. The Indian Diabetes Prevention Program (IDPP) was a smaller prospective study of 30 months mean duration comparing intensive lifestyle or standard lifestyle advice, each with and without metformin (1,000 mg/day) in subjects with IGT [91]. Many of these subjects would have had metabolic syndrome, but they were not separated in the analysis. The 3-year cumulative incidences of diabetes were 55.0 %, 39.3 %,

40.5 % and 39.5 % in standard lifestyle (control), intensive lifestyle modification, standard plus metformin and intensive plus metformin, respectively. Thus, the study confirmed the benefit of metformin to reduce progression of IGT to new diabetes with standard lifestyle, but there was no extra benefit conferred by adding metformin to intensive lifestyle (Table 8.4).

A 3-year prospective study in China found that metformin (3 × 250 mg/day) or acarbose (3 × 50 mg/day) added to standard lifestyle each substantially reduced the risk of diabetes in IGT subjects (−77 % and −88 % for metformin and acarbose, respectively) compared with intensive lifestyle (−43 %) [92]. A prospective mechanistic study of 40 Finnish subjects with IGT noted that metformin (2 × 500 mg/day) for 6 months produced a 20 % improvement of insulin-stimulated glucose metabolism during a euglycaemic hyperinsulinaemic clamp compared with placebo [93].

8.7 Obesity and PCOS

Studies assessing the effectiveness of metformin on weight loss in non-diabetic obese subjects and on reproductive parameters in non-diabetic PCOS are likely to have included subjects who fit the criteria of metabolic syndrome. While these studies do not allow extraction of data specific to metabolic syndrome they consistently confirm the capacity for metformin to reduce body weight or prevent weight gain in non-diabetic insulin-resistant states [20, 94]. A meta-analysis of 31 such studies (>8 weeks duration, average 1.8 years) noted that metformin reduced BMI by 5.3 %, FPG by 4.5 %, fasting insulin by 14.4 %, HOMA-IR (measure of insulin resistance) by 22.6 %, blood triglyceride by 5.3 % and LDL cholesterol by 5.6 %, with an increase in HDL cholesterol by 5.0 % compared with placebo or no treatment. This was associated with a relative reduction in the incidence of new diabetes by 40 % (absolute reduction of 6 %) [94].

8.8 Conclusion

The constellation of cardiovascular risk factors that comprises metabolic syndrome is modifiable, at least in part by lifestyle interventions. The anti-hyperglycaemic agent metformin can improve many of the individual components of metabolic syndrome, notably a reduction in progression of IGT/IFG to type 2 diabetes, weight reduction and often an improvement in the blood lipid profile and lower fasting insulin. There is also evidence that metformin can reduce the progression of metabolic syndrome as a collective of these cardiovascular risk factors and reduce sufficient of them that these subjects may no longer qualify as having metabolic syndrome. Metformin can also delay and possibly prevent the emergence of metabolic syndrome in normoglycaemic subjects at increased risk of diabetes.

References

1. Bailey CJ, Day C (2004) Metformin: its botanical background. Practical Diabetes Int 21: 115–117
2. Watanabe CK (1918) Studies in the metabolic changes induced by administration of guanidine bases. Influence of injected guanidine hydrochloride upon blood sugar content. J Biol Chem 33:253–265
3. Bailey CJ (1992) Biguanides and NIDDM. Diabetes Care 15:755–772
4. Slotta KH, Tschesche R (1929) Uber Biguanide. Die blutzuckersenkende Wirkung der Biguanides. Berichte Deutschen Chemischen Gesellschaft 62:1398–1405
5. Sterne SJ (1957) Du nouveau dans les antidiabetiques. La NN dimetylamine guanyl guanidine (N.N.D.G.). Maroc Med 36:1295–1296
6. UK Prospective Diabetes Study (UKPDS) Group (1998) Effect of intensive blood glucose control with metformin on complications in overweight patients with type 2 diabetes (UKPDS 34). Lancet 352:854–865
7. Bailey CJ et al (eds) (2007) Metformin, the gold standard. A scientific handbook. Wiley, Chichester, p 288
8. Alberti KG et al (2009) Harmonizing the metabolic syndrome. A joint interim statement of the International Diabetes Federation Task Force on Epidemiology and Prevention; National Heart, Lung, and Blood Institute; American Heart Association; World Heart Federation; International Atherosclerosis Society; and International Association for the Study of Obesity. Circulation 120:1640–1645
9. Inzucchi SE et al (2012) Management of hyperglycaemia in type 2 diabetes: a patient-centred approach. Position statement of the American Diabetes Association (ADA) and the European Association for the Study of Diabetes (EASD). Diabetes Care 35(6):1364–1379
10. IDF Clinical Guidelines Task Force (2005) Global guideline for type 2 diabetes. International Diabetes Federation, Brussels
11. Bailey CJ, Turner RC (1996) Drug therapy: metformin. N Engl J Med 334:574–579
12. DeFronzo RA, Goodman AM, Multicenter Metformin Study Group (1995) Efficacy of metformin in patients with non-insulin-dependent diabetes mellitus. N Engl J Med 333:541–549
13. Krentz AJ, Bailey CJ (2005) Oral antidiabetic agents: current role in type 2 diabetes mellitus. Drugs 65:384–411
14. Hirst JA et al (2012) Quantifying the effect of metformin treatment and dose on glycemic control. Diabetes Care 35:446–454
15. Fruehwald-Schultes B et al (2001) Metformin does not adversely affect hormonal and symptomatic responses to recurrent hypoglycemia. J Clin Endocrinol Metab 86:4187–4192
16. DeFronzo RA et al (1991) Mechanism of metformin action in obese and lean noninsulin dependent diabetic subjects. J Clin Endol Metab 73:1294–1301
17. Stumvoll M et al (1995) Metabolic effects of metformin in non-insulin dependent diabetes mellitus. N Engl J Med 333:550–554
18. Hundal RS et al (2000) Mechanism by which metformin reduces glucose production in type 2 diabetes. Diabetes 49:2063–2069
19. Mannucci E et al (2004) Effects of metformin on glucagon-like peptide-1 levels in obese patients with and without Type 2 diabetes. Diabetes Nutr Metab 17:336–342
20. Golay A (2008) Metformin and body weight. Int J Obes 32:61–72
21. Wiernsperger NF, Bailey CJ (1999) The antihyperglycaemic effect of metformin: therapeutic and cellular mechanisms. Drugs 58(Suppl 1):31–39
22. Cusi K, DeFronzo RA (1998) Metformin: a review of its metabolic effects. Diabetes Rev 6: 89–130
23. Bailey CJ (2008) Metformin: effects on micro and macrovascular complications of type 2 diabetes. Cardiovasc Drugs Ther 22:215–224

24. Evans JM et al (2006) Risk of mortality and adverse cardiovascular outcomes in type 2 diabetes: a comparison of patients treated with sulphonylureas and metformin. Diabetologia 49: 930–936
25. Nichols GA et al (2005) The incidence of congestive heart failure associated with antidiabetic therapies. Diabetes Metab Res Rev 21:51–57
26. McAfee AT et al (2007) Coronary heart disease outcomes in patients receiving antidiabetic agents. Pharmacoepidemiol Drug Saf 16:711–725
27. Johnson JA et al (2005) Reduced cardiovascular morbidity and mortality associated with metformin use in subjects with type 2 diabetes. Diabetic Med 22:497–502
28. Eurich DT et al (2005) Improved clinical outcomes associated with metformin in patients with diabetes and heart failure. Diabetes Care 28:2345–2351
29. Masudi FA et al (2005) Thiazolidinediones, metformin, and outcomes in older patients with diabetes and heart failure: an observational study. Circulation 111:583–590
30. Eurich DT et al (2007) Benefits and harms of antidiabetic agents in patients with diabetes and heart failure: systematic review. Br Med J 335(7618):497. doi:10.1136/bmj.39314.620174.80
31. Kao J et al (2004) Relation of metformin treatment to clinical events in diabetic patients undergoing percutaneous intervention. Am J Cardiol 93:1347–1350
32. Katakami N et al (2004) Metformin and gliclazide rather than glibenclamide attenuate progression of carotid intima-media thickness in subjects with type 2 diabetes. Diabetologia 47:1906–1913
33. Matsumoto K et al (2004) Metformin attenuates progression of carotid arterial wall thickness in patients with type 2 diabetes. Diabetes Res Clin Pract 64:2205–2208
34. Vague PH et al (1987) Metformin decreases the high plasminogen activation inhibitor activity, plasma insulin and triglyceride levels in non-diabetic obese subjects. Thromb Haemost 57: 326–328
35. Grant PJ et al (1991) Metformin causes a reduction in basal and post-venous occlusion plasminogen activator inhibitor-1 in type 2 diabetic patients. Diabet Med 8:361–365
36. Nagi DK, Yudkin JS (1993) Effects of metformin on insulin resistance, risk factors for cardiovascular disease, and plasminogen activator inhibitor in NIDDM subjects. Diabetes Care 16: 621–629
37. Grant PJ (1996) The effect of high- and medium-dose metformin therapy on cardiovascular risk factors in patients with type II diabetes. Diabetes Care 19:64–66
38. He G et al (2003) Metformin, but not thiazolidinediones, inhibits plasminogen activator inhibitor-1 production in human adipose tissue. Horm Metab Res 35:18–23
39. Grant PJ (1998) Metformin reduces circulating factor VII concentrations in patients with type 2 diabetes mellitus. Thromb Haemost 80:209
40. Standeven KF et al (2002) The effect of dimethyl biguanide on thrombin activity FXIII activation, fibrin polymerization and fibrin clot formation. Diabetes 51:189–197
41. Grant PJ (2003) Beneficial effects of metformin on haemostasis and vascular function in man. Diabetes Metab 29(Suppl 6):6S44–6S52
42. Sirtori CR et al (1984) Metformin improves peripheral vascular in nonhyperlipidemic patients with arterial disease. J Cardiovasc Pharmacol 6:914–923
43. Mather KJ et al (2001) Improved endothelial function with metformin in type 2 diabetes mellitus. J Am Coll Cardiol 37:1344–1350
44. De Aguiar LG et al (2006) Metformin improves endothelial vascular reactivity in first degree relatives of type 2 diabetic patients with metabolic syndrome and normal glucose tolerance. Diabetes Care 29:1083–1089
45. Vitale C et al (2005) Metformin improves endothelial function in patients with metabolic syndrome. J Intern Med 258:250–256
46. Marfella R et al (1996) Metformin improves hemodynamic and rheological responses to L-arginine in NIDDM patients. Diabetes Care 19:934–939
47. Asagami T et al (2002) Metformin treatment lowers asymmetric dimethylarginine concentrations in patients with type 2 diabetes. Metabolism 51:843–846

48. Natale A et al (2004) Vascular effects of improving metabolic control with metformin or rosiglitazone in type 2 diabetes. Diabetes Care 27:1349–1357
49. Kautzky-Willer A et al (2006) Insulin sensitivity during oral glucose tolerance test and its relation to parameters of glucose metabolism and endothelial function in type 2 diabetes subjects under metformin of thiazolidinedione. Diabetes Obes Metab 8:561–567
50. Mamputu JC et al (2003) Metformin inhibits monocyte adhesion to endothelial cells and foam cell formation. Br J Diabetes Vasc Dis 3:302–310
51. Caballero AE, Degado A, Aguillar-Salinas CA et al (2004) The differential effects of metformin on markers of endothelial activation and inflammation in subjects with impaired glucose tolerance: a placebo-controlled, randomized clinical trial. J Clin Endocrinol Metab 89: 3943–3948
52. Carter AM et al (2005) Metformin reduces C-reactive protein but not complement factor C3 in overweight patients with type 2 diabetes mellitus. Diabete Med 22:1282–1284
53. Akbar DH (2005) Effect of metformin and sulfonylurea on C-reactive protein level in well-controlled type 2 diabetics with metabolic syndrome. Endocrine 20:215–218
54. Morin-Papunen L et al (2003) Metformin reduces serum C-reactive protein levels in women with polycystic ovary syndrome. J Clin Endocrinol Metab 88:4649–4654
55. Tan BK et al (2011) The anti-atherogenic aspect of metformin treatment in insulin resistant women with polycystic ovary syndrome: role of the newly established pro-inflammatory adipokine acute-phase serum amyloid A; evidence of an adipose tissue-monocyte axis. Atherosclerosis 216:402–408
56. Chakraborty A et al (2011) Effect of metformin on oxidative stress, nitrosative stress and inflammatory biomarkers intype 2 diabetes patients. Diabetes Res Clin Pract 93:56–62
57. Wiernsperger NF (2007) 50 years later: is metformin a vascular drug with antidiabetic properties? Br J Diabetes Vasc Dis 7:204–210
58. Beisswenger P et al (1999) Metformin reduces systemic methylglyoxal levels in type 2 diabetes. Diabetes 48:198–202
59. Ouslimani N et al (2005) Metformin decreases intracellular production of reactive oxygen species in aortic endothelial cells. Metabolism 54:829–834
60. Mahrouf M et al (2006) Metformin reduces angiotensin-mediated intracellular production of reactive oxygen species in endothelial cells through the inhibition of protein kinase C. Biochem Pharmacol 72:176–183
61. Onaran I et al (2006) Metformin does not prevent DNA damage in lymphocytes despite its antioxidant properties against cumene hydroperoxide-induced oxidative stress. Mutat Res 611: 1–8
62. Lipska KJ et al (2011) Use of metformin in the setting of mild-to-moderate renal insufficiency. Diabetes Care 34:1431–1437
63. Tang T, et al (2009) Insulin sensitising drugs (metformin, rosiglitazone, pioglitazone, D-chiro-inositol) for women with polycystic ovary syndrome, oligo amenorrhoea and subfertility. Cochrane Database Syst Rev (4):CD003053
64. Rowan JA et al (2008) Metformin versus Insulin for the treatment of gestational diabetes. N Engl J Med 358(19):2003–15
65. Rakoski MO et al (2010) Meta-analysis: insulin sensitizers for the treatment of non-alcoholic steatohepatitis. Aliment Pharmacol Therapeut 32:1211–1221
66. Vigneri P et al (2009) Diabetes and cancer. Endocr Relat Cancer 16:1103–1123
67. Wilcock C, Bailey CJ (1994) Accumulation of metformin by tissues of the normal and diabetic mouse. Xenobiotica 24:49–57
68. Wang DS et al (2002) Involvement of organic cation transporter 1 in hepatic and intestinal distribution of metformin. J Pharmacol Exp Ther 302:510–515
69. El-Mir MY et al (2000) Dimethylbiguanide inhibits cell respiration via an indirect effect targeted on the respiratory chain complex i. J Biol Chem 275:223–228
70. Detaille D et al (1999) Cellular and molecular mechanisms involved in insulin's potentiation of glycogen synthase activity by metformin. Biochem Pharmacol 58:1475–1486

71. Zhou G et al (2001) Role of AMP-activated protein kinase in mechanism of metformin action. J Clin Invest 108:1167–1174
72. Shaw RJ et al (2005) The kinase LKB1 mediates glucose homeostasis in liver and therapeutic effects of metformin. Science 310:1642–1646
73. Stephenne X et al (2011) Metformin activate AMP-activated protein kinase in primary human hepatocytes by decreasing cellular energy status. Diabetologia 54:3101–3110
74. Liu Y et al (2008) A fast inducible switch modulates gluconeogenesis via activator/coactivator exchange. Nature 456:269–273
75. Hardie DG (2008) AMPK: a key regulator of energy balance in the single cell and the whole organism. Int J Obes 32:S7–S12
76. Zhang BB et al (2009) AMPK: an emerging drug target for diabetes and the metabolic syndrome. Cell Metab 9:407–416
77. Dowling RJO et al (2011) Understanding the benefit of metformin use in cancer treatment. BMC Med 9:33
78. Gillies CL et al (2007) Pharmacological and lifestyle interventions to prevent or delay type 2 diabetes in people with impaired glucose tolerance: systematic review and meta-analysis. Br Med J 334:299
79. Hussain A et al (2007) Prevention of type 2 diabetes: a review. Diabetes Res Clin Pract 76: 317–326
80. Fontbonne A et al (1996) The effect of metformin on the metabolic abnormalities associated with upper-body fat distribution. Diabetes Care 19:920–926
81. Charles MA et al (2000) Treatment with metformin of non-diabetic men with hypertension, hypertriglyceridaemia and central fat distribution: the BIGPRO 1.2 trial. Diabetes Metab Res Rev 16:2–7
82. Diabetes Prevention Program Research Group (2002) Reduction in the incidence of type 2 diabetes with lifestyle intervention or metformin. N Engl J Med 346:393–403
83. Lachim JM et al (2007) Factors associated with diabetes onset during metformin versus placebo therapy in the Diabetes Prevention Program. Diabetes 56:1153–1159
84. Diabetes Prevention Program Research Group (2005) Impact of intensive lifestyle and metformin therapy on cardiovascular disease risk factors in the Diabetes Prevention Program. Diabetes Care 28:888–894
85. Diabetes Prevention Program Research Group (2005) Intensive lifestyle intervention or metformin on inflammation and coagulation in participants with impaired glucose tolerance. Diabetes 54:1566–1572
86. Orchard TJ et al (2005) The effect of metformin and intensive lifestyle intervention on the metabolic syndrome: the Diabetes Prevention Program randomized trial. Ann Intern Med 142: 611–619
87. Diabetes Prevention Program Research Group (2003) Effects of withdrawal from metformin on the development of diabetes in the Diabetes Prevention Program. Diabetes Care 26: 977–980
88. Diabetes Prevention Program Research Group (2009) 10-year follow-up of diabetes incidence and weight loss in the Diabetes Prevention Program outcomes study. Lancet 374:1677–1686
89. The Diabetes Prevention Program Research Group (2012) Long-term safety, tolerability, and weight loss associated with metformin in the Diabetes Prevention Program Outcomes Study. Diabetes Care 35:731–737
90. The Diabetes Prevention Program Research Group (2012) The 10-year cost-effectiveness of lifestyle intervention or metformin for diabetes prevention. An intent to treat analysis of the DPP/DPPOS. Diabetes Care 35:663–5
91. Ramachandran A et al (2006) The Indian Diabetes Prevention Programme shows that lifestyle modification and metformin prevent type 2 diabetes in Asian Indian subjects with impaired glucose tolerance (IDPP-1). Diabetologia 49:289–297

92. Wenying J et al (2001) The preventive effect of acarbose and metformin on the IGT population from becoming diabetes mellitus: a 3-year multicentral prospective study. Chin J Endocrinol Metab 17:131–134
93. Lehtovirta M et al (2001) Metabolic effects of metformin in patients with impaired glucose tolerance. Diabetic Med 18:578–583
94. Salpeter SR et al (2008) Meta-analysis: metformin treatment in persons at risk for diabetes mellitus. Am J Med 121:149–157

9 Treatment with Thiazolidinediones

Seda Suvag, Kristina M. Utzschneider, and Steven E. Kahn

9.1 Introduction

Thiazolidinediones are peroxisome proliferator-activated receptor (PPAR)-gamma agonists that have been commonly used in the treatment of type 2 diabetes. They have also been considered for use in individuals with metabolic syndrome as they target a number of components of the syndrome through their multiple actions that include improvements in insulin sensitivity and glycaemic control, adipocyte maturation, and lipid metabolism. However, the thiazolidinediones have also been associated with a number of adverse outcomes, including effects on the cardiovascular system and bone, which have limited their use in clinical practice.

Given that at the time of writing, the keyword "thiazolidinedione" yielded 9,667 PubMed articles and combining it with "metabolic syndrome" resulted in 628 citations, it is clear that this class of medications has been extensively studied. This expansive literature also means that neither every aspect can be covered nor can all relevant studies be mentioned. Therefore, we have purposefully narrowed the scope of our discussions and have been selective in citing relevant studies. This chapter will review the mechanisms of actions of thiazolidinediones, highlight their effects on various aspects of the metabolic syndrome, and discuss the adverse clinical outcomes associated with their use.

S. Suvag • K.M. Utzschneider • S.E. Kahn (✉)
Division of Metabolism, Endocrinology and Nutrition, Department of Medicine, VA Puget Sound Health Care System and University of Washington, 1660 South Columbian Way (151), Seattle, WA 98108, USA
e-mail: skahn@u.washington.edu

H. Beck-Nielsen (ed.), *The Metabolic Syndrome*,
DOI 10.1007/978-3-7091-1331-8_9, © Springer-Verlag Wien 2013

9.2 History of the Thiazolidinediones

Troglitazone, the first thiazolidinedione used for the treatment of type 2 diabetes, was approved in 1997 but was withdrawn from the market in 2000 due to hepatotoxicity [1]. The two thiazolidinediones currently being employed clinically are pioglitazone and rosiglitazone, which were introduced in the late 1990s. However, in 2010 access to rosiglitazone was suspended by the European Medicines Agency (EMA) and restricted by the United States Food and Drug Administration (FDA) because of reports that it was associated with a higher risk of cardiovascular events [2]. As a result, rosiglitazone use has dropped dramatically. Recently, there have been concerns about the possible association of pioglitazone with bladder cancer. As a result, the use of pioglitazone has been suspended in certain European countries [3]. The FDA recommends against use of pioglitazone in patients with active bladder cancer and to use it with caution in patients with a history of bladder cancer.

Troglitazone and rosiglitazone are selective peroxisome proliferator-activated receptor (PPAR)-gamma agonists, whereas pioglitazone is more of a dual agonist as it binds and activates both PPAR-gamma and PPAR-alpha [4]. The glitazars, which are currently in development, also act as dual PPAR-gamma and PPAR-alpha agonists [5]. One of these agents, muraglitazar, was associated with adverse cardiovascular outcomes, including myocardial infarction, and therefore its development was suspended in 2006 [6, 7]. Another dual PPAR-gamma and PPAR-alpha agonist, aleglitazar, is now in phase III clinical trials [7]. Full or partial PPAR-alpha agonists such as the fibrates (fenofibrate, bezafibrate, ciprofibrate, and gemfibrozil) are commonly used in the treatment of dyslipidaemia as they reduce triglyceride levels and increase high-density lipoprotein (HDL) cholesterol levels [8].

9.3 PPARs and the Mechanism of Action of Thiazolidinediones

PPARs are nuclear hormone receptors and transcription factors [9], of which three subtypes have been identified: alpha [10], gamma [11], and delta (also known as beta) [12]. The two that have been harnessed clinically are gamma and alpha. PPAR-gamma is most abundantly expressed in adipose tissue [13], but is also present in pancreatic beta-cells [14], vascular endothelium [15], macrophages [16], and the central nervous system [17], whereas PPAR-alpha is found mostly in the liver, heart, vascular wall, and skeletal muscle [18, 19]. PPAR-gamma agonists have multiple effects, including promotion of adipocyte differentiation and improvement in insulin sensitivity. The major role of PPAR-alpha agonists is the regulation of genes that are involved with lipoprotein metabolism and free fatty acid oxidation [20]. PPAR-delta is also expressed in multiple tissues, including the skin [21], adipose tissue [20], and brain [22], and regulates genes that are involved with oxidation of fatty acids and storage of lipids [23].

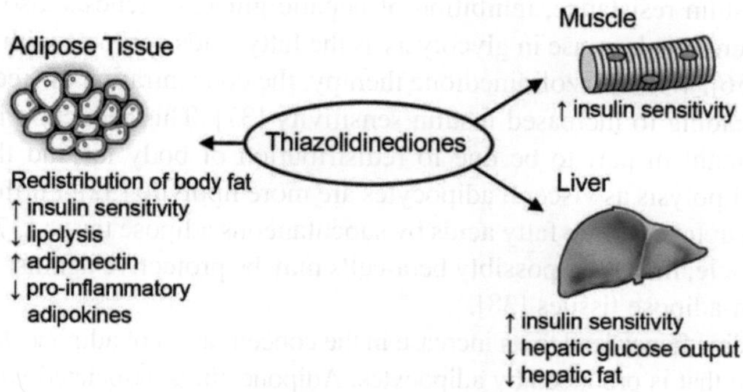

Fig. 9.1 Metabolic effects of thiazolidinediones. The effects of thiazolidinediones on adipose tissue include adipogenesis, differentiation and proliferation of adipocytes, and redistribution of visceral to subcutaneous adipose tissue, which leads to improvements in insulin sensitivity and reduction in lipolysis. With thiazolidinedione therapy there is an increase in adipocyte production of adiponectin and decrease in various pro-inflammatory adipokines, which also contribute to the improvement in insulin sensitivity. Thiazolidinediones also improve glucose metabolism by decreasing hepatic glucose output and hepatic fat accumulation as well as improving skeletal muscle insulin sensitivity

Thiazolidinediones bind and modulate the activity of one or more PPARs. As they activate the PPARs, they heterodimerise with the retinoid-X receptor and bind specific deoxyribonucleic acid (DNA) elements, which are known as peroxisome proliferator response elements (PPREs) [24]. This leads to the regulation of expression of over one hundred genes that are mainly involved in glucose and lipid metabolism and to the induction of a transcription cascade that results in the differentiation and proliferation of adipocytes, adipogenesis, uptake and storage of fatty acids into fat tissue, and enhancement in insulin action via increased insulin sensitivity [25, 26].

They also redistribute adipose tissue resulting in an increase in subcutaneous fat and a decrease in visceral adipose tissue (Fig. 9.1); however, the exact mechanism for this body fat redistribution is not entirely clear [27]. In addition, they may selectively promote pre-adipocyte differentiation in the subcutaneous fat, but not in the visceral fat via differential gene regulation [28]. Increased visceral adipose tissue has been associated with insulin resistance [29], and therefore the reduction of visceral adipose tissue may explain in part the increase in insulin sensitivity seen with thiazolidinedione treatment [30, 31].

In obesity, lipolysis of adipose tissue results in excessive circulating free fatty acids, which are deposited in the liver and skeletal muscle. Excess visceral adipose tissue may be particularly deleterious due to increased lipolytic activity within this fat depot compared with subcutaneous adipose tissue [32]. Excessive amounts of free fatty acids have been implicated in the development of insulin resistance via accumulation of toxic intermediates such as diacylglycerol (DAG) and ceramide, which activate serine and threonine kinases [33]. This in turn leads to serine instead of tyrosine phosphorylation of the insulin receptor and insulin receptor substrate proteins, which results in the attenuation of insulin signalling [34]. With the resultant insulin resistance, inhibition of hepatic gluconeogenesis also diminishes [35], and there is a decrease in glycolysis as the fatty acids compete with glucose for oxidation [36]. With thiazolidinedione therapy, the concentration of free fatty acids decreases leading to increased insulin sensitivity [37]. This reduction in free fatty acids is thought in part to be due to redistribution of body fat and the resultant decrease in lipolysis as visceral adipocytes are more lipolytic [32]. Furthermore, the preferential uptake of free fatty acids by subcutaneous adipose tissue [37] instead of skeletal muscle, liver, and possibly beta-cells may be protective against lipotoxicity in these non-adipose tissues [38].

Thiazolidinediones lead to an increase in the concentration of adiponectin (Fig. 9.1), an adipokine that is produced by adipocytes. Adiponectin is associated with increased insulin sensitivity [39] and appears to be protective against atherosclerosis [40]. Levels of adiponectin are decreased in patients with obesity, insulin resistance, metabolic syndrome, type 2 diabetes, and coronary artery disease [41, 42]. Adiponectin has also been shown to downregulate the production of other adipokines that have been associated with insulin resistance, including tumour necrosis factor (TNF)-alpha, interleukin (IL)-6, and resistin [43].

Thus, thiazolidinediones have a number of effects that lead to improvements in insulin sensitivity and contribute to improved glucose and fatty acid metabolism.

9.4 Effects of Thiazolidinediones on Altered Glucose Metabolism and Insulin Resistance

Insulin resistance is strongly associated with obesity and components of the metabolic syndrome [44] and is a cardinal feature of impaired glucose tolerance and type 2 diabetes [45]. Thus, thiazolidinediones have been used in the treatment of type 2 diabetes and have also been demonstrated to prevent the progression from impaired glucose tolerance to type 2 diabetes [46–48]. Through their ability to decrease hepatic glucose output [47] and improve glucose utilisation in insulin-sensitive tissues, thiazolidinediones reduce both fasting and postprandial glucose concentrations [49]. As they do not directly stimulate insulin release from the beta-cell, when used alone they do not increase the risk of hypoglycaemia.

9.4.1 Thiazolidinediones for the Prevention of Type 2 Diabetes

Elevated fasting glucose is one manifestation of the metabolic syndrome and reflects impaired glucose metabolism. It is a risk factor for the future development of type 2 diabetes and cardiovascular disease [50]. Thus, a number of clinical studies have investigated the effects of thiazolidinediones in patients with impaired glucose metabolism as a means to reduce the risk of developing type 2 diabetes.

One of the largest randomised clinical trials addressing this concept was the Diabetes REduction Assessment with ramipril and rosiglitazone Medication (DREAM) Study [46]. In this study, 5,269 adults with impaired fasting glucose and/or impaired glucose tolerance received either rosiglitazone or placebo for a median of 3 years. Type 2 diabetes was diagnosed in 25 % of those in the placebo group and only in 10.6 % of those in the rosiglitazone group. Thus, treatment with rosiglitazone reduced the risk of conversion to diabetes by 62 %. Furthermore, in subjects receiving rosiglitazone, normal fasting glucose (defined as <6.1 mmol/l; <110 mg/dl) was achieved in 50.5 % of participants compared with only 30.3 % on placebo. In a follow-up study, a subset of participants underwent an oral glucose tolerance test 1–2 years after the active treatment phase of DREAM ended. The incidence of type 2 diabetes and regression to normoglycaemia were found to be similar in both rosiglitazone and placebo groups, indicating that ongoing treatment with rosiglitazone was necessary in order to have a persistent effect in preventing type 2 diabetes [51].

Prior to examination of the effect of rosiglitazone in DREAM, two studies examined the effect of troglitazone to reduce the progression to type 2 diabetes in high-risk individuals. TRoglitazone In the Prevention of Diabetes (TRIPOD) involved a relatively small cohort of 266 individuals with a history of gestational diabetes, half of whom received troglitazone [52]. In this study, following a median of 30 months of treatment, the annual incidence rate of diabetes was 12.1 % in those women receiving placebo and 5.4 % in those assigned to troglitazone. The second study was the Diabetes Prevention Program (DPP), which studied individuals with impaired glucose tolerance [47]. In the DPP, the troglitazone arm was discontinued due to hepatotoxicity, at which time participants had been treated for a mean of only 0.9 years. During this period, the diabetes incidence rate in those treated with troglitazone was 3.0 cases/100 person years compared with 12.0, 6.7, and 5.1 cases/100 person years in the placebo, metformin, and intensive lifestyle intervention groups in the study, respectively. These findings represented a 75 % reduction in the diabetes incidence rate in troglitazone-treated participants compared with placebo. Following withdrawal of the intervention, subjects were followed for a number of years. This follow-up provided some additional interesting observations. Following withdrawal of the active intervention, the incidence rate of new cases of diabetes was not different to that in the placebo group. Thus, during this period of additional follow-up, the overall number of new cases of diabetes in those who had received troglitazone remained lower than in those who had no active intervention, suggesting that troglitazone delayed the onset of diabetes during the period of active treatment and that this difference was maintained following its withdrawal.

Most recently, ACTos NOW for Prevention of Diabetes (ACT NOW) investigated whether pioglitazone can prevent the progression to diabetes in participants with impaired glucose tolerance [48]. Six hundred and two patients were randomly assigned to take pioglitazone or placebo and were followed for a median of 2.4 years. Annual incidence rates for type 2 diabetes were 2.1 % in the pioglitazone group versus 7.6 % in the placebo group, representing a 72 % reduction in the risk of developing type 2 diabetes. The intervention reduced both fasting and 2-h glucose levels so that at the end of the study, 48 % of those receiving pioglitazone had achieved a state of normal glucose tolerance compared with 28 % in those assigned to placebo. These findings were in keeping with the other studies, suggesting that thiazolidinediones are effective in reducing progression to type 2 diabetes in individuals at increased risk.

Lastly, the combination of low-dose rosiglitazone and metformin was compared with placebo in the CAnadian Normoglycemia Outcomes Evaluation (CANOE) study that recruited 207 participants with impaired glucose tolerance [53]. Over a median treatment period of 3.9 years, diabetes was diagnosed in only 14 % of those in the combination therapy group as opposed to 39 % in the placebo group. Regression to normal glucose tolerance was again more common in the group receiving thiazolidinedione, occurring in 80 % of participants compared with 53 % in the placebo group.

In summary, there is good evidence from these large, randomised, placebo-controlled clinical trials that the thiazolidinedione class of medications delays progression to type 2 diabetes in individuals who are at high risk by virtue of the fact that they have impaired glucose tolerance or a history of gestational diabetes. These findings when compared with those with other interventions such as lifestyle changes, which emphasised diet and exercise (reduced type 2 diabetes by 29–58 % [54–57]) or pharmacological (reduced type 2 diabetes by 26–31 % with metformin [55, 56], by 25 % with acarbose [58], and by 28 % with glargine [59]), suggest that thiazolidinediones are the most effective in slowing progression to diabetes.

9.4.2 Thiazolidinediones in the Treatment of Type 2 Diabetes

The metabolic syndrome is a well-recognised risk factor for the development of type 2 diabetes [60]. As thiazolidinediones target insulin resistance, which plays a central role in the pathogenesis of type 2 diabetes, they have been used commonly for the treatment of this disorder [61]. They have been approved for use as monotherapy as well as in combination with most other oral agents as well as insulin [62–67]. The magnitude of the glucose response when thiazolidinedione therapy is instituted is, in general, dependent on the fasting glucose concentration, with a greater absolute decline being observed in individuals with higher glucose levels [68]. Given that the thiazolidinediones do not stimulate insulin release, when used alone they do not typically cause hypoglycaemia. However, when combined with insulin or agents that stimulate the beta-cell such as sulfonylureas, the risk of hypoglycaemia is increased above that with either agent alone [69, 70].

The greatest insight on the relative effectiveness of thiazolidinediones compared with other glucose-lowering agents comes from A Diabetes Outcome Progression Trial (ADOPT), in which the effect of rosiglitazone therapy was compared with metformin and glyburide [71]. Patients in this study were drug-naïve and had diabetes for less than 3 years. They were randomised to treatment with one of the medications with the primary outcome being monotherapy failure, defined as a fasting plasma glucose >10.0 mmol/l (>180 mg/dl). After 5 years, the incidence of monotherapy failure was 15 % with rosiglitazone, 21 % with metformin, and 34 % with glyburide. In comparison with metformin and glyburide, rosiglitazone reduced the risk of monotherapy failure by 32 and 63 %, respectively. In the patients in whom the

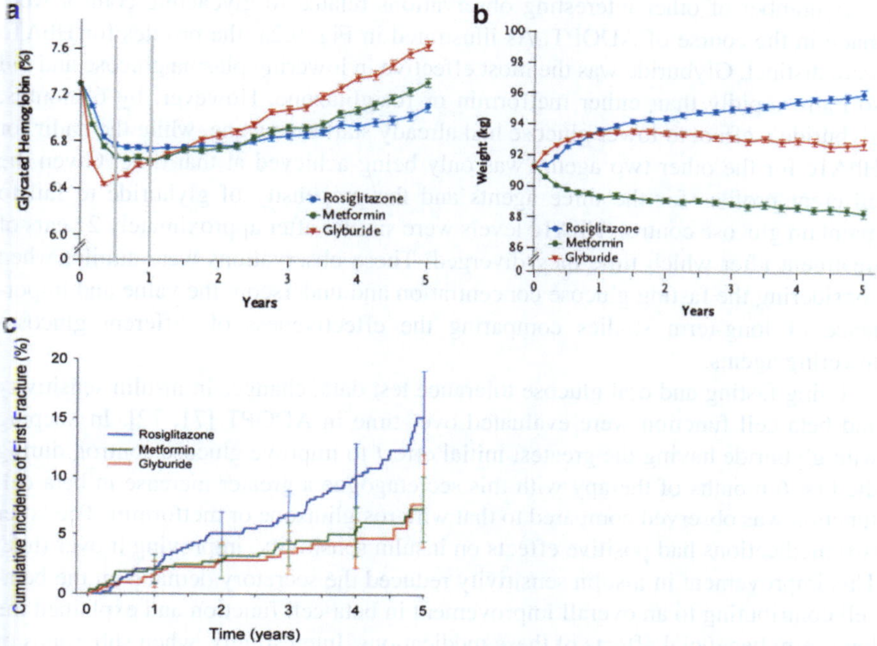

Fig. 9.2 Changes in HbA1c (*Panel a*) and weight (*Panel b*), and cumulative incidence of fractures (in women; *Panel c*) over time with rosiglitazone, metformin, and glyburide in the ADOPT study. As shown in *Panel a*, greater reductions in HbA1c levels occurred with glyburide during the first 6 months compared to metformin and rosiglitazone. However, after 6 months HbA1c levels steadily rose in the glyburide group, whereas reductions in HbA1c levels were maintained in the rosiglitazone and metformin groups for over 1 year. HbA1c levels diverged at around 2 years of therapy. At 5 years, the lowest HbA1c level was achieved with rosiglitazone followed by metformin. As illustrated in *Panel b*, a steady increase in weight was seen in those taking rosiglitazone throughout the study, while weight gain with glyburide occurred in the first year after which no further increase. Metformin therapy was associated with more favourable changes in weight. As shown in *Panel c*, an increased incidence of bone fractures was observed in women taking rosiglitazone beyond 1 year. Data are shown as mean ± SE. *Vertical lines* in *Panel a* represent 6 and 12 months of therapy. Reproduced with permission from ([71]; *Panels a and b*) and ([153] *Panel c*)

mean HbA1c level was 7.4 % at entry into the study, a level <7 % was maintained until 57 months with rosiglitazone, 45 months with metformin, and 33 months with glyburide (Fig. 9.2a). Given this differential effect on HbA1c, at the end of 4 years 40 % of patients taking rosiglitazone had an HbA1c level less than 7 % compared with 36 % using metformin and 26 % on glyburide. Subgroup analyses showed that rosiglitazone was more effective than glyburide in all subgroups, whereas rosiglitazone was found to be more effective than metformin in patients who were at least 50 years old and in patients with a waist circumference greater than 110 cm. Based on this work it was concluded that rosiglitazone was clinically superior to glyburide, but less so compared with metformin.

A number of other interesting observations related to glycaemic control were made in the course of ADOPT. As illustrated in Fig. 9.2a, the profiles for HbA1c were distinct. Glyburide was the most effective in lowering plasma glucose and did so more rapidly than either metformin or rosiglitazone. However, by 6 months, glyburide's effect to lower glucose had already started to wane, while the nadir for HbA1c for the other two agents was only being achieved at that time. Given the different profiles for the three agents and the propensity of glyburide to fail to maintain glucose control, HbA1c levels were similar after approximately 2 years of treatment after which time they diverged. These observations were similar when considering the fasting glucose concentration and underscore the value and importance of long-term studies comparing the effectiveness of different glucose-lowering agents.

Using fasting and oral glucose tolerance test data, changes in insulin sensitivity and beta-cell function were evaluated over time in ADOPT [71, 72]. In keeping with glyburide having the greatest initial effect to improve glucose control, during the first 6 months of therapy with this secretagogue a greater increase in beta-cell function was observed compared to that with rosiglitazone or metformin. The latter two medications had positive effects on insulin sensitivity, improving it over time. This improvement in insulin sensitivity reduced the secretory demand on the beta-cell contributing to an overall improvement in beta-cell function and explained the long-term beneficial effects of these medications. Interestingly, when subgroups of participants who did or did not respond well to the glucose-lowering therapies were compared, the findings were quite different. At the time they entered the study, all participants were drug-naïve. However, the group that met the primary outcome, which was monotherapy failure, had poorer beta-cell function at baseline. Irrespective of their treatment assignment, those who failed therapy showed a progressive loss of beta-cell function, all reaching a similar degree of dysfunction when their fasting glucose levels exceeded 10.0 mmol/l (180 mg/dl). Thus, it appears that the loss of beta-cell function is not only a critical determinant of the failure of glucose-lowering therapy to maintain glycaemic control, but importantly interventions aimed at retaining beta-cell function in patients with type 2 diabetes have to be commenced very early in the course of the disease [71, 72].

As mentioned, thiazolidinediones have also proven to be very useful in combination with other agents when treating adult patients with type 2 diabetes. The Treatment Options for Type 2 Diabetes in Adolescents and Youth (TODAY) study provided interesting insight into treatment approaches in children between the ages of 10 and 17 years who were recently diagnosed with type 2 diabetes [73]. As in adults, the use of two medications proved to be better than a single agent; thus, addition of rosiglitazone to metformin was more efficacious in improving glycaemic control than was metformin alone. Of further interest, combining an intensive lifestyle with metformin did not provide the same difference in glucose control as did the combination of metformin and rosiglitazone. Whether this was simply a function of the children's difficulty to adequately modify their lifestyles or represents possible differences in the response of different age groups to interventions cannot be easily discerned. Further, the fact that more than half the children progressed to therapeutic failure, defined as an HbA1c of 8 % or more for 6 months or a need for insulin, suggests that the disease may run a somewhat different course in children. The findings from studies addressing these issues will be of great interest in the future.

9.5 Effects of Thiazolidinediones on Blood Pressure

Elevated blood pressure is a metabolic syndrome criterion and well-recognised risk factor for cardiovascular disease [74]. Hypertension is also associated with insulin resistance [75]. Insulin induces vasodilatation in various vascular beds via the release of endothelium-derived nitric oxide, which lowers blood pressure [76]. In insulin-resistant states, the vasodilatory effect of insulin is impaired and is thought therefore to predispose to hypertension. The hyperinsulinaemia resulting from insulin resistance can also lead to stimulation of sympathetic activity resulting in renal sodium and water retention, which may then also contribute to the development of hypertension [77, 78]. With thiazolidinedione therapy, reductions in blood pressure occur and are felt to be due to improvements in insulin sensitivity and endothelial function [79], resulting from increased endothelial nitric oxide production and endothelial-mediated vasodilatation [80].

Treatment with thiazolidinediones has been shown to protect against the development of hypertension and to reduce blood pressure in animal models of hypertension or insulin resistance [81]. In studies of patients with hypertension and type 2 diabetes, a blood pressure lowering effect of thiazolidinediones has also been observed [82–88]. This effect is relatively modest (2.0–10.2 mmHg for systolic blood pressure and 2.3–8 mmHg for diastolic blood pressure) and has been demonstrated to be independent of glucose lowering. Further, it has been associated with a reduction in microalbuminuria, suggesting additional beneficial effects of thiazolidinedione therapy in the kidney. Whether there is a difference in the magnitude of the response with rosiglitazone or pioglitazone is not that clear. One small study has suggested a marginal advantage with pioglitazone [89], while another failed to find such an effect [90]. Either way, the effect is small and, given the debatable beneficial and possible adverse effect of thiazolidinediones on the risk of cardiovascular disease, is not an important consideration in the decision to treat patients with this class of agents.

9.6 Thiazolidinediones and Lipids

Two classical components of the metabolic syndrome are elevated triglycerides and reduced HDL cholesterol levels, with dyslipidaemia being a major risk factor for cardiovascular disease in individuals with or without diabetes. As an example, in the Fenofibrate Intervention and Event Lowering in Diabetes (FIELD) study of patients with type 2 diabetes, the combination of low HDL cholesterol levels along with marked hypertriglyceridaemia (>2.3 mmol/l) increased cardiovascular disease risk by 41 % [91].

The dyslipidaemia of the metabolic syndrome can be impacted by thiazolidinediones as these medications have favourable effects on both HDL cholesterol and triglyceride levels [92–94]. In general, pioglitazone leads to greater increases in HDL cholesterol levels and more commonly reductions in triglyceride levels than rosiglitazone, in part because of its greater PPAR-alpha effect [95]. In one study directly comparing these two agents in a large number of patients with type 2 diabetes and dyslipidaemia, treatment for 24 weeks with pioglitazone was associated with nearly 15 % increase in HDL cholesterol, while rosiglitazone only increased HDL cholesterol by about half that amount [92]. Triglyceride levels decreased by 12 % with pioglitazone, while they increased 14.9 % with rosiglitazone. Both agents increased LDL cholesterol, although the increase was smaller with pioglitazone, being just below 16 %. Similar findings were recently reported in the Thiazolidinedione Intervention with Vitamin D Evaluation (TIDE) trial, which randomised patients with type 2 diabetes to either rosiglitazone or pioglitazone. The study was stopped prior to the planned completion date because of the regulatory concerns with rosiglitazone [96]. At that time, nearly 400 subjects had received treatment with one of the thiazolidinediones, while over 500 had been taking placebo for an average of just over 5 months. Compared to placebo, pioglitazone treatment was associated with significant beneficial directional changes in triglycerides and HDL cholesterol, effects not observed with rosiglitazone. Neither medication was associated with significant changes in LDL cholesterol.

Another major trial that used pioglitazone was the Prospective Pioglitazone Clinical Trial in Macrovascular Events (PROACTIVE), in which the effect of this agent on all-cause mortality, non-fatal myocardial infarction, and stroke was compared with placebo in 5,238 patients with type 2 diabetes and macrovascular disease [94]. In this study, the beneficial effect of pioglitazone on plasma lipids was again apparent. Over an average follow-up of just under 3 years, treatment with pioglitazone was associated with an 11.4 % reduction in triglyceride levels compared with an increase of 1.8 % in the placebo group. The change in HDL cholesterol was also superior with pioglitazone, increasing by 19.0 % against a 10.1 % increase with placebo. However, the LDL cholesterol changes were less favourable, increasing by 7.2 % in the pioglitazone group as opposed to a 4.9 % increase in those receiving placebo. At baseline the percentage of patients on glucose-lowering therapy (metformin, sulfonylureas, insulin, various combinations of these three medications, and diet) and cardiovascular medications (statins, fibrates, thiazides and loop diuretics, beta blockers, angiotensin-converting enzyme inhibitors, angiotensin II antagonists, calcium-channel blockers, nitrates, and anti-platelet agents) was similar. During the study, the concomitant use of insulin and metformin increased in the placebo group, but that of sulfonylureas, thiazide and loop diuretics, anti-platelet agents, statins, and fibrates did not differ between the pioglitazone and placebo. Of note, the favourable changes in lipids with pioglitazone occurred in the absence of equipoise in glucose control and, therefore, what degree of the effect can be ascribed to differences in glucose control cannot really be discerned.

In the Pioglitazone Effect on Regression of Intravascular Sonographic Coronary Obstruction Prospective Evaluation (PERISCOPE) study, where the effects of pioglitazone and glimepiride on progression of coronary atherosclerosis were compared using intravascular ultrasonography in patients with type 2 diabetes and coronary heart disease, the attained glucose levels were more similar than in PROACTIVE. Under these circumstances, where differences in glucose concentrations were less likely to be influential, at the end of 18 months of treatment HDL cholesterol levels increased 0.15 mmol/l (5.7 mg/dl) with pioglitazone compared with 0.023 mmol/l (0.9 mg/dl) with glimepiride. The impact on triglycerides also favoured pioglitazone, with which they decreased 0.18 mmol/l (16.3 mg/dl) whereas they increased 0.037 mmol/l (3.3 mg/dl) with glimepiride. LDL cholesterol levels increased minimally in both groups, with the change from baseline level not being significant [93].

In ADOPT, the lipid profiles differed after an average of 4 years of intervention with the three different glucose-lowering medications. Again, however, glucose levels were not comparable, being lower with rosiglitazone than either metformin or glyburide. Furthermore, a greater proportion of patients receiving rosiglitazone were receiving lipid-lowering therapy, with just over half the participants in this group receiving statins compared with a little more than 40 % in the other two treatment groups. Under these conditions, LDL cholesterol levels were still significantly greater in the rosiglitazone-treated participants compared with the cohorts receiving either metformin or glyburide. HDL cholesterol levels were significantly higher in the rosiglitazone group, with the difference being greater compared with glyburide than metformin. The levels of triglycerides were lower with rosiglitazone than glyburide, but not different to those observed with metformin [71]. Thus, collectively these data also suggest that the effect of rosiglitazone on plasma lipids likely differs from that of pioglitazone.

The lack of a major beneficial effect of rosiglitazone on plasma lipids in the absence of diabetes has been examined in individuals with low HDL cholesterol levels. In two small studies of patients with metabolic syndrome and low HDL cholesterol levels, treatment with rosiglitazone for 8 or 12 weeks was not associated with significant changes in HDL cholesterol, triglyceride, or LDL cholesterol levels [43, 97]. Thus, it would appear that in individuals with the dyslipidaemia that is characteristic of the metabolic syndrome, there does not appear to be a true beneficial effect of rosiglitazone on plasma lipids. In a small study of patients with metabolic syndrome, 12 weeks of pioglitazone therapy resulted in a small increase in HDL cholesterol compared with placebo, while triglyceride levels were unchanged [98]. Adding pioglitazone to statin therapy in individuals with metabolic syndrome and without diabetes increased HDL cholesterol and decreased triglyceride levels over a period of a year [99]. Thus, in general pioglitazone has a more favourable effect on HDL cholesterol and triglyceride levels in patients with metabolic syndrome compared with rosiglitazone.

In the metabolic syndrome LDL cholesterol levels are not typically elevated; however, there are increases in the number of small LDL particles and apoB levels [100]. An increased number of small LDL particles have been associated with increased triglycerides, decreased HDL cholesterol, and increased apoB levels [101]. Small LDL particles are denser compared with larger LDL particles and more atherogenic [102, 103]. Treatment with rosiglitazone has been shown to change the phenotype of LDL from small and dense to large and less dense despite increasing LDL cholesterol levels modestly [103, 104]. Pioglitazone treatment has also been associated with reductions in small LDL particles in the face of no change in LDL cholesterol levels [98].

In summary, dependent somewhat on the patient population, both pioglitazone and rosiglitazone produce changes in lipids that are not entirely favourable. The change in LDL cholesterol, which increases with both, is the least favourable. The changes in HDL cholesterol and triglycerides are more favourable with pioglitazone, likely as it has partial PPAR-alpha agonist activity. This difference in the lipid response is perhaps one reason why pioglitazone may be associated with better cardiovascular outcomes compared with rosiglitazone [25, 105].

9.7 Effects of Thiazolidinediones on Waist Circumference and Body Fat Distribution

Increased waist circumference is also a metabolic syndrome criterion, being included as it provides an estimate of central adiposity. The cut points for this measure vary by population, but in all instances central body fat distribution has been demonstrated to be associated with increased risks of type 2 diabetes and cardiovascular disease [106]. Further, it has been demonstrated that these outcomes are related more to the visceral fat compartment than the subcutaneous region [107, 108], with increased visceral fat portending deleterious changes in all features of the metabolic syndrome [109]. Thus, redistributing fat from the intra-abdominal to the subcutaneous depots would likely have a positive effect on metabolic outcomes.

Treatment with thiazolidinediones typically leads to increases in body weight, the magnitude of which varies [110]. Marked weight gain has also been reported, but this may be the result of fluid retention particularly in those patients receiving insulin [111]. The variation in weight gain observed with thiazolidinediones may be in part related to the duration of therapy, as it has been demonstrated in patients with type 2 diabetes that while both thiazolidinediones and sulfonylureas increase body weight, the patterns differ. With thiazolidinediones weight gain is continuous during active therapy (for at least a period of 4 years) while that with the sulfonylurea glyburide has been shown to increase over the first year and then to plateau [71] (Fig. 9.2b).

While the changes in body weight with thiazolidinediones are not necessarily desirable, their use appears to be associated with a favourable redistribution of body fat assessed using waist and hip circumferences as well as with imaging modalities [30, 112–114]. In ADOPT there was an increase in both the waist and hip circumferences resulting in a stable waist-to-hip ratio, while in DREAM there was no change in waist but an increase in hip circumference resulting in a lower waist-to-hip ratio with thiazolidinedione therapy, indicating either a neutral [71] or favourable effect on fat distribution [46]. Imaging approaches to examine fat distribution have been used in small studies. In one, 13 patients with type 2 diabetes treated with either diet or a stable dose of sulfonylurea were studied using magnetic resonance imaging, which demonstrated that 16 weeks of pioglitazone therapy decreased the ratio of visceral to subcutaneous fat due to an increase in subcutaneous and decrease in visceral fat area [30]. A similar finding has been reported in another study using computed tomography in 12 overweight or obese insulin-resistant patients without diabetes treated for 12 weeks with pioglitazone [114]. This effect of the thiazolidinediones to redistribute and simultaneously increase subcutaneous fat appears to be related in part to their ability to stimulate adipogenesis [114]. In some instances it would appear that the degree of weight gain and adipogenesis is a determinant of therapeutic effectiveness on insulin sensitivity, particularly in women [37]. This same effect on adipogenesis likely explains the observation of an increase in adiponectin, the fat-derived protein associated with insulin sensitivity [39], which is discussed in greater detail in the following section.

9.8 Effects of Thiazolidinediones on Inflammatory Markers

The metabolic syndrome, obesity, and insulin resistance have all been associated with chronic subacute inflammation that may contribute to cardiovascular disease [115]. In these conditions, levels of pro-inflammatory mediators such as C-reactive protein (CRP), TNF-alpha, IL-1 and IL-6, serum amyloid A (SAA), leptin, resistin, retinol-binding protein-4 (RBP-4), plasminogen activator inhibitor-1 (PAI-1) [116], and matrix metalloproteinase-9 (MMP-9) [117] have all been shown to be increased, whereas the levels of plasma adiponectin, which has anti-inflammatory properties, are decreased [116]. Further, in subcutaneous adipose tissue biopsies, protein levels of CRP, IL-1, IL-6 and IL-8, leptin, SAA, RBP-4, PAI-1, and monocyte chemotactic protein-1 (MCP-1) have all been found to be significantly greater in those with metabolic syndrome compared with controls [118].

CRP has been a major focus of investigation as it is associated with the metabolic syndrome [119] and carries with it an increased risk of type 2 diabetes [120], cardiovascular disease, and stroke [121]. It is produced mainly by the liver, but can also be made by adipocytes [122]. A number of studies have examined the effect of thiazolidinedione therapy on CRP as well as some of the other inflammatory markers, the concept being that reducing inflammation may result in a decrease in cardiovascular events. One of the largest cohorts studied was the ADOPT participants. At baseline in these individuals, who were drug-naïve in terms of glucose-lowering agents, levels of CRP increased with increasing number of metabolic syndrome components [123]. The increase in these patients was shown to be determined by body adiposity, rather than insulin sensitivity or glucose control. With all three interventions, rosiglitazone, metformin, and glyburide, CRP levels decreased over time. While the change in absolute levels was greater in women than in men, the proportionate change was similar in both genders.

Comparison of the treatment effect of the three agents demonstrated that the CRP-lowering effect of rosiglitazone was 48 % greater than that of glyburide and 31 % more than metformin. Given that the weight changes in the three treatment groups were quite disparate, it appears that while body size is an important determinant of inflammation, it is not a critical determinant of the impact of therapy.

In keeping with their effects to downregulate the expression of the pro-inflammatory mediators and upregulate the anti-inflammatory adipokine adiponectin [116], treatment of patients with metabolic syndrome with thiazolidinediones has beneficial effects on inflammation. In different studies, all with relatively small numbers of individuals, different inflammatory markers have been examined. Thus, for example, 12 weeks of rosiglitazone treatment of individuals with the metabolic syndrome, low HDL cholesterol levels, and without diabetes resulted in improvements in CRP, IL-6, and TNF-alpha receptor-2 profiles [43], while in another study in which this thiazolidinedione was administered for 12 months, favourable changes in CRP, IL-6, and IL-18 were observed [124]. Also, in keeping with a beneficial effect, adiponectin levels increased with rosiglitazone treatment of patients with metabolic syndrome [124–126].

Studies with pioglitazone have similarly demonstrated favourable effects on inflammatory markers in individuals with the metabolic syndrome, although some of the markers that have been examined differ. For example, in a study involving 60 patients with metabolic syndrome and low HDL cholesterol, pioglitazone treatment for 12 weeks led to reductions in CRP and resistin and an increase in adiponectin compared with placebo [98]. It has also been demonstrated in obese, insulin-resistant subjects without diabetes that pioglitazone has a more favourable effect to increase adiponectin than diet and exercise, increasing it by 75 % compared with 15 % with the lifestyle intervention after 19 weeks [127]. Overall, while thiazolidinedione treatment leads to reductions in pro-inflammatory markers such as CRP and an increase in the adipokine adiponectin, these changes that were hypothesised to underlie a cardioprotective effect of these agents have, unfortunately, not translated into such benefit. The lack of demonstrable cardiovascular disease protection with thiazolidinedione treatment [128–130] despite improvements in the inflammatory profile also highlights the general need for caution in ascribing to these inflammatory markers the same relative status as other markers of cardiovascular risk.

9.9 Effects of Thiazolidinediones on Non-Alcoholic Fatty Liver Disease and Non-Alcoholic Steatohepatitis

Non-alcoholic fatty liver disease (NAFLD), the ectopic accumulation of fat in the liver in the absence of significant alcohol intake, has been associated with insulin resistance, type 2 diabetes, obesity, dyslipidaemia, and hypertension [131, 132]. In some patients NAFLD can progress to non-alcoholic steatohepatitis (NASH), which is characterised by hepatic inflammation, injury, and fibrosis, and which in turn can progress to cirrhosis and end-stage liver disease [131].

Insulin resistance is thought to be one of the major factors contributing to excessive fat deposition in the liver. Thus, targeting insulin resistance with thiazolidinediones has been a therapeutic approach employed in patients with NAFLD [133]. While insulin sensitisation of the liver occurs, changes in adipose tissue also appear to play an important role [31, 134]. Thiazolidinediones modulate the expression in adipose tissue not only of PPAR-gamma, but also of lipoprotein lipase and adiponectin, resulting in lower free fatty acid levels and increased circulating adiponectin concentrations. The net result is an enhancement of insulin action in the liver and decreased substrate availability for ectopic lipid deposition in the hepatocyte.

Pioglitazone has been studied in patients with biopsy-confirmed NASH who had either impaired glucose tolerance or type 2 diabetes. In combination with a hypocaloric diet in order to reduce weight gain, it increased hepatic sensitivity and improved glycaemic control [135]. Hepatic fat content decreased by 54 %, whereas it did not change in those assigned to the placebo arm. Importantly, the decrease in liver fat in the pioglitazone arm was associated with improvements in histological features. Finally, in line with these beneficial effects, transaminase levels decreased to a greater extent in those taking the PPAR agonist. That the combination of these changes was not likely to be simply the effect of improving glycaemia comes from another study in which a cohort of 247 non-diabetic adults with NASH were randomised to receive pioglitazone, vitamin E, or placebo for 96 weeks. Again pioglitazone was associated with benefit, documented as reductions in hepatic steatosis, lobular inflammation, and serum transaminases compared with placebo. Vitamin E treatment compared with placebo resulted in a higher rate of improvement in histological features of NASH, along with improvements in transaminases, hepatic steatosis, and lobular inflammation [136].

These positive outcomes with pioglitazone have also been observed with rosiglitazone, suggesting that they are not necessarily dependent on the PPAR-alpha effect of pioglitazone. Rosiglitazone treatment of individuals with biopsy-proven NASH for a year was associated with histological evidence of improvement in steatosis and reductions in transaminase levels [133].

While thiazolidinediones have a beneficial effect to improve the histological disturbances seen with NAFLD or NASH, this effect has been shown to disappear with discontinuation of therapy. In a study in which nine patients with biopsy-proven NASH were treated for 48 weeks with pioglitazone and followed up after 48 weeks off treatment [137], while liver enzymes normalised and hepatic volume and fat content decreased on therapy, after discontinuation of treatment hepatic volume increased, and the quantity of fat in the liver increased above baseline. Also, while on therapy only one patient still met the histological criteria for NASH, after withdrawal of pioglitazone therapy the histological diagnosis of NASH was again made in seven patients with some features such as ballooning cell injury being worse after stopping therapy. One possible explanation given for these troubling findings was weight gain and the increase in total body fat. In keeping with the recurrence of fatty liver following withdrawal of therapy, other studies have reported return of liver enzymes to baseline within several months after discontinuation of thiazolidinedione therapy [133, 138].

In summary, the thiazolidinediones have been shown to decrease liver fat and improve histological disturbances in non-alcoholic liver diseases by actions in the hepatocyte and the peripheral tissues. However, it would seem that their continued use is required if these beneficial effects are likely to be maintained long term.

9.10 Adverse Effects of Thiazolidinediones

As with most medications, thiazolidinediones have been found to have clinically relevant adverse effects (Fig. 9.3). These include weight gain, fluid retention resulting in peripheral oedema and congestive heart failure, an increased risk of bone fractures especially in women, and a potential increased risk of certain malignancies. Evidence suggesting an increased risk of myocardial infarction and cardiovascular mortality with rosiglitazone therapy prompted severe restrictions on the use of this medication. These adverse effects are discussed in more detail and have limited the use of thiazolidinediones in clinical practice.

9.10.1 Cardiovascular Side Effects

A major concern with rosiglitazone that led to its suspension in a number of countries and marked restrictions in its use in others was an increased risk of cardiovascular events. In a meta-analysis that included 42 randomised clinical trials that lasted for at least 24 weeks, rosiglitazone was associated with an increased risk of myocardial infarction (odds ratio of 1.43; 95 % CI, 1.03–1.98) [2]. These findings resulted in a furious debate as they were not a consistent observation, especially in the long-term studies. The ensuing discussions also resulted in the requirement imposed by the United States Food and Drug Administration that future registration of glucose-lowering medications will require a formal assessment of the risk for cardiovascular events [139]. With pioglitazone this same observation has not been made. In fact, based on the results of the PROACTIVE study, pioglitazone was felt to provide protection against coronary and peripheral vascular events. In this study of over 5,000 patients randomised to pioglitazone or placebo, active treatment was associated with a tendency towards a reduction in the primary composite outcome, which included all-cause mortality, acute coronary syndrome, non-fatal myocardial infarction, stroke, endovascular or surgical intervention in the coronary or leg arteries, and amputation above the ankle (hazard ratio 0.90, 95 % confidence interval (CI) 0.80–1.02, $p = 0.095$). The major secondary endpoint was the composite of all-cause mortality, non-fatal myocardial infarction, and stroke, and this decreased significantly with pioglitazone (hazard ratio 0.84, 95 % CI 0.72–0.98, $p = 0.027$) [94]. The statistical approach used in this study to conclude that pioglitazone was protective was also mired in controversy [140]. Despite a meta-analysis performed by the same group that had performed the one with rosiglitazone, suggesting that pioglitazone was associated with a lower risk of

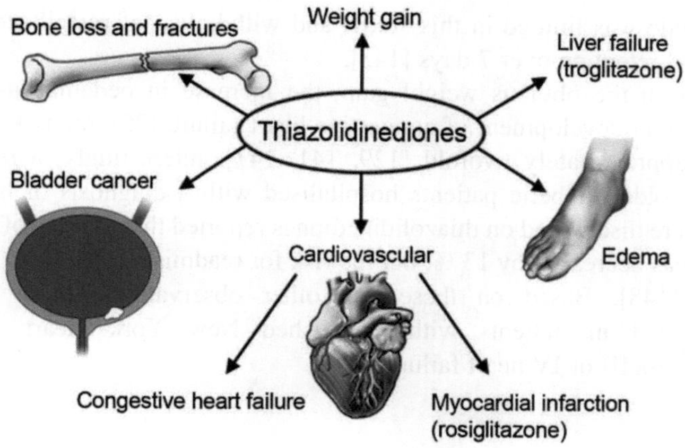

Fig. 9.3 Adverse effects of thiazolidinediones. Most common adverse effects of thiazolidinediones include weight gain, oedema, and congestive heart failure. Bone loss and fractures, especially in the lower and upper limbs of women treated with thiazolidinediones for over 1 year, have been observed and thought to be due to increased osteoclastic activity. Liver failure due to troglitazone led to its withdrawal from the market. An increased risk of myocardial infarction has been associated with rosiglitazone, which resulted in restrictions in its use. Most recently, concern over a possible increased risk of bladder cancer has limited clinical use of pioglitazone

mortality, myocardial infarction, or stroke [141], this agent is not generally accepted to provide cardiovascular protection.

9.10.2 Fluid Retention, Oedema, and Congestive Heart Failure

Fluid retention leading to weight gain, oedema, and, on occasion, congestive heart failure had been recognised as an adverse effect of treatment with these agents soon after their introduction. The mechanism by which fluid retention occurs is felt to be due to increased renal sodium and fluid reabsorption resulting from the activation of the PPAR-gamma receptors in the collecting ducts of nephrons, which in turn leads to upregulation of sodium transporter expression and translocation [142, 143]. This end result of sodium and fluid retention is enhanced by the fact that both hyperglycaemia and thiazolidinediones increase the expression of PPAR-gamma in the nephron [144]. PPAR-gamma activation of endothelial cells and vascular smooth muscle cells may also increase capillary permeability contributing to increased fluid reabsorption [145]. This causes expansion in plasma volume, which leads to a fall in the haematocrit level and can result in clinical oedema [143].

The occurrence of peripheral oedema with thiazolidinedione therapy is thought to be dose-dependent, occurring in about 4–8 % of patients taking thiazolidinediones [63, 143, 146]. A clinical study showed reversal of fluid retention induced by rosiglitazone with spironolactone or hydrochlorothiazide, resulting in an increase in the haematocrit and decrease in extracellular fluid volume. The effect of furosemide was limited in this study, and withdrawal of rosiglitazone did not reverse fluid retention over 7 days [143].

Aside from the obvious weight gain, the increase in oedema has also been associated with development of congestive heart failure [25], the risk of which is increased approximately twofold [129, 141, 147]. Interestingly, a retrospective analysis of older diabetic patients hospitalised with a diagnosis of heart failure and who were discharged on thiazolidinediones reported that the risk of subsequent mortality was decreased by 13 %, but the risk for readmission for heart failure was increased [148]. Based on these and other observations, these agents are contraindicated in patients with established New York Heart Association (NYHA) Class III or IV heart failure.

9.10.3 Weight Gain

One of the most vexing adverse effects of thiazolidinediones is weight gain (2.0–4.3 kg on average) [110], which often is greater in those with the greatest improvement of their glucose control [48, 149, 150]. For every 1 % decrease in the HbA1c value with thiazolidinedione therapy, there is a 2–3 kg increase in body weight [25]. Unfortunately, the weight gained is typically preserved despite discontinuation of thiazolidinedione therapy [137, 138].

There are several possible mechanisms that may be playing a role in weight gain with thiazolidinedione therapy, including body fat redistribution with an increase in the amount of subcutaneous adipose tissue, alterations in adipokine release patterns including decreased synthesis of leptin, which in turn leads to less suppression of appetite [151], fluid retention [30], and decreased glycosuria with improved glycaemic control [28]. In addition, central effects on body weight control mechanisms may also play a role as activation of PPAR-gamma in the central nervous system promotes increased feeding [152].

9.10.4 Bone Fractures

The occurrence of bone fractures with thiazolidinedione therapy was first reported with rosiglitazone in ADOPT [71]. This outcome was probably not noted before as the increase in fracture risk only manifests after a year of therapy (Fig. 9.2c) [153], underscoring the value of long-term studies for examining the pros and cons of glucose-lowering medications. Subsequently, a retrospective examination of the data obtained during studies with pioglitazone demonstrated the same outcome [154], in keeping with this being a class effect. The risk of bone fractures is increased approximately twofold in women using thiazolidinediones as compared with that observed with other glucose-lowering medications. Whether the risk is increased in men is debatable, with most studies not observing such. Interestingly, these fractures more frequently involve the upper limbs, including the humerus and hand, and the lower limbs, including the foot. While in younger women no increased occurrence of hip or vertebral fractures has been noted [71], observational and case–control studies suggest the possibility that in older women the risk for hip fractures is increased [155, 156]. It is possible that the increased risk of fractures in this more traditional location may be related to the presence of decreased bone mineral density in these women [155].

While it is clear that chronic thiazolidinedione exposure is associated with an increased risk of fractures, the mechanism by which this occurs remains unclear. In animal studies, activation of PPAR-gamma has been shown to cause a shift in the flow of mesenchymal precursor cells from osteoblastic to adipogenic lineages [157]. Activation of PPAR-gamma may also decrease insulin-like growth factor (IGF)-1 levels in bone, thereby decreasing new osteoblast formation [158]. Thus, it appears that PPAR-gamma activation can decrease new bone formation while increasing fat content in bone marrow leading to bone loss [156].

In humans, thiazolidinedione therapy has been associated with increased bone resorption as well as decreased bone formation, resulting in decreased bone density in healthy postmenopausal women and men with type 2 diabetes [159, 160]. In ADOPT, women taking rosiglitazone had an increase in C-terminal telopeptide, a marker for osteoclast activity, which was not observed in women treated with metformin or glyburide or in men taking any of the three agents [161]. Markers for osteoblastic activity, including procollagen type 1 N-propeptide and bone alkaline phosphatase, decreased in both genders with the decline being greater with metformin than rosiglitazone. These findings suggest that thiazolidinediones may increase fracture risk in women primarily via an increase in osteoclastic activity, leading to greater bone resorption [161].

Given the increased risk of bone fractures with chronic thiazolidinedione therapy, risk factors for bone fractures should be taken into account prior to initiating or continuing thiazolidinediones, especially in women. This assessment could include a formal determination of bone mineral density as an estimate of potential increased fracture risk.

9.10.5 Bladder Cancer

A more recent concern is the possibly increased risk of urinary bladder cancer with pioglitazone. While an increase in the number of cases was first noted in PROACTIVE, this difference occurred very early in the trial and so was felt to most likely represent a chance finding [94]. Since 2011 there have been reports of an increase in the risk of bladder cancer in publications that have used databases in the United States [162], France [163], and United Kingdom [164]. In these reports, the hazard ratio ranged from 1.2 to 1.83, with longer and greater exposure being associated with a greater risk [162, 164].

What are possible mechanisms responsible for the increase in bladder cancer with thiazolidinediones? In humans, the only real knowledge is that the PPAR-gamma receptor is expressed in normal bladder as well as in bladder tumours [165]. In studies in rats, bladder tumours have been observed predominantly in males [166]. In these animal studies, changes in urinary composition include a decrease in the level of urinary citrate that protects against lithogenesis and increases in amounts of urinary calcium and magnesium precipitates and in microcalculi [167]. Fluid retention that results from the use of these pharmacological agents leads to an increase in urine volume and bladder enlargement as well as urothelial cell hypertrophy [166]. Morphological changes such as urothelial irritation, proliferation, and neoplasia have also been noted in animal studies with long-term use of these agents [167].

While these database studies suggest an increased risk and animal studies propose mechanisms by which thiazolidinediones may produce changes in bladder morphology, these approaches clearly cannot substitute for a long-term clinical trial with adjudicated events. However, such a study would be an impossibility given the number of participants that would be required and the extremely long duration that would be needed. Thus, based on current knowledge, the French and German Medicines Agencies suspended the use of pioglitazone in June 2011 [168]. EMA concluded that pioglitazone was associated with a small increased risk of bladder cancer, and the FDA recommends that pioglitazone should be used with caution in patients with a history of bladder cancer and should not be used in patients with active bladder cancer.

9.11 Conclusions

Thiazolidinediones target multiple components of the metabolic syndrome, including glucose and lipid metabolism. They reduce insulin resistance and can prevent diabetes in individuals with impaired glucose tolerance. Further, they have been shown to reduce inflammatory markers as well as lead to an improvement in some aspects of the lipid profile. However, they have been associated with a number of adverse effects such as congestive heart failure, oedema, weight gain, and bone fractures and evidence suggesting a small increase in the risk of developing bladder cancer. Weighing the benefits and risks associated with the use of this class of compounds, a number of regulatory agencies have severely restricted the use of rosiglitazone while others have limited the availability of pioglitazone. Further, for many of the same reasons, clinicians in numerous countries are reducing the volume of prescriptions they write for thiazolidinediones. Whether new and improved more selective thiazolidinediones that have the benefits without the current plethora of risks will be forthcoming is something we can hope for, but we may have to wait a while before our wish is realised.

Acknowledgements The writing of this chapter was supported in part by the United States Department of Veterans Affairs and NIH grant T32 DK007247.

References

1. Tjokroprawiro A (2006) New approach in the treatment of T2DM and metabolic syndrome (focus on a novel insulin sensitizer). Acta Med Indones 38(3):160–166
2. Nissen SE, Wolski K (2007) Effect of rosiglitazone on the risk of myocardial infarction and death from cardiovascular causes. N Engl J Med 356(24):2457–2471
3. Update on ongoing European review of pioglitazone–containing medicines. 2011 [cited 2012 September 28]; Available from: http://www.ema.europa.eu/docs/en_GB/document_library/Press_release/2011/06/WC500107515.pdf.
4. Sakamoto J, Kimura H, Moriyama S, Odaka H, Momose Y, Sugiyama Y et al (2000) Activation of human peroxisome proliferator-activated receptor (PPAR) subtypes by pioglitazone. Biochem Biophys Res Commun 278(3):704–711
5. Kendall DM, Rubin CJ, Mohideen P, Ledeine JM, Belder R, Gross J et al (2006) Improvement of glycemic control, triglycerides, and HDL cholesterol levels with muraglitazar, a dual (alpha/gamma) peroxisome proliferator-activated receptor activator, in patients with type 2 diabetes inadequately controlled with metformin monotherapy: a double-blind, randomized, pioglitazone-comparative study. Diabetes Care 29(5):1016–1023
6. Nissen SE, Wolski K, Topol EJ (2005) Effect of muraglitazar on death and major adverse cardiovascular events in patients with type 2 diabetes mellitus. JAMA 294(20):2581–2586
7. Wilding JP (2012) PPAR agonists for the treatment of cardiovascular disease in patients with diabetes. Diabetes Obes Metab 14(11):973–982
8. Berger JP, Akiyama TE, Meinke PT (2005) PPARs: therapeutic targets for metabolic disease. Trends Pharmacol Sci 26(5):244–251
9. Tyagi S, Gupta P, Saini AS, Kaushal C, Sharma S (2011) The peroxisome proliferator-activated receptor: a family of nuclear receptors role in various diseases. J Adv Pharm Technol Res 2(4):236–240
10. Issemann I, Green S (1990) Activation of a member of the steroid hormone receptor superfamily by peroxisome proliferators. Nature 347(6294):645–650
11. Greene ME, Blumberg B, McBride OW, Yi HF, Kronquist K, Kwan K et al (1995) Isolation of the human peroxisome proliferator activated receptor gamma cDNA: expression in hematopoietic cells and chromosomal mapping. Gene Expr 4(4–5):281–299
12. Hansen JB, Zhang H, Rasmussen TH, Petersen RK, Flindt EN, Kristiansen K (2001) Peroxisome proliferator-activated receptor delta (PPARdelta)-mediated regulation of preadipocyte proliferation and gene expression is dependent on cAMP signaling. J Biol Chem 276(5): 3175–3182
13. Vidal-Puig AJ, Considine RV, Jimenez-Linan M, Werman A, Pories WJ, Caro JF et al (1997) Peroxisome proliferator-activated receptor gene expression in human tissues. Effects of obesity, weight loss, and regulation by insulin and glucocorticoids. J Clin Invest 99(10): 2416–2422
14. Dubois M, Pattou F, Kerr-Conte J, Gmyr V, Vandewalle B, Desreumaux P et al (2000) Expression of peroxisome proliferator-activated receptor gamma (PPARgamma) in normal human pancreatic islet cells. Diabetologia 43(9):1165–1169
15. Wang N, Verna L, Chen NG, Chen J, Li H, Forman BM et al (2002) Constitutive activation of peroxisome proliferator-activated receptor-gamma suppresses pro-inflammatory adhesion molecules in human vascular endothelial cells. J Biol Chem 277(37):34176–34181
16. Chinetti G, Griglio S, Antonucci M, Torra IP, Delerive P, Majd Z et al (1998) Activation of proliferator-activated receptors alpha and gamma induces apoptosis of human monocyte-derived macrophages. J Biol Chem 273(40):25573–25580
17. Sarruf DA, Yu F, Nguyen HT, Williams DL, Printz RL, Niswender KD et al (2009) Expression of peroxisome proliferator-activated receptor-gamma in key neuronal subsets regulating glucose metabolism and energy homeostasis. Endocrinology 150(2):707–712
18. Mukherjee R, Jow L, Noonan D, McDonnell DP (1994) Human and rat peroxisome proliferator activated receptors (PPARs) demonstrate similar tissue distribution but different responsiveness to PPAR activators. J Steroid Biochem Mol Biol 51(3–4):157–166

19. Barbier O, Torra IP, Duguay Y, Blanquart C, Fruchart JC, Glineur C et al (2002) Pleiotropic actions of peroxisome proliferator-activated receptors in lipid metabolism and atherosclerosis. Arterioscler Thromb Vasc Biol 22(5):717–726
20. Loviscach M, Rehman N, Carter L, Mudaliar S, Mohadeen P, Ciaraldi TP et al (2000) Distribution of peroxisome proliferator-activated receptors (PPARs) in human skeletal muscle and adipose tissue: relation to insulin action. Diabetologia 43(3):304–311
21. Kang HY, Chung E, Lee M, Cho Y, Kang WH (2004) Expression and function of peroxisome proliferator-activated receptors in human melanocytes. Br J Dermatol 150(3):462–468
22. Chattopadhyay N, Singh DP, Heese O, Godbole MM, Sinohara T, Black PM et al (2000) Expression of peroxisome proliferator-activated receptors (PPARS) in human astrocytic cells: PPAR gamma agonists as inducers of apoptosis. J Neurosci Res 61(1):67–74
23. Ooi EM, Watts GF, Sprecher DL, Chan DC, Barrett PH (2011) Mechanism of action of a peroxisome proliferator-activated receptor (PPAR)-delta agonist on lipoprotein metabolism in dyslipidemic subjects with central obesity. J Clin Endocrinol Metab 96(10):E1568–E1576
24. Kliewer SA, Umesono K, Noonan DJ, Heyman RA, Evans RM (1992) Convergence of 9-cis retinoic acid and peroxisome proliferator signalling pathways through heterodimer formation of their receptors. Nature 358(6389):771–774
25. Yki-Jarvinen H (2004) Thiazolidinediones. N Engl J Med 351(11):1106–1118
26. Oberfield JL, Collins JL, Holmes CP, Goreham DM, Cooper JP, Cobb JE et al (1999) A peroxisome proliferator-activated receptor gamma ligand inhibits adipocyte differentiation. Proc Natl Acad Sci USA 96(11):6102–6106
27. Laplante M, Festuccia WT, Soucy G, Gelinas Y, Lalonde J, Berger JP et al (2006) Mechanisms of the depot specificity of peroxisome proliferator-activated receptor gamma action on adipose tissue metabolism. Diabetes 55(10):2771–2778
28. Kang JG, Park CY, Ihm SH, Yoo HJ, Park H, Rhee EJ et al (2010) Mechanisms of adipose tissue redistribution with rosiglitazone treatment in various adipose depots. Metabolism 59(1):46–53
29. de Souza CJ, Eckhardt M, Gagen K, Dong M, Chen W, Laurent D et al (2001) Effects of pioglitazone on adipose tissue remodeling within the setting of obesity and insulin resistance. Diabetes 50(8):1863–1871
30. Miyazaki Y, Mahankali A, Matsuda M, Mahankali S, Hardies J, Cusi K et al (2002) Effect of pioglitazone on abdominal fat distribution and insulin sensitivity in type 2 diabetic patients. J Clin Endocrinol Metab 87(6):2784–2791
31. Tiikkainen M, Hakkinen AM, Korsheninnikova E, Nyman T, Makimattila S, Yki-Jarvinen H (2004) Effects of rosiglitazone and metformin on liver fat content, hepatic insulin resistance, insulin clearance, and gene expression in adipose tissue in patients with type 2 diabetes. Diabetes 53(8):2169–2176
32. Wajchenberg BL (2000) Subcutaneous and visceral adipose tissue: their relation to the metabolic syndrome. Endocr Rev 21(6):697–738
33. Bajaj M, Baig R, Suraamornkul S, Hardies LJ, Coletta DK, Cline GW et al (2010) Effects of pioglitazone on intramyocellular fat metabolism in patients with type 2 diabetes mellitus. J Clin Endocrinol Metab 95(4):1916–1923
34. Boura-Halfon S, Zick Y (2009) Phosphorylation of IRS proteins, insulin action, and insulin resistance. Am J Physiol Endocrinol Metab 296(4):E581–E591
35. Barthel A, Schmoll D (2003) Novel concepts in insulin regulation of hepatic gluconeogenesis. Am J Physiol Endocrinol Metab 285(4):E685–E692
36. Boden G, Shulman GI (2002) Free fatty acids in obesity and type 2 diabetes: defining their role in the development of insulin resistance and beta-cell dysfunction. Eur J Clin Invest 32(Suppl 3):14–23
37. Bays H, Mandarino L, DeFronzo RA (2004) Role of the adipocyte, free fatty acids, and ectopic fat in pathogenesis of type 2 diabetes mellitus: peroxisomal proliferator-activated receptor agonists provide a rational therapeutic approach. J Clin Endocrinol Metab 89(2): 463–478

38. Freedland ES (2004) Role of a critical visceral adipose tissue threshold (CVATT) in metabolic syndrome: implications for controlling dietary carbohydrates: a review. Nutr Metab (Lond) 1(1):12
39. Yu JG, Javorschi S, Hevener AL, Kruszynska YT, Norman RA, Sinha M et al (2002) The effect of thiazolidinediones on plasma adiponectin levels in normal, obese, and type 2 diabetic subjects. Diabetes 51(10):2968–2974
40. Hajer GR, van Haeften TW, Visseren FL (2008) Adipose tissue dysfunction in obesity, diabetes, and vascular diseases. Eur Heart J 29(24):2959–2971
41. Weyer C, Funahashi T, Tanaka S, Hotta K, Matsuzawa Y, Pratley RE et al (2001) Hypoadiponectinemia in obesity and type 2 diabetes: close association with insulin resistance and hyperinsulinemia. J Clin Endocrinol Metab 86(5):1930–1935
42. Ai M, Otokozawa S, Asztalos BF, White CC, Cupples LA, Nakajima K et al (2011) Adiponectin: an independent risk factor for coronary heart disease in men in the Framingham Offspring Study. Atherosclerosis 217(2):543–548
43. Samaha FF, Szapary PO, Iqbal N, Williams MM, Bloedon LT, Kochar A et al (2006) Effects of rosiglitazone on lipids, adipokines, and inflammatory markers in nondiabetic patients with low high-density lipoprotein cholesterol and metabolic syndrome. Arterioscler Thromb Vasc Biol 26(3):624–630
44. Haffner SM, Valdez RA, Hazuda HP, Mitchell BD, Morales PA, Stern MP (1992) Prospective analysis of the insulin-resistance syndrome (syndrome X). Diabetes 41(6):715–722
45. Weyer C, Bogardus C, Mott DM, Pratley RE (1999) The natural history of insulin secretory dysfunction and insulin resistance in the pathogenesis of type 2 diabetes mellitus. J Clin Invest 104(6):787–794
46. Gerstein HC, Yusuf S, Bosch J, Pogue J, Sheridan P, Dinccag N et al (2006) Effect of rosiglitazone on the frequency of diabetes in patients with impaired glucose tolerance or impaired fasting glucose: a randomised controlled trial. Lancet 368(9541):1096–1105
47. Knowler WC, Hamman RF, Edelstein SL, Barrett-Connor E, Ehrmann DA, Walker EA et al (2005) Prevention of type 2 diabetes with troglitazone in the Diabetes Prevention Program. Diabetes 54(4):1150–1156
48. DeFronzo RA, Tripathy D, Schwenke DC, Banerji M, Bray GA, Buchanan TA et al (2011) Pioglitazone for diabetes prevention in impaired glucose tolerance. N Engl J Med 364(12): 1104–1115
49. Ravikumar B, Gerrard J, Dalla Man C, Firbank MJ, Lane A, English PT et al (2008) Pioglitazone decreases fasting and postprandial endogenous glucose production in proportion to decrease in hepatic triglyceride content. Diabetes 57(9):2288–2295
50. Goldberg RB, Temprosa M, Haffner S, Orchard TJ, Ratner RE, Fowler SE et al (2009) Effect of progression from impaired glucose tolerance to diabetes on cardiovascular risk factors and its amelioration by lifestyle and metformin intervention. Diabetes Care 32(4):726–732
51. Gerstein HC, Mohan V, Avezum A, Bergenstal RM, Chiasson JL, Garrido M et al (2011) Long-term effect of rosiglitazone and/or ramipril on the incidence of diabetes. Diabetologia 54(3):487–495
52. Buchanan TA, Xiang AH, Peters RK, Kjos SL, Marroquin A, Goico J et al (2002) Preservation of pancreatic beta-cell function and prevention of type 2 diabetes by pharmacological treatment of insulin resistance in high-risk Hispanic women. Diabetes 51(9):2796–2803
53. Zinman B, Harris SB, Neuman J, Gerstein HC, Retnakaran RR, Raboud J et al (2010) Low-dose combination therapy with rosiglitazone and metformin to prevent type 2 diabetes mellitus (CANOE trial): a double-blind randomised controlled study. Lancet 376(9735): 103–111
54. Pan XR, Li GW, Hu YH, Wang JX, Yang WY, An ZX et al (1997) Effects of diet and exercise in preventing NIDDM in people with impaired glucose tolerance. The Da Qing IGT and Diabetes Study. Diabetes Care 20(4):537–544
55. Ramachandran A, Snehalatha C, Mary S, Mukesh B, Bhaskar AD, Vijay V et al (2006) The Indian Diabetes Prevention Programme shows that lifestyle modification and metformin

prevent type 2 diabetes in Asian Indian subjects with impaired glucose tolerance (IDPP-1). Diabetologia 49(2):289–297
56. Knowler WC, Barrett-Connor E, Fowler SE, Hamman RF, Lachin JM, Walker EA et al (2002) Reduction in the incidence of type 2 diabetes with lifestyle intervention or metformin. N Engl J Med 346(6):393–403
57. Tuomilehto J, Lindstrom J, Eriksson JG, Valle TT, Hamalainen H, Ilanne-Parikka P et al (2001) Prevention of type 2 diabetes mellitus by changes in lifestyle among subjects with impaired glucose tolerance. N Engl J Med 344(18):1343–1350
58. Chiasson JL, Josse RG, Gomis R, Hanefeld M, Karasik A, Laakso M et al (2002) Acarbose for prevention of type 2 diabetes mellitus: the STOP-NIDDM randomised trial. Lancet 359(9323):2072–2077
59. Gerstein HC, Bosch J, Dagenais GR, Diaz R, Jung H, Maggioni AP et al (2012) Basal insulin and cardiovascular and other outcomes in dysglycemia. N Engl J Med 367(4):319–328
60. Lorenzo C, Williams K, Hunt KJ, Haffner SM (2007) The National Cholesterol Education Program—Adult Treatment Panel III, International Diabetes Federation, and World Health Organization definitions of the metabolic syndrome as predictors of incident cardiovascular disease and diabetes. Diabetes Care 30(1):8–13
61. Pittas AG, Greenberg AS (2002) Thiazolidinediones in the treatment of type 2 diabetes. Expert Opin Pharmacother 3(5):529–540
62. Lebovitz HE, Dole JF, Patwardhan R, Rappaport EB, Freed MI, Rosiglitazone Clinical Trials Study Group (2001) Rosiglitazone monotherapy is effective in patients with type 2 diabetes. J Clin Endocrinol Metab 86(1):280–288
63. Aronoff S, Rosenblatt S, Braithwaite S, Egan JW, Mathisen AL, Schneider RL, The Pioglitazone 001 Study Group (2000) Pioglitazone hydrochloride monotherapy improves glycemic control in the treatment of patients with type 2 diabetes: a 6-month randomized placebo-controlled dose–response study. Diabetes Care 23(11):1605–1611
64. Zinman B, Gerich J, Buse JB, Lewin A, Schwartz S, Raskin P et al (2009) Efficacy and safety of the human glucagon-like peptide-1 analog liraglutide in combination with metformin and thiazolidinedione in patients with type 2 diabetes (LEAD-4 Met+TZD). Diabetes Care 32(7): 1224–1230
65. Einhorn D, Rendell M, Rosenzweig J, Egan JW, Mathisen AL, Schneider RL (2000) Pioglitazone hydrochloride in combination with metformin in the treatment of type 2 diabetes mellitus: a randomized, placebo-controlled study. Clin Ther 22(12):1395–1409
66. Papanas N, Katsiki N, Hatzitolios AI, Maltezos E (2011) Pioglitazone: a valuable component of combination therapy for type 2 diabetes mellitus. Expert Opin Pharmacother 12(10): 1457–1461
67. Shah PK, Mudaliar S, Chang AR, Aroda V, Andre M, Burke P et al (2011) Effects of intensive insulin therapy alone and in combination with pioglitazone on body weight, composition, distribution and liver fat content in patients with type 2 diabetes. Diabetes Obes Metab 13(6):505–510
68. Goldstein BJ (2002) Differentiating members of the thiazolidinedione class: a focus on efficacy. Diabetes Metab Res Rev 18(Suppl 2):S16–S22
69. Bennett WL, Maruthur NM, Singh S, Segal JB, Wilson LM, Chatterjee R et al (2011) Comparative effectiveness and safety of medications for type 2 diabetes: an update including new drugs and 2-drug combinations. Ann Intern Med 154(9):602–613
70. Raskin P, Rendell M, Riddle MC, Dole JF, Freed MI, Rosenstock J et al (2001) A randomized trial of rosiglitazone therapy in patients with inadequately controlled insulin-treated type 2 diabetes. Diabetes Care 24(7):1226–1232
71. Kahn SE, Haffner SM, Heise MA, Herman WH, Holman RR, Jones NP et al (2006) Glycemic durability of rosiglitazone, metformin, or glyburide monotherapy. N Engl J Med 355(23): 2427–2443
72. Kahn SE, Lachin JM, Zinman B, Haffner SM, Aftring RP, Paul G et al (2011) Effects of rosiglitazone, glyburide, and metformin on beta-cell function and insulin sensitivity in ADOPT. Diabetes 60(5):1552–1560

73. Group TS, Zeitler P, Hirst K, Pyle L, Linder B, Copeland K et al (2012) A clinical trial to maintain glycemic control in youth with type 2 diabetes. N Engl J Med 366(24):2247–2256
74. Weycker D, Nichols GA, O'Keeffe-Rosetti M, Edelsberg J, Khan ZM, Kaura S et al (2007) Risk-factor clustering and cardiovascular disease risk in hypertensive patients. Am J Hypertens 20(6):599–607
75. Ferrannini E, Buzzigoli G, Bonadonna R, Giorico MA, Oleggini M, Graziadei L et al (1987) Insulin resistance in essential hypertension. N Engl J Med 317(6):350–357
76. Potenza MA, Gagliardi S, Nacci C, Carratu MR, Montagnani M (2009) Endothelial dysfunction in diabetes: from mechanisms to therapeutic targets. Curr Med Chem 16(1):94–112
77. Walker AB, Chattington PD, Buckingham RE, Williams G (1999) The thiazolidinedione rosiglitazone (BRL-49653) lowers blood pressure and protects against impairment of endothelial function in Zucker fatty rats. Diabetes 48(7):1448–1453
78. El-Atat FA, Stas SN, McFarlane SI, Sowers JR (2004) The relationship between hyperinsulinemia, hypertension and progressive renal disease. J Am Soc Nephrol 15(11): 2816–2827
79. Martens FM, Visseren FL, de Koning EJ, Rabelink TJ (2005) Short-term pioglitazone treatment improves vascular function irrespective of metabolic changes in patients with type 2 diabetes. J Cardiovasc Pharmacol 46(6):773–778
80. Horio T, Suzuki M, Takamisawa I, Suzuki K, Hiuge A, Yoshimasa Y et al (2005) Pioglitazone-induced insulin sensitization improves vascular endothelial function in nondiabetic patients with essential hypertension. Am J Hypertens 18(12 Pt 1):1626–1630
81. Sarafidis PA, Lasaridis AN (2006) Actions of peroxisome proliferator-activated receptors-gamma agonists explaining a possible blood pressure-lowering effect. Am J Hypertens 19(6): 646–653
82. Raji A, Seely EW, Bekins SA, Williams GH, Simonson DC (2003) Rosiglitazone improves insulin sensitivity and lowers blood pressure in hypertensive patients. Diabetes Care 26(1): 172–178
83. Yosefy C, Magen E, Kiselevich A, Priluk R, London D, Volchek L et al (2004) Rosiglitazone improves, while glibenclamide worsens blood pressure control in treated hypertensive diabetic and dyslipidemic subjects via modulation of insulin resistance and sympathetic activity. J Cardiovasc Pharmacol 44(2):215–222
84. Li GW, Wang JP, Li CM, Chen YY, Yang WY, Xing XY et al (2004) Anti-hypertensive effect of rosiglitazone in non-diabetic essential hypertension. CJIM 43(12):907–910
85. Sarafidis PA, Lasaridis AN, Nilsson PM, Pagkalos EM, Hitoglou-Makedou AD, Pliakos CI et al (2004) Ambulatory blood pressure reduction after rosiglitazone treatment in patients with type 2 diabetes and hypertension correlates with insulin sensitivity increase. J Hypertens 22(9):1769–1777
86. Gerber P, Lubben G, Heusler S, Dodo A (2003) Effects of pioglitazone on metabolic control and blood pressure: a randomised study in patients with type 2 diabetes mellitus. Curr Med Res Opin 19(6):532–539
87. Langenfeld MR, Forst T, Hohberg C, Kann P, Lubben G, Konrad T et al (2005) Pioglitazone decreases carotid intima-media thickness independently of glycemic control in patients with type 2 diabetes mellitus: results from a controlled randomized study. Circulation 111(19):2525–2531
88. Fullert S, Schneider F, Haak E, Rau H, Badenhoop K, Lubben G et al (2002) Effects of pioglitazone in nondiabetic patients with arterial hypertension: a double-blind, placebo-controlled study. J Clin Endocrinol Metab 87(12):5503–5506
89. Derosa G, Cicero AF, Dangelo A, Gaddi A, Ragonesi PD, Piccinni MN et al (2005) Thiazolidinedione effects on blood pressure in diabetic patients with metabolic syndrome treated with glimepiride. Hypertens Res 28(11):917–924
90. Derosa G, Fogari E, Cicero AF, D'Angelo A, Ciccarelli L, Piccinni MN et al (2007) Blood pressure control and inflammatory markers in type 2 diabetic patients treated with pioglitazone or rosiglitazone and metformin. Hypertens Res 30(5):387–394

91. Scott R, Donoghoe M, Watts GF, O'Brien R, Pardy C, Taskinen MR et al (2011) Impact of metabolic syndrome and its components on cardiovascular disease event rates in 4900 patients with type 2 diabetes assigned to placebo in the FIELD randomised trial. Cardiovasc Diabetol 10:102
92. Goldberg RB, Kendall DM, Deeg MA, Buse JB, Zagar AJ, Pinaire JA et al (2005) A comparison of lipid and glycemic effects of pioglitazone and rosiglitazone in patients with type 2 diabetes and dyslipidemia. Diabetes Care 28(7):1547–1554
93. Nissen SE, Nicholls SJ, Wolski K, Nesto R, Kupfer S, Perez A et al (2008) Comparison of pioglitazone vs glimepiride on progression of coronary atherosclerosis in patients with type 2 diabetes: the PERISCOPE randomized controlled trial. JAMA 299(13):1561–1573
94. Dormandy JA, Charbonnel B, Eckland DJ, Erdmann E, Massi-Benedetti M, Moules IK et al (2005) Secondary prevention of macrovascular events in patients with type 2 diabetes in the PROactive Study (PROspective pioglitAzone Clinical Trial In macroVascular Events): a randomised controlled trial. Lancet 366(9493):1279–1289
95. Vijay SK, Mishra M, Kumar H, Tripathi K (2009) Effect of pioglitazone and rosiglitazone on mediators of endothelial dysfunction, markers of angiogenesis and inflammatory cytokines in type-2 diabetes. Acta Diabetol 46(1):27–33
96. Punthakee Z, Bosch J, Dagenais G, Diaz R, Holman R, Probstfield J et al (2012) Design, history and results of the Thiazolidinedione Intervention with vitamin D Evaluation (TIDE) randomised controlled trial. Diabetologia 55(1):36–45
97. Millar JS, Ikewaki K, Bloedon LT, Wolfe ML, Szapary PO, Rader DJ (2011) Effect of rosiglitazone on HDL metabolism in subjects with metabolic syndrome and low HDL. J Lipid Res 52(1):136–142
98. Szapary PO, Bloedon LT, Samaha FF, Duffy D, Wolfe ML, Soffer D et al (2006) Effects of pioglitazone on lipoproteins, inflammatory markers, and adipokines in nondiabetic patients with metabolic syndrome. Arterioscler Thromb Vasc Biol 26(1):182–188
99. Murdock DK, Jansen D, Juza RM, Kersten M, Olson K, Hendricks B (2006) Benefit of adding pioglitazone to statin therapy in non-diabetic patients with the metabolic syndrome. WMJ 105(5):22–25
100. Brunzell JD, Ayyobi AF (2003) Dyslipidemia in the metabolic syndrome and type 2 diabetes mellitus. Am J Med 115(Suppl 8A):24S–28S
101. Kathiresan S, Otvos JD, Sullivan LM, Keyes MJ, Schaefer EJ, Wilson PW et al (2006) Increased small low-density lipoprotein particle number: a prominent feature of the metabolic syndrome in the Framingham Heart Study. Circulation 113(1):20–29
102. Brunzell JD (2005) Increased ApoB in small dense LDL particles predicts premature coronary artery disease. Arterioscler Thromb Vasc Biol 25(3):474–475
103. Yu D, Murdoch SJ, Parikh SJ, Marcovina SM, Cobitz A, Chen H et al (2006) Rosiglitazone increases LDL particle size and buoyancy and decreases C-reactive protein in patients with type 2 diabetes on statin therapy. Diab Vasc Dis Res 3(3):189–196
104. Freed MI, Ratner R, Marcovina SM, Kreider MM, Biswas N, Cohen BR et al (2002) Effects of rosiglitazone alone and in combination with atorvastatin on the metabolic abnormalities in type 2 diabetes mellitus. Am J Cardiol 90(9):947–952
105. Winkelmayer WC, Setoguchi S, Levin R, Solomon DH (2008) Comparison of cardiovascular outcomes in elderly patients with diabetes who initiated rosiglitazone vs pioglitazone therapy. Arch Intern Med 168(21):2368–2375
106. Despres JP (2012) Body fat distribution and risk of cardiovascular disease: an update. Circulation 126(10):1301–1313
107. Pou KM, Massaro JM, Hoffmann U, Vasan RS, Maurovich-Horvat P, Larson MG et al (2007) Visceral and subcutaneous adipose tissue volumes are cross-sectionally related to markers of inflammation and oxidative stress: the Framingham Heart Study. Circulation 116(11): 1234–1241
108. Liu J, Fox CS, Hickson DA, May WD, Hairston KG, Carr JJ et al (2010) Impact of abdominal visceral and subcutaneous adipose tissue on cardiometabolic risk factors: the Jackson Heart Study. J Clin Endocrinol Metab 95(12):5419–5426

109. Carr DB, Utzschneider KM, Hull RL, Kodama K, Retzlaff BM, Brunzell JD et al (2004) Intra-abdominal fat is a major determinant of the National Cholesterol Education Program Adult Treatment Panel III criteria for the metabolic syndrome. Diabetes 53(8): 2087–2094
110. Kushner RF, Sujak M (2009) Prevention of weight gain in adult patients with type 2 diabetes treated with pioglitazone. Obesity 17(5):1017–1022
111. Charbonnel B, DeFronzo R, Davidson J, Schmitz O, Birkeland K, Pirags V et al (2010) Pioglitazone use in combination with insulin in the prospective pioglitazone clinical trial in macrovascular events study (PROactive19). J Clin Endocrinol Metab 95(5):2163–2171
112. Smith SR, De Jonge L, Volaufova J, Li Y, Xie H, Bray GA (2005) Effect of pioglitazone on body composition and energy expenditure: a randomized controlled trial. Metabolism 54(1): 24–32
113. Moon JH, Kim HJ, Kim SK, Kang ES, Lee BW, Ahn CW et al (2011) Fat redistribution preferentially reflects the anti-inflammatory benefits of pioglitazone treatment. Metabolism 60(2):165–172
114. McLaughlin TM, Liu T, Yee G, Abbasi F, Lamendola C, Reaven GM et al (2010) Pioglitazone increases the proportion of small cells in human abdominal subcutaneous adipose tissue. Obesity 18(5):926–931
115. Romeo GR, Lee J, Shoelson SE (2012) Metabolic syndrome, insulin resistance, and roles of inflammation—mechanisms and therapeutic targets. Arterioscler Thromb Vasc Biol 32(8): 1771–1776
116. Tontonoz P, Spiegelman BM (2008) Fat and beyond: the diverse biology of PPARgamma. Annu Rev Biochem 77:289–312
117. Unal R, Yao-Borengasser A, Varma V, Rasouli N, Labbate C, Kern PA et al (2010) Matrix metalloproteinase-9 is increased in obese subjects and decreases in response to pioglitazone. J Clin Endocrinol Metab 95(6):2993–3001
118. Bremer AA, Devaraj S, Afify A, Jialal I (2011) Adipose tissue dysregulation in patients with metabolic syndrome. J Clin Endocrinol Metab 96(11):E1782–E1788
119. Rutter MK, Meigs JB, Sullivan LM, D'Agostino RB Sr, Wilson PW (2004) C-reactive protein, the metabolic syndrome, and prediction of cardiovascular events in the Framingham Offspring Study. Circulation 110(4):380–385
120. Dehghan A, van Hoek M, Sijbrands EJ, Stijnen T, Hofman A, Witteman JC (2007) Risk of type 2 diabetes attributable to C-reactive protein and other risk factors. Diabetes Care 30(10): 2695–2699
121. Shishehbor MH, Bhatt DL, Topol EJ (2003) Using C-reactive protein to assess cardiovascular disease risk. Cleve Clin J Med 70(7):634–640
122. Kahn SE, Haffner SM, Viberti G, Herman WH, Lachin JM, Kravitz BG et al (2010) Rosiglitazone decreases C-reactive protein to a greater extent relative to glyburide and metformin over 4 years despite greater weight gain: observations from a Diabetes Outcome Progression Trial (ADOPT). Diabetes Care 33(1):177–183
123. Kahn SE, Zinman B, Haffner SM, O'Neill MC, Kravitz BG, Yu D et al (2006) Obesity is a major determinant of the association of C-reactive protein levels and the metabolic syndrome in type 2 diabetes. Diabetes 55(8):2357–2364
124. Esposito K, Ciotola M, Carleo D, Schisano B, Saccomanno F, Sasso FC et al (2006) Effect of rosiglitazone on endothelial function and inflammatory markers in patients with the metabolic syndrome. Diabetes Care 29(5):1071–1076
125. Bahia L, Aguiar LG, Villela N, Bottino D, Godoy-Matos AF, Geloneze B et al (2007) Adiponectin is associated with improvement of endothelial function after rosiglitazone treatment in non-diabetic individuals with metabolic syndrome. Atherosclerosis 195(1): 138–146
126. Kim SG, Ryu OH, Kim HY, Lee KW, Seo JA, Kim NH et al (2006) Effect of rosiglitazone on plasma adiponectin levels and arterial stiffness in subjects with prediabetes or non-diabetic metabolic syndrome. Eur J Endocrinol 154(3):433–440

127. Shadid S, Stehouwer CD, Jensen MD (2006) Diet/exercise versus pioglitazone: effects of insulin sensitization with decreasing or increasing fat mass on adipokines and inflammatory markers. J Clin Endocrinol Metab 91(9):3418–3425
128. Lipscombe LL, Gomes T, Levesque LE, Hux JE, Juurlink DN, Alter DA (2007) Thiazolidinediones and cardiovascular outcomes in older patients with diabetes. JAMA 298(22): 2634–2643
129. Singh S, Loke YK, Furberg CD (2007) Long-term risk of cardiovascular events with rosiglitazone: a meta-analysis. JAMA 298(10):1189–1195
130. Kaul S, Bolger AF, Herrington D, Giugliano RP, Eckel RH (2010) Thiazolidinedione drugs and cardiovascular risks: a science advisory from the American Heart Association and American College of Cardiology Foundation. Circulation 121(16):1868–1877
131. Utzschneider KM, Kahn SE (2006) Review: the role of insulin resistance in nonalcoholic fatty liver disease. J Clin Endocrinol Metab 91(12):4753–4761
132. Hamaguchi MKT, Takeda N, Nakagawa T, Taniguchi H, Fujii K et al (2005) The metabolic syndrome as a predictor of nonalcoholic fatty liver disease. Ann Intern Med 143(10):722–728
133. Ratziu V, Giral P, Jacqueminet S, Charlotte F, Hartemann-Heurtier A, Serfaty L et al (2008) Rosiglitazone for nonalcoholic steatohepatitis: one-year results of the randomized placebo-controlled Fatty Liver Improvement with Rosiglitazone Therapy (FLIRT) Trial. Gastroenterology 135(1):100–110
134. Mayerson AB, Hundal RS, Dufour S, Lebon V, Befroy D, Cline GW et al (2002) The effects of rosiglitazone on insulin sensitivity, lipolysis, and hepatic and skeletal muscle triglyceride content in patients with type 2 diabetes. Diabetes 51(3):797–802
135. Belfort R, Harrison SA, Brown K, Darland C, Finch J, Hardies J et al (2006) A placebo-controlled trial of pioglitazone in subjects with nonalcoholic steatohepatitis. N Engl J Med 355(22):2297–2307
136. Sanyal AJ, Chalasani N, Kowdley KV, McCullough A, Diehl AM, Bass NM et al (2010) Pioglitazone, vitamin E, or placebo for nonalcoholic steatohepatitis. N Engl J Med 362(18): 1675–1685
137. Lutchman G, Modi A, Kleiner DE, Promrat K, Heller T, Ghany M et al (2007) The effects of discontinuing pioglitazone in patients with nonalcoholic steatohepatitis. Hepatology 46(2): 424–429
138. Neuschwander-Tetri BA, Brunt EM, Wehmeier KR, Oliver D, Bacon BR (2003) Improved nonalcoholic steatohepatitis after 48 weeks of treatment with the PPAR-gamma ligand rosiglitazone. Hepatology 38(4):1008–1017
139. Guidance for Industry: Diabetes Mellitus—Evaluating Cardiovascular Risk in New Antidiabetic Therapies to Treat Type 2 Diabetes. 2008 [cited 2012 September 12 2012]; Available from: http://www.fda.gov/downloads/Drugs/GuidanceComplianceRegulatoryInformation/Guidances/ucm071627.pdf
140. Ryder RE (2011) Pioglitazone: an agent which reduces stroke, myocardial infarction and death and is also a key component of the modern paradigm for the optimum management of type 2 diabetes. Br J Diabetes Vasc Dis 11(3):113–120
141. Lincoff AM, Wolski K, Nicholls SJ, Nissen SE (2007) Pioglitazone and risk of cardiovascular events in patients with type 2 diabetes mellitus: a meta-analysis of randomized trials. JAMA 298(10):1180–1188
142. Berlie HD, Kalus JS, Jaber LA (2007) Thiazolidinediones and the risk of edema: a meta-analysis. Diabetes Res Clin Pract 76(2):279–289
143. Karalliedde J, Buckingham R, Starkie M, Lorand D, Stewart M, Viberti G et al (2006) Effect of various diuretic treatments on rosiglitazone-induced fluid retention. J Am Soc Nephrol 17(12):3482–3490
144. Panchapakesan U, Pollock C, Saad S (2009) Review article: importance of the kidney proximal tubular cells in thiazolidinedione-mediated sodium and water uptake. Nephrology 14(3):298–301

145. Yang T, Soodvilai S (2008) Renal and vascular mechanisms of thiazolidinedione-induced fluid retention. PPAR Res 2008:943614
146. Wainstein J, Katz L, Engel SS, Xu L, Golm GT, Hussain S et al (2012) Initial therapy with the fixed-dose combination of sitagliptin and metformin results in greater improvement in glycaemic control compared with pioglitazone monotherapy in patients with type 2 diabetes. Diabetes Obes Metab 14(5):409–418
147. Lago RM, Singh PP, Nesto RW (2007) Congestive heart failure and cardiovascular death in patients with prediabetes and type 2 diabetes given thiazolidinediones: a meta-analysis of randomised clinical trials. Lancet 370(9593):1129–1136
148. Masoudi FA, Inzucchi SE, Wang Y, Havranek EP, Foody JM, Krumholz HM (2005) Thiazolidinediones, metformin, and outcomes in older patients with diabetes and heart failure: an observational study. Circulation 111(5):583–590
149. Lebovitz HE (2002) Differentiating members of the thiazolidinedione class: a focus on safety. Diabetes Metab Res Rev 18(Suppl 2):S23–S29
150. Gastaldelli A, Ferrannini E, Miyazaki Y, Matsuda M, Mari A, DeFronzo RA (2007) Thiazolidinediones improve beta-cell function in type 2 diabetic patients. Am J Physiol Endocrinol Metab 292(3):E871–E883
151. Kissileff HR, Thornton JC, Torres MI, Pavlovich K, Mayer LS, Kalari V et al (2012) Leptin reverses declines in satiation in weight-reduced obese humans. Am J Clin Nutr 95(2): 309–317
152. Ryan KK, Li B, Grayson BE, Matter EK, Woods SC, Seeley RJ (2011) A role for central nervous system PPAR-gamma in the regulation of energy balance. Nat Med 17(5):623–626
153. Kahn SE, Zinman B, Lachin JM, Haffner SM, Herman WH, Holman RR et al (2008) Rosiglitazone-associated fractures in type 2 diabetes: an analysis from A Diabetes Outcome Progression Trial (ADOPT). Diabetes Care 31(5):845–851
154. Takeda Pharmaceuticals Company (2007) Observation of an increased incidence of fractures in female patients who received long-term treatment with ACTOS (pioglitazone HCl) tablets for type 2 diabetes mellitus. 2007 [cited 2012 September 11 212]; Available from: http://www.fda.gov/downloads/Safety/MedWatch/SafetyInformation/SafetyAlertsforHumanMedicalProducts/UCM153896.pdf
155. Loke YKSS, Furberg CD (2009) Long-term use of thiazolidinediones and fractures in type 2 diabetes: a meta-analysis. CMAJ 180(1):32–39
156. Meier CKM, Bodmer M, Jick SS, Jick H, Meier CR (2008) Use of thiazolidinediones and fracture risk. Arch Intern Med 168(8):820–825
157. Ali AA, Weinstein RS, Stewart SA, Parfitt AM, Manolagas SC, Jilka RL (2005) Rosiglitazone causes bone loss in mice by suppressing osteoblast differentiation and bone formation. Endocrinology 146(3):1226–1235
158. Lecka-Czernik B, Ackert-Bicknell C, Adamo ML, Marmolejos V, Churchill GA, Shockley KR et al (2007) Activation of peroxisome proliferator-activated receptor gamma (PPARgamma) by rosiglitazone suppresses components of the insulin-like growth factor regulatory system in vitro and in vivo. Endocrinology 148(2):903–911
159. Grey A, Bolland M, Gamble G, Wattie D, Horne A, Davidson J et al (2007) The peroxisome proliferator-activated receptor-gamma agonist rosiglitazone decreases bone formation and bone mineral density in healthy postmenopausal women: a randomized, controlled trial. J Clin Endocrinol Metab 92(4):1305–1310
160. Yaturu S, Bryant B, Jain SK (2007) Thiazolidinedione treatment decreases bone mineral density in type 2 diabetic men. Diabetes Care 30(6):1574–1576
161. Zinman B, Haffner SM, Herman WH, Holman RR, Lachin JM, Kravitz BG et al (2010) Effect of rosiglitazone, metformin, and glyburide on bone biomarkers in patients with type 2 diabetes. J Clin Endocrinol Metab 95(1):134–142
162. Lewis JD, Ferrara A, Peng T, Hedderson M, Bilker WB, Quesenberry CP Jr et al (2011) Risk of bladder cancer among diabetic patients treated with pioglitazone: interim report of a longitudinal cohort study. Diabetes Care 34(4):916–922

163. Neumann A, Weill A, Ricordeau P, Fagot JP, Alla F, Allemand H (2012) Pioglitazone and risk of bladder cancer among diabetic patients in France: a population-based cohort study. Diabetologia 55(7):1953–1962
164. Azoulay L, Yin H, Filion KB, Assayag J, Majdan A, Pollak MN, Suissa S (2012) The use of pioglitazone and the risk of bladder cancer in people with type 2 diabetes: nested case–control study. BMJ 344:e3645
165. Yoshimura R, Matsuyama M, Segawa Y, Hase T, Mitsuhashi M, Tsuchida K et al (2003) Expression of peroxisome proliferator-activated receptors (PPARs) in human urinary bladder carcinoma and growth inhibition by its agonists. Int J Cancer 104(5):597–602
166. Cohen SM (2005) Effects of PPARgamma and combined agonists on the urinary tract of rats and other species. Toxicol Sci 87(2):322–327
167. Dominick MA, White MR, Sanderson TP, Van Vleet T, Cohen SM, Arnold LE et al (2006) Urothelial carcinogenesis in the urinary bladder of male rats treated with muraglitazar, a PPAR alpha/gamma agonist: evidence for urolithiasis as the inciting event in the mode of action. Toxicol Pathol 34(7):903–920
168. Ryder RE (2011) Pioglitazone and bladder cancer. Lancet 378(9802):1544

The Role of Statins in the Metabolic Syndrome

10

Peter M. Nilsson

10.1 Introduction

The so-called 3-hydroxy-3-methyl-glutaryl-CoA (HMGCoA) reductase inhibitors, or the statins, represent a class of drugs that has been developed successfully over almost 30 years and are now widely used all over the world for cardiovascular prevention. The popularity of these drugs is based on the fact that not only they are clinically effective, but also some leading brands are now cheap when generics have been introduced. The statins can be classified into the drugs which are more effective per mg, such as rosuvastatin and atorvastatin, and the more common statins such as simvastatin, pravastatin, and fluvastatin. The first one, lovastatin, is not in use anymore. Newer drugs are being developed such as pivastatin, but one drug, cerivastatin, was withdrawn due to hepatotoxicity. All the statins use the same kind of metabolic mechanisms even if they differ in potency and pharmacological properties.

Most of the statins are well-documented lipid-lowering drugs for cardiovascular prevention and protection, based on evidence, both for primary [1, 2] and secondary prevention [3, 4]. A number of trials have been summarised in meta-analyses showing clinical benefits in both genders [5] and in patients with type 2 diabetes [6]. The main lipid-modifying effects of this class of drugs consist of a reduction of low-density lipoprotein (LDL) cholesterol proportionate to dosage and differing with the type of statin used, as well as a modest reduction of triglycerides in combination with a modest elevation of high-density lipoprotein (HDL) cholesterol [7]. Statins may be used in monotherapy or in combination with other lipid-lowering drugs for a more pronounced effect on lipid control, for example in combination with fibrates, resins, or cholesterol uptake inhibitors such as ezetimibe. Based on one meta-analysis the reduction of coronary risk is in general

P.M. Nilsson (✉)
Department of Clinical Sciences, Lund University, University Hospital, Entrance 33, 205 02 Malmö, Sweden
e-mail: Peter.Nilsson@med.lu.se

H. Beck-Nielsen (ed.), *The Metabolic Syndrome*,
DOI 10.1007/978-3-7091-1331-8_10, © Springer-Verlag Wien 2013

proportionate to the reduction in LDL cholesterol [8]. Also stroke events are prevented by statin therapy, both in primary prevention [9] and in secondary prevention [10], although the exact mechanisms are not fully known.

10.2 Clinical Effects in Patients with Metabolic Syndrome

In subjects showing features of the metabolic syndrome, statins alone or in combination treatment have been shown to modify lipid levels in a favourable way [11–15] and also to reduce cardiovascular events, for example, in the follow-up of the large-scale Heart Protection Study (HPS) [16] and in the Justification for the Use of Statins in Prevention: an Intervention Trial Evaluating Rosuvastatin (JUPITER) study [17]. There are no indications that the preventive effects differ to a substantial degree in patients with or without metabolic syndrome. It is more a question of the pre-treatment total cardiovascular risk level—i.e. the higher this risk is, the higher the benefits. In the JUPITER study, for the composite end-point of myocardial infarction, stroke, revascularisation, or death, the 5-year numbers needed to treat were 20 (95 % confidence interval (CI), 14–34), in general, compared with 19 and 22 for those with and without metabolic syndrome [17]. In a separate analysis of JUPITER, as requested by European authorities, primary prevention in patients with elevated high sensitive C-reactive protein (hsCRP), who had high global cardiovascular risk (10-year Framingham risk score >20 % or SCORE risk ≥5 %), but LDL cholesterol levels not requiring pharmacologic treatment, rosuvastatin 20 mg significantly reduced major cardiovascular events versus placebo [18].

The Effects of Simvastatin and Rosiglitazone Combination in patients with the metabolic syndrome (SIROCCO) study showed that in patients with metabolic syndrome prescribed a statin/thiazolidinedione (TZD) combination manifested greater reductions in markers of vascular inflammation and oxidant stress, 24-h ambulatory blood pressure, and increases in adiponectin as well as improved glycaemic indices [19]. In the Treat to New Targets (TNT) study the statin effect was proportional to the dosage used when comparing atorvastatin 80 mg and 10 mg in secondary prevention [20].

10.3 Side Effects and Risk of New Onset Diabetes

Among adverse effects associated with statin therapy, muscular pain and rhabdomyolysis, although a rare condition, are well-known examples along with some other less common side effects including elevation of hepatic enzymes. Less studied are the influences on glucose metabolism and the increased risk of new onset diabetes by statin treatment, as has been documented in a recent meta-analysis [21]. Based on data from five statin intervention trials with 32,752 participants without diabetes at baseline, 2,749 developed diabetes (1,449 assigned intensive-dose therapy and 1,300 assigned moderate-dose therapy, representing 2.0 additional cases in the intensive-dose group per 1,000 patient-years) and 6,684 experienced cardiovascular events (3,134 and 3,550, respectively, representing 6.5 fewer cases in the intensive-dose group per 1,000 patient-years) over a mean period of 4.9 years. Odds ratios were 1.12 (95 % CI, 1.04–1.22) for new onset diabetes and 0.84 (95 % CI, 0.75–0.94) for cardiovascular events for participants receiving intensive therapy compared with moderate-dose therapy [21]. As compared with moderate-dose statin therapy, the number needed to harm per year for intensive-dose statin therapy was calculated to be 498 for new onset diabetes, while the number needed to treat per year for intensive-dose statin therapy was 155 for cardiovascular events according to the meta-analysis [21].

This detrimental effect on glucose metabolism is thus overshadowed by the beneficial effects on cardiovascular prevention and protection as also documented in other meta-analyses [1–6]. In addition, it has been suggested that there may exist differences between the statins, but this has to be further investigated [22]. Clinical studies including large-scale randomised, controlled trials demonstrate potential differences between individual statins, with pravastatin even promoting some risk reduction for new onset of diabetes. Conversely, other statins including atorvastatin, rosuvastatin, and simvastatin all promote a significant increase in this risk. This may reflect the overall potency of the statins or other pleiotropic effects of the drugs. Given the frequent concordance of metabolic diseases including diabetes, obesity, and metabolic syndrome with cardiovascular diseases associated with hyperlipidaemia, it is important to understand the potential metabolic risks and benefits of therapies with distinct statins [22]. If this should influence the choice of statin therapy for a certain patient is, however, less clear and not tested in randomised studies.

10.4 Statin Effects on Blood Pressure Levels

One interesting aspect of statin therapy is the potential for blood pressure lowering. Several studies have documented a small but significant reducing effect associated with statin therapy, although it was not shown in all studies. This effect could be due to positive effects on endothelial function with vasodilation or based on other unknown mechanisms. One meta-analysis included patients from 20 randomised, controlled trials of statin therapy (828 patients) in which concomitant antihypertensive treatment (if any) remained unchanged throughout the study. A total of 291 and 272 patients were given a statin or placebo, respectively, in parallel group trials, whereas 265 took part in crossover trials receiving a statin and placebo [23]. Systolic blood pressure was significantly lower in patients on statin than in those on placebo or control hypolipidaemic drug (mean difference: −1.9 mmHg; 95 % CI: −3.8 to −0.1). The effect was greater when the analysis was restricted to studies with a baseline systolic blood pressure >130 mmHg (systolic blood pressure reduction: −4.0; 95 % CI: −5.8 to −2.2 mmHg). In general, the higher the baseline blood pressure, the greater the effect of statins on blood pressure lowering ($p = 0.066$ for systolic blood pressure and $p = 0.023$ for diastolic blood pressure).

Table 10.1 Summary of dyslipidaemia in the metabolic syndrome and in type 2 diabetes

• Dyslipidaemia in MetS represents a cluster of lipid and lipoprotein abnormalities including elevation of both fasting and postprandial TGs, apo B, and small dense LDL, and low HDL-C and apo AI.
• Non-HDL-C or apo B are good surrogate markers of TRLs and remnants and are a secondary objective of therapy. Non-HDL-C <3.3 mmol/L (less than ~130 mg/dL) or apo B <100 mg/dL is desirable.
• Increased waist circumference and elevation of TGs seems to be a simple tool to capture the high risk subjects with MetS.
• Atherogenic dyslipidaemia is one of the major risk factors for CVD in people with type 2 diabetes.

From: European Association for Cardiovascular Prevention & Rehabilitation, Reiner Z, Catapano AL, De Backer G, Graham I, Taskinen MR, Wiklund O, et al. (2011) ESC/EAS Guidelines for the management of dyslipidaemias: the Task Force for the management of dyslipidaemias of the European Society of Cardiology (ESC) and the European Atherosclerosis Society (EAS). Eur Heart J 32:1769–818

Apo apolipoprotein, *CVD* cardiovascular disease, *HDL-C* high-density lipoprotein-cholesterol, *LDL* low-density lipoprotein, *MetS* metabolic syndrome, *TG* triglyceride, *TRLs* trigyceride-rich lipoproteins

The blood pressure response to statins was unrelated to age, changes in serum cholesterol, or length of the trial. It was concluded from the meta-analysis [23] that statin therapy has a relatively small but statistically significant and clinically meaningful effect on blood pressure.

10.5 European Guidelines on Dyslipidaemia Treatment Strategies

During 2011 the European Society of Cardiology (ESC) and the European Atherosclerosis Society (EAS) published joint guidelines on treatment of dyslipidaemia [24], a common feature of patients with metabolic syndrome and associated with insulin resistance (Table 10.1). It was stated that lifestyle therapy to improve the atherogenic lipid profile should be recommended to all subjects with metabolic syndrome and dietary advice should be tailored according to individual needs. Statins are recommended as first-line lipid-lowering drugs, but if targets are not achieved on maximally tolerated doses of statins, drug combinations may offer additional lowering of LDL cholesterol; the evidence from outcome studies is, however, limited. This is similar to recommendations in patients with type 2 diabetes where the evidence is stronger due to more studies.

The concept of raising HDL cholesterol seems attractive based on the strength of the relationship between low HDL cholesterol and increased cardiovascular risk in observational studies. The available tools to raise HDL cholesterol in clinical practice are limited, lifestyle modification providing the first option. Statins generally tend to increase HDL cholesterol but to a low degree. However, at present nicotinic acid provides the best drug strategy to raise HDL cholesterol, although fibrates can also be used. Glycaemic control may deteriorate by nicotinic acid at high doses. Both atorvastatin and fenofibrate exhibit pleiotropic effects to improve cardiovascular risk factors in patients with pre-diabetes or metabolic syndrome [25], but these effects have to be validated in long-term randomised studies in such patients.

10.6 Conclusions

In conclusion, statin therapy for patients with metabolic syndrome and dyslipidaemia in combination with elevated levels of small, dense LDL cholesterol particles should be prescribed if the total cardiovascular risk is sufficiently elevated to motivate drug therapy and if lifestyle interventions are not sufficient to correct the risk factor profile [26]. Recent European guidelines advocate the use of statin therapy in these patients [24], but fibrates may be considered in some patients with more pronounced dyslipidaemia associated with the metabolic syndrome. In a few high-risk patients a statin and a fibrate can be used in combination, but this takes extra precautions to safeguard from side effects, especially liver toxicity [24, 27]. Statins can also be combined with ezetimibe, a cholesterol reabsorption blocker, for a more ambitious lowering of LDL cholesterol in high-risk patients. Ezetimibe is currently tested for independent cardiovascular effects in patient with coronary heart disease or following acute coronary syndromes in the Improved Reduction of Outcomes: Vytorin Efficacy International Trial (IMPROVE-IT) [28]. The risk of new onset diabetes associated with statin therapy [21] reveals new mechanisms but should not detract from the use of statins in risk patients with pre-diabetes or metabolic syndrome as the benefits far outweigh the risks. It is also of importance to investigate statin effects in patients with metabolic syndrome from different ethnic groups, as currently being investigated in the Reversal Intervention for Metabolic Syndrome (TRIMS) study [29]. One special risk group of importance is patients with hypertension and metabolic syndrome where statin therapy is often indicated based on views from the European Society of Hypertension [30, 31]. These patients are often undertreated for their metabolic abnormalities if the focus is only put on blood pressure control per se.

References

1. Taylor F, Ward K, Moore TH, Burke M, Davey Smith G, Casas JP, Ebrahim S (2011) Statins for the primary prevention of cardiovascular disease. Cochrane Database Syst Rev (1): CD004816
2. Tonelli M, Lloyd A, Clement F, Conly J, Husereau D, Hemmelgarn B et al (2011) Alberta Kidney Disease Network. Efficacy of statins for primary prevention in people at low cardiovascular risk: a meta-analysis. Can Med Assoc J 183:E1189–E1202
3. Yusuf S, Islam S, Chow CK, Rangarajan S, Dagenais G, Diaz R et al (2011) Prospective Urban Rural Epidemiology (PURE) Study Investigators. Use of secondary prevention drugs for

cardiovascular disease in the community in high-income, middle-income, and low-income countries (the PURE Study): a prospective epidemiological survey. Lancet 378:1231–1243
4. Spector R, Snapinn SM (2011) Statins for secondary prevention of cardiovascular disease: the right dose. Pharmacology 87:63–69
5. Kostis WJ, Cheng JQ, Dobrzynski JM, Cabrera J, Kostis JB (2012) Meta-analysis of statin effects in women versus men. J Am Coll Cardiol 59:572–582
6. Chen YH, Feng B, Chen ZW (2012) Statins for primary prevention of cardiovascular and cerebrovascular events in diabetic patients without established cardiovascular diseases: a meta-analysis. Exp Clin Endocrinol Diabetes 120:116–120
7. Yamashita S, Tsubakio-Yamamoto K, Ohama T, Nakagawa-Toyama Y, Nishida M (2010) Molecular mechanisms of HDL-cholesterol elevation by statins and its effects on HDL functions. J Atheroscler Thromb 17:436–451
8. Cholesterol Treatment Trialists' (CTT) Collaboration, Baigent C, Blackwell L, Emberson J, Holland LE, Reith C, Bhala N (2010) Efficacy and safety of more intensive lowering of LDL cholesterol: a meta-analysis of data from 170,000 participants in 26 randomised trials. Lancet 376:1670–1681
9. Paciaroni M, Bogousslavsky J (2009) Statins and stroke prevention. Expert Rev Cardiovasc Ther 7:1231–1243
10. Callahan A, Amarenco P, Goldstein LB, Sillesen H, Messig M, Samsa GP et al (2011) SPARCL Investigators. Risk of stroke and cardiovascular events after ischemic stroke or transient ischemic attack in patients with type 2 diabetes or metabolic syndrome: secondary analysis of the Stroke Prevention by Aggressive Reduction in Cholesterol Levels (SPARCL) trial. Arch Neurol 68(10):1245–1251
11. Lundbye JB, Thompson PD (2005) Statin use in the metabolic syndrome. Curr Atheroscler Rep 7:17–21
12. Ooi EM, Watts GF, Chan DC, Chen MM, Nestel PJ, Sviridov D, Barrett PH (2008) Dose-dependent effect of rosuvastatin on VLDL-apolipoprotein C-III kinetics in the metabolic syndrome. Diabetes Care 31:1656–1661
13. Rosenson RS, Otvos JD, Hsia J (2009) Effects of rosuvastatin and atorvastatin on LDL and HDL particle concentrations in patients with metabolic syndrome: a randomized, double-blind, controlled study. Diabetes Care 32:1087–1091
14. Athyros VG, Ganotakis E, Kolovou GD, Nicolaou V, Achimastos A, Bilianou E et al (2011) Assessing the treatment effect in metabolic syndrome without perceptible diabetes (ATTEMPT) collaborative. Assessing the treatment effect in metabolic syndrome without perceptible diabetes (ATTEMPT): a prospective-randomized study in middle aged men and women. Curr Vasc Pharmacol 9:647–657
15. Robinson JG, Ballantyne CM, Hsueh W, Rosen J, Lin J, Shah A, Lowe RS et al (2011) Achievement of specified low-density lipoprotein cholesterol, non-high-density lipoprotein cholesterol apolipoprotein B, and high-sensitivity C-reactive protein levels with ezetimibe/simvastatin or atorvastatin in metabolic syndrome patients with and without atherosclerotic vascular disease (from the VYMET study). J Clin Lipidol 5:474–482
16. Heart Protection Study Collaborative Group, Bulbulia R, Bowman L, Wallendszus K, Parish S, Armitage J, Peto R et al (2011) Effects on 11-year mortality and morbidity of lowering LDL cholesterol with simvastatin for about 5 years in 20,536 high-risk individuals: a randomised controlled trial. Lancet 378:2013–2020
17. JUPITER Study Group, Ridker PM, MacFadyen JG, Fonseca FA, Genest J, Gotto AM, Kastelein JJ et al (2009) Number needed to treat with rosuvastatin to prevent first cardiovascular events and death among men and women with low low-density lipoprotein cholesterol and elevated high-sensitivity C-reactive protein: justification for the use of statins in prevention: an intervention trial evaluating rosuvastatin (JUPITER). Circ Cardiovasc Qual Outcomes 2:616–623
18. Koenig W, Ridker PM (2011) Rosuvastatin for primary prevention in patients with European systematic coronary risk evaluation risk ≥5 % or Framingham risk >20 %: post hoc analyses of the JUPITER trial requested by European health authorities. Eur Heart J 32:75–83

19. Lazich I, Sarafidis P, de Guzman E, Patel A, Oliva R, Bakris G (2012) Effects of combining simvastatin with rosiglitazone on inflammation, oxidant stress and ambulatory blood pressure in patients with the metabolic syndrome: the SIROCO study. Diabetes Obes Metab 14:181–186
20. LaRosa JC, Deedwania PC, Shepherd J, Wenger NK, Greten H, DeMicco DA et al (2010) TNT Investigators. Comparison of 80 versus 10 mg of atorvastatin on occurrence of cardiovascular events after the first event (from the Treating to New Targets [TNT] trial). Am J Cardiol 105:283–287
21. Preiss D, Seshasai SR, Welsh P, Murphy SA, Ho JE, Waters DD et al (2011) Risk of incident diabetes with intensive-dose compared with moderate-dose statin therapy: a meta-analysis. JAMA 305:2556–2564
22. Koh KK, Sakuma I, Quon MJ (2011) Differential metabolic effects of distinct statins. Atherosclerosis 215:1–8
23. Strazzullo P, Kerry SM, Barbato A, Versiero M, D'Elia L, Cappuccio FP (2007) Do statins reduce blood pressure? - a meta-analysis of randomized, controlled trials. Hypertension 49:792–798
24. European Association for Cardiovascular Prevention & Rehabilitation, Reiner Z, Catapano AL, De Backer G, Graham I, Taskinen MR, Wiklund O et al (2011) ESC/EAS Guidelines for the management of dyslipidaemias: the Task Force for the management of dyslipidaemias of the European Society of Cardiology (ESC) and the European Atherosclerosis Society (EAS). Eur Heart J 32:1769–1818
25. Krysiak R, Gdula-Dymek A, Bachowski R, Okopien B (2010) Pleiotropic effects of atorvastatin and fenofibrate in metabolic syndrome and different types of pre-diabetes. Diabetes Care 33:2266–2270
26. Ott C, Schmieder RE (2009) The role of statins in the treatment of the metabolic syndrome. Curr Hypertens Rep 11:143–149
27. Hermans MP (2010) Impact of fenofibrate on type 2 diabetes patients with features of the metabolic syndrome: subgroup analysis from FIELD. Curr Cardiol Rev 6:112–118
28. Cannon CP, Giugliano RP, Blazing MA, Harrington RA, Peterson JL, Sisk CM et al (2008) IMPROVE-IT investigators. Rationale and design of IMPROVE-IT (IMProved Reduction of Outcomes: Vytorin Efficacy International Trial): comparison of ezetimbe/simvastatin versus simvastatin monotherapy on cardiovascular outcomes in patients with acute coronary syndromes. Am Heart J 156:826–832
29. Dunkley AJ, Davies MJ, Stone MA, Taub NA, Troughton J, Yates T, Khunti K (2011) The Reversal Intervention for Metabolic Syndrome (TRIMS) study: rationale, design, and baseline data. Trials 12:107
30. Redon J, Cifkova R, Laurent S, Nilsson P, Narkiewicz K, Erdine S, Mancia G (2008) Scientific Council of the European Society of Hypertension. The metabolic syndrome in hypertension: European society of hypertension position statement. J Hypertens 26:1891–1900
31. Cífková R, Nilsson PM (2009) Statins and hypertension. J Hypertens 27:662–665

The Indication for Antithrombotic Primary Prophylaxis and Treatment in Case of Thromboembolic Complications in Patients with Metabolic Syndrome

11

Steen Husted

11.1 Introduction

In the literature, guidelines for the use of antithrombotic drugs in patients with metabolic syndrome exclusively describe risk-modifying treatment in the subpopulation of patients with diabetes mellitus. In the setting of antithrombotic treatment strategy in primary prevention, patients with diabetes mellitus are also considered, as cardiovascular disease is the leading cause of morbidity and mortality in patients with diabetes mellitus. Diabetes mellitus is associated with a two- to fourfold risk of developing coronary artery disease (CAD), peripheral arterial disease (PAD) and stroke [1].

Patients with diabetes mellitus have a long-term cardiovascular risk similar to that observed among patients without diabetes mellitus, but who have had a prior myocardial infarction (MI) [2]. Furthermore, patients with diabetes mellitus, who already suffered an ischaemic event, have a higher rate of recurrence than patients without diabetes mellitus [3].

The prevalence of diabetes mellitus in individuals with CAD is estimated to be around 15 % in developed countries, and among patients presenting with acute coronary syndrome (ACS) or undergoing percutaneous coronary intervention (PCI) the prevalence is estimated to be 30 % and 26 %, respectively [4, 5].

Patients with diabetes mellitus have inferior outcomes compared with patients without diabetes mellitus across the spectrum of cardiovascular presentations and procedures with a significant increased 30-day and 1-year mortality in both non-ST-elevation (NSTE)-ACS and ST-elevation (STE)-MI [6].

Following stent implantation in relation to PCI, patients with diabetes mellitus have a higher risk of stent thrombosis than patients without diabetes mellitus [7].

S. Husted (✉)
Region Hospital West, Aarhus, Denmark
e-mail: steehust@rm.dk

H. Beck-Nielsen (ed.), *The Metabolic Syndrome*,
DOI 10.1007/978-3-7091-1331-8_11, © Springer-Verlag Wien 2013

Several factors account for the increased atherothrombotic risk in patients with diabetes mellitus, who frequently have other cardiovascular risk factors like hypertension, dyslipidaemia or obesity [1–3]. However, this risk accounts for no more than 25 % of their excess cardiovascular risk [8]. Other factors specific for the diabetic population contribute to their atherothrombotic risk, which includes hyperglycaemia, insulin resistance and proinflammatory as well as prothrombotic states [9, 10].

The prothrombotic state is related to endothelial dysfunction, impaired fibrinolysis, increased coagulation factors and increased platelet reactivity.

The endothelium of patients with diabetes mellitus has increased "stickiness" from greater expression of adhesion molecules, decreased nitric oxide (NO) generation and increased interaction between the endothelium and inflammatory leucocytes [11]. Patients with diabetes mellitus have higher levels of fibrinogen, von Willebrand factor (vWF), factor VII, factor VIII and thrombin generation [12, 13], while tissue plasminogen activator (t-PA) is low and plasminogen activator inhibitor-1(PAI-1) is high [14, 15].

Platelet dysfunction in patients with diabetes mellitus leads to hyperresponsiveness to platelet agonists and subsequent increases in pathological platelet activation and aggregation [16].

Given this prothrombotic state and increased baseline risk, randomised trials and meta-analyses have generally documented greater absolute benefit from both oral and parenteral antiplatelet therapy in patients with diabetes mellitus and ACS compared with patients without diabetes mellitus.

11.2 Antithrombotic Drugs

In primary prevention and secondary prevention after atherothrombotic events in patients with diabetes mellitus, antiplatelet drugs are very important (Fig. 11.1). In addition, platelet activation and subsequent aggregation play a dominant role in the propagation of arterial thrombosis and are the key therapeutic targets in the management of acute atherothrombotic events.

Acetylsalicylic acid (aspirin) targets cyclo-oxygenase (COX-1), inhibiting thromboxane A_2 formation inducing a functional permanent inhibition of platelets. Aspirin is the basic antiplatelet therapy in most clinical situations.

In high-risk situations additional complementary platelet aggregation pathways must be inhibited to ensure effective treatment and prevention of thrombosis formation or propagation. Adenosine diphosphate (ADP) binding to the $P2Y_{12}$ receptor plays an important role in platelet activation and aggregation amplifying the initial platelet response to vascular damage. Several antagonists of the $P2Y_{12}$ receptor are available. The thienopyridine prodrugs clopidogrel and prasugrel, both administered orally, are actively biotransformed into molecules that bind irreversibly to the $P2Y_{12}$ receptor. The use of ticlopidine, another thienopyridine, is not recommended because of the risk of severe side effects (neutropaenia).

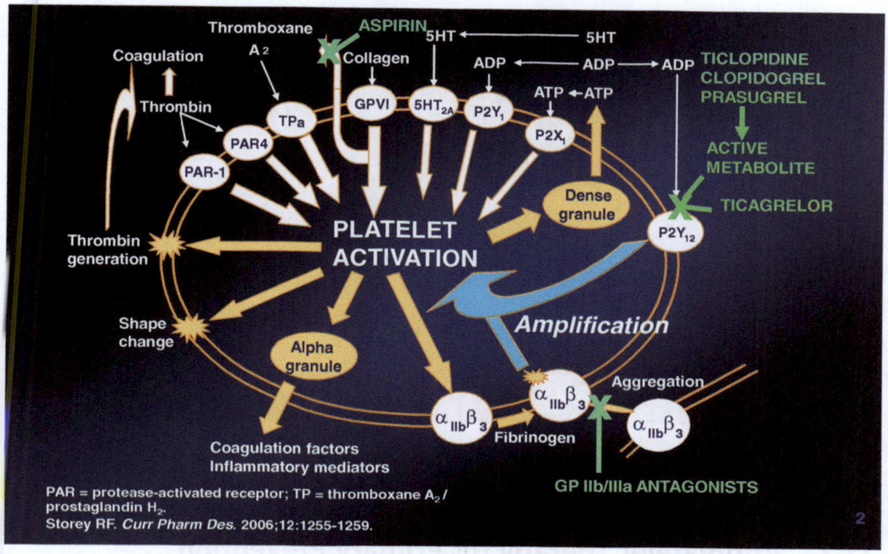

Fig. 11.1 Platelet receptors and pharmacological platelet inhibition

Ticagrelor is a pyrimidine derivative for oral administration and belongs to a new class of antiplatelet drugs, which without biotransformation bind reversibly to the $P2Y_{12}$ receptor, thus antagonising ADP signalling and platelet activation.

Glycoprotein IIb/IIIa (GP) receptor antagonists (abciximab, eptifibatide and tirofiban) target the final common pathway of platelet aggregation (Fig. 11.1).

Anticoagulants are used in the acute phase of ACS and the oral drugs are used for long-term treatment in patients with a risk of cardioembolic events. This may be atrial fibrillation and severe dysfunction of the left ventricle of the heart.

There is evidence that anticoagulation is effective in addition to platelet inhibition in ACS and that the combination of the two is more effective than either treatment alone. The anticoagulants act either as indirect or direct inhibitors of coagulation (Fig. 11.2).

Unfractionated heparin (UFH), low-molecular weight heparin (LMWH) and fondaparinux need antithrombin for their action and are administered parentally. UFH and LMWH inhibit both factor Xa and thrombin, while fondaparinux only inhibits factor Xa.

Of the oral anticoagulants the vitamin-K antagonists act on formation of coagulation factors II, VII, IX and X, while the new drugs apixaban, rivaroxaban and dabigatran etexilate (prodrug) act directly on activated coagulation factors and both apixaban and rivaroxaban inhibit factor Xa, while dabigatran (the active metabolite of dabigatran etexilate) acts on thrombin. Bivalirudin is also a direct inhibitor of thrombin, but can only be administered parentally.

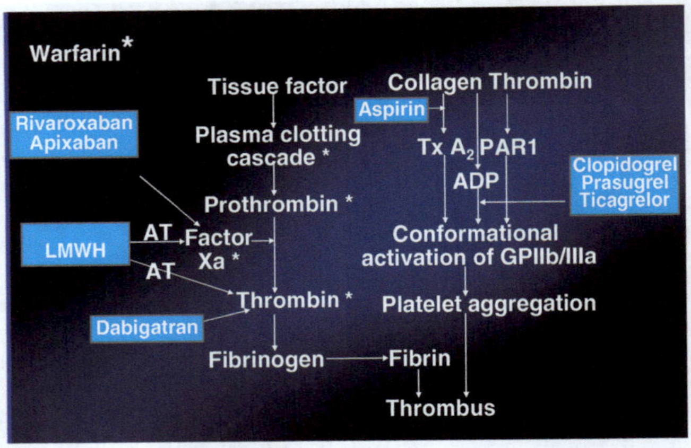

Fig. 11.2 Targets for long-term antithrombotic treatment

11.3 Antiplatelet Therapy for Primary Prevention

Aspirin is the only antiplatelet drug so far tested in primary prevention in major trials with subpopulations of patients with diabetes mellitus. The Antithrombotic Trialists' Collaboration showed among 4,000 patients with diabetes mellitus, but without cardiovascular disease (CVD), an absolute risk reduction in serious vascular events by aspirin of 0.07 % per year [relative risk (RR) 0.88; 5 % confidence interval (CI) 0.82–0.94] [3]. In the Prevention of Progression of Arterial Disease and Diabetes (POPADAD) trial in patients with diabetes mellitus and asymptomatic PAD, aspirin therapy failed to demonstrate a risk reduction in cardiovascular events [17]. In a meta-analysis of the effect of aspirin for primary prevention a reduction in nonfatal MI, but not in cardiovascular death, was demonstrated [18]. In the analysis, the risk of major bleeding complications was significantly increased.

Important major trials testing aspirin in patients with diabetes mellitus are ongoing and until the results of these studies are reported low-dose aspirin (75–162 mg) may be used in diabetic men aged ≥50 years or women aged ≥60 years with at least one additional CVD risk factor and who are at low risk for major bleeding (i.e. no history of previous gastrointestinal bleeding or peptic ulcer disease or concurrent use of other medications that increase bleeding risk) [19, 20].

11.4 Antithromboic Therapy in Patients with Diabetes Mellitus and with Thromboembolic Complications

11.4.1 Acute Coronary Syndrome

Patients with diabetes mellitus suffering from ACS are older, are more often female, more often have co-morbidities such as hypertension and renal failure, more often present with atypical symptoms and are more prone to develop complications, particularly heart failure and bleeding [21]. Diabetes mellitus is an independent predictor of mortality in ACS [22, 23].

The Euro Heart Survey showed that 37 % of patients with NSTE-ACS had established or newly discovered diabetes mellitus [21]. Though this big subpopulation of patients with diabetes mellitus is at higher risk for short- and long-term cardiovascular events they are suboptimally treated compared with patients without diabetes mellitus. In registries, reperfusion therapies (including revascularisation), thienopyridines (especially clopidogrel) and GP receptor antagonists are used less frequently among patients with diabetes mellitus than among patients without diabetes mellitus, with a clear impact on in-hospital and long-term mortality [21, 23]. As patients with diabetes mellitus are high-risk patients they require aggressive pharmacological as well as invasive management in the acute setting of an atherothrombotic event and in secondary prevention.

The two more recent guidelines on NSTE-ACS [24] and STEMI [25] from The European Society of Cardiology give recommendations for the use of antiplatelet drugs and anticoagulants including the new drugs now available on the market. It is evaluated if the high-risk subpopulation of patients with diabetes mellitus should be offered specific strategies to reduce the risk of recurrent ischaemic events and death.

Though revascularisation in patients with diabetes mellitus causes specific problems with typical diffuse and extensive CAD and a higher risk of restenosis as well as thrombotic occlusion of grafts and stents, an early invasive approach has been shown to be beneficial with a greater benefit in patients with diabetes mellitus than in non-diabetic patients [26]. It is unclear if coronary artery bypass grafting (CABG) offers better outcome than PCI in patients with diabetes mellitus and ACS similar to what is seen in stable patients with diabetes mellitus and CAD [27].

There is no evidence that the antithrombotic regimen should differ between patients with diabetes mellitus and non-diabetic patients [24, 25]. Two major trials, the Trial to Assess Improvement in Therapeutic Outcomes by Optimizing Platelet InhibitioN with Prasugrel-Thrombolysis in Myocardial Infarction (TRITON-TIMI) 38 [28] and the Platelet Inhibition and Patient Outcomes trial (PLATO) [29], showed that treatment with prasugrel or ticagrelor, respectively, in combination with aspirin is superior to dual platelet inhibition with clopidogrel and aspirin. In patients with diabetes mellitus prasugrel vs. clopidogrel reduced the risk of the composite endpoint of cardiovascular death, MI or stroke without excess major bleeding [30]. Ticagrelor vs. clopidogrel in patients with diabetes mellitus reduced the rate of ischaemic events in ACS patients irrespective of diabetic status and glycaemic control without an increase in major bleeding events [31]. In addition ticagrelor reduced all-cause mortality in patients with HbA1c above the median (>6 %).

Independent of the choice of treatment strategy dual platelet inhibition is recommended in all patients with ACS for a period of 12 months followed by monotherapy with either aspirin or clopidogrel (specific indications; see below).

Prior studies indicated a beneficial effect of intravenous administration of GP receptor antagonists in patients with diabetes mellitus, but on top of the potent $P2Y_{12}$-blocking agents the benefit is limited and routine use cannot be recommended [24, 25].

In the acute setting of ACS parentally administered anticoagulants like UFH, LMWH, fondaparinux and bivalirudin may be used similarly in patients with or without diabetes mellitus. With an indication for long-term anticoagulation in case of atrial fibrillation or severe dysfunction of the left ventricle, warfarin in combination with dual platelet inhibition is the drug of choice because of lack of data in this setting with the new oral anticoagulants (dabigatran etexilate, apixaban and rivaroxaban).

11.5 Secondary Prophylaxis in Patients with Diabetes Mellitus and with Stable Atherosclerotic Disease

The use of aspirin in secondary prevention was supported by the meta-analysis performed by the Antithrombotic Trialists' Collaboration involving 212,000 high-risk patients with acute or previous vascular disease or some other predisposing condition with an increased risk of occlusive vascular disease [3]. Antiplatelet agents, mainly aspirin, reduced the incidence of vascular events from 22.3 % to 18.5 % in the cohort of patients with diabetes mellitus and from 16.4 % to 12.8 % in patients without diabetes mellitus, indicating a higher risk in patients with diabetes mellitus, but consistent benefit of therapy. Aspirin low dose (75–150 mg daily) was at least as effective as higher doses and showed a lower risk of bleeding complications.

Patients with diabetes mellitus have a high rate of inadequate response to aspirin, when assessed by non-COX-1-specific methods, and in these patients increasing aspirin dose has been suggested to overcome resistance [32]. A recent study demonstrated that platelet cyclo-oxygenase activity recovered faster in patients with diabetes mellitus vs. patients without diabetes mellitus receiving aspirin once daily [33]. This difference in recovery was completely reversed by a twice-daily dosing of aspirin. These findings have not been addressed in major clinical studies in patients with diabetes mellitus.

Of the $P2Y_{12}$ receptor antagonists clopidogrel is the only drug besides ticlopidine tested in stable atherosclerotic patients for long-term use. The Clopidogrel Versus Aspirin in Patients at Risk of Ischaemic Events (CAPRIE) trial evaluated the efficacy of clopidogrel 75 mg daily vs. aspirin 325 mg daily in 19,185 patients with recent stroke, recent MI or established PAD [34]. The patients were followed for a mean of 1.9 years and 20 % had diabetes mellitus. The annual incidence of vascular death, MI or ischaemic stroke was 5.32 % with clopidogrel and 5.83 % with aspirin (RR 8.7 %; $p = 0.043$). In the diabetic subpopulation the incidence was 15.6 % for clopidogrel and 17.7 % for aspirin ($p = 0.042$) [35]. This led to 21 vascular events prevented for every 1,000 patients with diabetes mellitus treated, which for insulin-dependent patients increased to 38. In the CAPRIE trial 11,592 patients were identified with PAD and in these high-risk patients the combined primary endpoint was reduced by 24 % ($p = 0.0028$) by clopidogrel, indicating a benefit of clopidogrel over aspirin especially in high-risk atherosclerotic patients.

Currently, the American Diabetes Association recommends the use of clopidogrel in very high-risk patients with diabetes mellitus or as an alternative therapy in patients intolerant to aspirin [36].

The Clopidogrel for High Atherothrombotic Risk and Ischaemic Stabilization, Management, and Avoidance (CHARISMA) trial patients ($n = 15{,}603$) with either clinically evident CVD (non-ACS patients) or multiple risk factors were randomised to clopidogrel 75 mg daily in combination with aspirin (75–162 mg daily) or aspirin monotherapy [37]. Dual platelet inhibition was no more effective than aspirin alone against cardiovascular death, MI or stroke both in the entire cohort and in the subpopulation (42 %) of patients with diabetes mellitus. Therefore, long-term dual antiplatelet therapy with aspirin and clopidogrel cannot be advocated, not even in patients with diabetes mellitus except in the ACS/PCI setting.

PCI with stent placement in the coronary artery demands the use of dual platelet inhibition with aspirin in combination with a $P2Y_{12}$ receptor antagonist. The duration of therapy with the $P2Y_{12}$ receptor antagonist depends on the type of stent used. A bare metal stent demands one month of therapy, and a drug-eluting stent, which releases drugs with antiproliferative properties, demands 3–6 months dependent on the type of stent. Aspirin must continue indefinitely.

11.6 Diabetes Mellitus in Other Populations of Patients with Atherothrombotic Disease

In patients with ischaemic stroke or transient ischaemic attack dual platelet inhibition with clopidogrel 75 mg daily in combination with aspirin 75 mg daily was tested against clopidogrel monotherapy in a treatment period of 18 months [38]. No effect of dual platelet inhibition on major ischaemic events could be demonstrated in the whole cohort or the 2/3 of patients with diabetes mellitus, but the risk of major bleeding was significantly increased. In the Prevention Regimen for Effectively Avoiding Second Strokes (PRoFESS) study, clopidogrel 75 mg daily was tested against aspirin 25 mg plus dipyridamole 200 mg twice daily in 22,332 patients with ischaemic stroke with a follow-up of median 2.5 years [39]. The study showed no difference in major ischaemic events in the two treatment groups, but more major bleedings including intracranial bleeding in the group receiving aspirin plus dipyridamole. Similar effect and risk patterns were demonstrated for the 25 % patients with diabetes mellitus included in the study.

Based on the results from the PRoFESS trials, long-term treatment with clopidogrel or aspirin plus dipyridamole in patients with diabetes mellitus following ischaemic stroke is equally effective and the choice of therapy is made on individual basis. With other vascular beds involved in the atherosclerotic disease, CAD or PAD, clopidogrel will be the best option.

11.7 Diabetes Mellitus and Cardioembolic Risk in Atrial Fibrillation

Diabetes mellitus is an independent risk factor for stroke and systemic embolism in patients with atrial fibrillation [40]. In the most recent update of the European Society for Cardiology guidelines for the management of atrial fibrillation, a new risk score, the CHA_2DS_2-VASc score, has been introduced as basis for allocation of patients to antithrombotic prophylaxis [40]. A score of just 1 (diabetes mellitus alone gives a score of 1) results in an indication for anticoagulant therapy with a vitamin-K antagonist or one of the new direct-acting oral anticoagulants (dabigatran etexilate, rivaroxaban and apixaban). Aspirin use as an alternative is not recommended and the choice between a vitamin-K antagonist and the new oral anticoagulants is on an individual basis with a preference in the guidelines for the new drugs. Patients with diabetes mellitus have a risk-benefit ratio with the new drugs similar to patients without diabetes mellitus.

11.8 Concluding Remarks

Patients with diabetes mellitus have a high risk of developing atherosclerosis and thrombotic complications. In case of thrombotic complications the prognosis is worse in patients with diabetes mellitus as compared with patients without diabetes mellitus. Registries have shown that patients with diabetes mellitus do not receive an optimal reperfusion therapy as well as pharmacotherapy though the absolute risk reduction with an aggressive therapy is higher than in patients without diabetes mellitus.

Aspirin therapy should be used in primary prophylaxis in patients with diabetes mellitus with high-risk features.

Clopidogrel instead of aspirin should be considered in secondary prophylaxis of patients with diabetes mellitus and previous ACS, ischaemic stroke or PAD especially in case of polyvascular disease. Dual platelet inhibition cannot be recommended in stable patients except in a limited period in case of treatment with coronary stents.

ACS patients with diabetes mellitus should be offered reperfusion with either PCI or CABG if indicated and antiplatelet therapy with one of the new $P2Y_{12}$ receptor antagonists, ticagrelor or prasugrel, instead of clopidogrel together with aspirin for 12 months. The choice of monotherapy with an antiplatelet drug beyond 12 months must be made on individual basis.

Independent of the new treatment options available, the risk of ischaemic events and mortality in atherosclerotic patients with diabetes mellitus is still very high. Continued scientific activity and clinical trials to optimise this therapy are highly recommended.

References

1. Laakso MLS (1997) Epidemiology of macrovascular disease in diabetes. Diabetes Rev 5:294–315
2. Haffner SM, Letho S, Ronnema T et al (1998) Mortality from coronary heart disease in subjects with type 2 diabetes and in nondiabetic subjects with and without prior myocardial infarction. N Engl J Med 39:229–234
3. Baigent C, Blackwell L, Collins R et al (2009) Aspirin in the primary and secondary prevention of vascular disease: collaborative meta-analysis of individual participant data from randomized trials. Lancet 373:1849–1860
4. Brieger D, Fox KA, Fitzgerald G et al (2009) Predicting freedom from clinical events in non-ST-elevation acute coronary syndromes. The Global Registry of Acute Coronary Events. Heart 95:888–894
5. Anderson HV, Shaw RE, Brindis RG et al (2002) A contemporary overview of percutaneous coronary interventions. The American College of Cardiology – National Cardiovascular Data Registry (ACC-NCDR). J Am Coll Cardiol 39:1096–1103
6. Donahoe SM, Stewart GC, McCabe CH et al (2007) Diabetes and mortality following acute coronary syndromes. JAMA 298:765–775
7. Machecourt J, Danchin N, Lablanche JM et al (2007) Risk factors for stent thrombosis after implantation of sirolimus-eluting stents in diabetic and nondiabetic patients: the EVASTENT Mached-Cohort Registry. J Am Coll Cardiol 50:501–508
8. Nesto RW (2004) Correlation between cardiovascular disease and diabetes mellitus: current concepts. Am J Med 116(Suppl 5A):11S–22S
9. Colwell JA, Nesto RW (2003) The platelet in diabetes: focus on prevention of ischemic events. Diabetes Care 26:2181–2188
10. Ferroni P, Basili S, Falco A, Davi G (2004) Platelet activation in type 2 diabetes mellitus. J Thromb Haemost 2:1282–1291
11. El Haouari M, Rosado JA (2008) Platelet signalling abnormalities in patients with type 2 diabetes mellitus: a review. Blood Cells Mol Dis 41:119–123
12. Meigs JB, Mittleman MA, Nathan DM et al (2000) Hyperinsulinemia, hyperglycemia, and impaired hemostasis: the Framingham Offspring Study. JAMA 282:221–228
13. Juhan-Vague I, Alessi MC, Vague P (1996) Thrombogenic and fibrinolytic factors and cardiovascular risk in non-insulin-dependent diabetes mellitus. Ann Med 28:371–380
14. Schneider DJ, Nordt TK, Sobel BE (1993) Attenuated fibrinolysis and accelerated atherogenesis in type II diabetic patients. Diabetes 42:1–7
15. Nordt TK, Bode C (2000) Impaired endogenous fibrinolysis in diabetes mellitus: mechanisms and therapeutic approaches. Semin Thromb Hemost 26:495–501
16. Natarajan A, Zaman AG, Marshall SM (2008) Platelet hyperactivity in type 2 diabetes: role of antiplatelet agents. Diab Vasc Dis Res 5:138–144
17. Belch J, MacCuish A, Campbell I et al (2008) The prevention of progression of arterial disease and diabetes (POPADAD) trial: factorial randomized placebo controlled trial of aspirin and antioxidants in patients with diabetes and asymptomatic peripheral arterial disease. Br Med J 337:a1840
18. Seshasai SR, Wijesuriya S, Sivakumaran R et al (2012) Effect of aspirin on vascular and nonvascular outcomes: meta-analysis of randomized controlled trials. Arch Intern Med 172:209–216
19. American Diabetes Association (2011) Executive Summary: Standards of Medical Care in Diabetes—2011. Diabetes Care 34(Suppl 1):S4–S10
20. Pignone M, Alberts MJ, Colwell JA et al (2010) Aspirin for primary prevention of cardiovascular events in people with diabetes: a position statement of the American Diabetes Association, a scientific statement of the American Heart Association, and an expert consensus document of the American College of Cardiology Foundation. Circulation 121:2694–2701

21. Doteval A, Hasdai D, Wallentin L, Battler A, Rosengren A (2005) Diabetes mellitus: clinical presentation and outcome in men and women with acute coronary syndromes. Data from the Euro Heart Survey ACS. Diabet Med 22:1542–1550
22. Donahoe SM, Stewart GC, McGabe CH et al (2007) Diabetes and mortality following acute coronary syndromes. JAMA 298:765–775
23. Hasin T, Hochadel M, Gitt AK et al (2009) Comparison of treatment and outcome of acute coronary syndrome in patients with versus patients without diabetes mellitus. Am J Cardiol 103:772–778
24. Hamm CW, Bassand J-P, Agewall S et al (2011) ESC guidelines for the management of acute coronary syndromes in patients presenting without persistent ST-segment elevation. Eur Heart J 32:2999–3054
25. Steg PG, James SK, Atar D et al (2012) ESC guidelines for the management of acute myocardial infarction in patients presenting with ST-segment elevation. Eur Heart J 33:2569–2619
26. Cannon CP, Weintraub WS, Demopoulos LA et al (2001) Comparison of early invasive and conservative strategies in patients with unstable coronary syndromes treated with the glycoprotein IIb/IIIa inhibitor tirofiban. N Engl J Med 344:1879–1887
27. Hatky MA, Boothroyd DB, Bravata DM et al (2009) Coronary artery bypass surgery compared with percutaneous coronary interventions for multivessel disease: a collaborative analysis of individual patient data from ten randomised trials. Lancet 373:1190–1197
28. Wiviott S, Braunwald E, McGabe C et al (2007) Prasugrel versus clopidogrel in patients with acute coronary syndromes. N Engl J Med 357:2001–2015
29. Wallentin L, Becker RC, Budaj A et al (2009) Ticagrelor versus clopidogrel in patients with acute coronary syndromes. N Engl J Med 361:1045–1057
30. Wiviott SD, Braunwald E, Angiolillo DJ et al (2008) Greater clinical benefit of more intensive oral antiplatelet therapy with prasugrel in patients with diabetes mellitus in the trial to assess improvement in therapeutic outcomes by optimizing platelet inhibition with prasugrel. Thrombolysis in Myocardial Infarction 38. Circulation 118:1626–1636
31. James S, Angiolillo DJ, Cornel JH et al (2010) Ticagrelor vs clopidogrel in patients with acute coronary syndromes and diabetes: a substudy from the PLATelet inhibition and patient Outcomes (PLATO) trial. Eur Heart J 31:3006–3016
32. DiChiara J, Bliden KP, Tantry US et al (2007) The effect of aspirin dosing on platelet function in diabetic and nondiabetic patients: an analysis from Aspirin-Induced Platelet Effect (ASPECT) study. Diabetes 56:3014–3019
33. Rocca B, Santilli F, Pitocco D et al (2012) The recovery of platelet cyclooxygenase activity explains interindividual variability in reponsiveness to low-dose aspirin in patients with and without diabetes. J Thromb Haemost 10:1220–1230
34. CAPRIE Steering Committee (1996) A randomized, blinded trial of clopidogrel versus aspirin in patients at risk of ischaemic events (CAPRIE). Lancet 348:1329–1339
35. Bhatt D, Marso S, Hirsch A et al (2002) Amplified benefit of clopidogrel versus aspirin in patients with diabetes mellitus. Am J Cardiol 90:625–628
36. American Diabetes Association, Colwell JA (2004) Aspirin therapy in diabetes. Diabetes Care 27(Suppl 1):S72–S73
37. Bhatt DL, Fox KA, Hacke W et al (2006) Clopidogrel and aspirin versus aspirin alone for the prevention of atherothrombotic events. N Engl J Med 354:1706–1717
38. Diener HC, Bogousslavsky J, Brass LM et al (2004) Aspirin and copidogrel compared with clopidogrel alone after recent ischaemic stroke or transient ischaemic attack in high-risk patients (MATCH): randomised, double-blind, placebo-controlled trial. Lancet 364:331–337
39. Sacco RL, Diener HC, Yusuf S et al (2008) Aspirin and extended release dipyridamole versus clopidogrel for recurrent stroke. N Engl J Med 359:1238–1251
40. Camm AJ, Lip GY, DeCaterina R et al (2012) Focused update of the ESC guidelines for the management of atrial fibrillation. An update of the 2010 ESC guideline for the management of atrial fibrillation. Developed with the special contribution of the European Heart Rhythm Association. Eur Heart J 33:2719–2747

The Role of Glucagon-like Receptor-1 Agonists in the Metabolic Syndrome

12

Tina Vilsbøll, Salvatore Calanna, and Filip K. Knop

12.1 Introduction to Incretin Hormones and Incretin Effect

The incretin hormones, glucagon-like peptide-1 (GLP-1) and glucose-dependent insulinotropic polypeptide (GIP), are intestinal hormones released in response to nutrient ingestion. Both hormones possess strong glucose-dependent insulinotropic properties and enhance glucose-induced insulin secretion from the beginning of a meal. They are responsible for the so-called incretin effect, which refers to the amplification of insulin secretion that occurs when glucose is ingested orally, as opposed to infused intravenously, in amounts that result in identical glucose excursions—isoglycaemia. The scientific history of the incretin effect extends back to the very early twentieth century, and the scientific interest surrounding it has intensified markedly over time. The incretin effect is defined as the beta-cell secretory response evoked by factors other than glucose itself and is represented by the difference in integrated responses of plasma insulin, plasma C-peptide, or insulin secretion rate, measured during oral glucose ingestion vs. isoglycaemic intravenous (i.v.) glucose infusion. In healthy subjects, the incretin effect accounts for up to 70 % of the total amount of insulin released in response to an oral glucose load (depending on the size of the glucose load: the more glucose ingested, the higher incretin effect elicited). GLP-1 and GIP have been established as important hormones in mimicry experiments in humans, where the hormones were infused

T. Vilsbøll (✉) • F.K. Knop
Diabetes Research Division, Department of Internal Medicine F, Gentofte Hospital, University of Copenhagen, Niels Andersens Vej 65, DK-2900 Hellerup, Denmark
e-mail: t.vilsboll@dadlnet.dk

S. Calanna
Diabetes Research Division, Department of Internal Medicine F, Gentofte Hospital, University of Copenhagen, Niels Andersens Vej 65, DK-2900 Hellerup, Denmark

Department of Clinical and Molecular Biomedicine, University of Catania, Catania, Italy

H. Beck-Nielsen (ed.), *The Metabolic Syndrome*,
DOI 10.1007/978-3-7091-1331-8_12, © Springer-Verlag Wien 2013

together with i.v. glucose to concentrations approximating those observed during oral glucose tolerance tests (OGTT). The action of both hormones is strictly glucose-dependent and consists of potentiation of glucose-induced insulin secretion. Therefore, neither hormone has insulinotropic activity at lower glucose concentrations (less than 4 mM). Nevertheless, experiments have demonstrated that hormones are active already from the beginning of a meal (even at fasting glucose levels) and that they contribute almost equally, but with the effect of GLP-1 predominating at higher glucose levels.

Besides stimulating insulin release (incretin effect), and thereby glucose-uptake, GLP-1 and GIP have several other actions; both hormones stimulate insulin gene transcription, increase pancreatic beta-cell mass, and protect against beta-cell apoptosis. Surprisingly, however, the two hormones exert opposing effects on glucagon secretion: GIP stimulates and GLP-1 inhibits glucagon secretion glucose-dependently. Moreover, only GLP-1 regulates body weight by inhibiting appetite and gastric emptying (possibly through a combination of direct and indirect effects including activation of central GLP-1 receptors) and, perhaps, stimulating resting energy expenditure. Because of these actions, GLP-1-based therapy was recently introduced to the market as a new therapy of type 2 diabetes.

The metabolic syndrome is a constellation of interrelated metabolic disorders that confer a higher risk of type 2 diabetes by reducing glucose sensitivity. It has been recognised as a pro-inflammatory, prothrombotic state, associated with elevated levels of C-reactive protein (CRP), interleukin (IL)-6, and plasminogen activator inhibitor (PAI)-1. The most accepted and unifying hypothesis to describe the pathophysiology of the metabolic syndrome is insulin resistance. As a consequence of excess central adiposity, insulin resistance has been thought to be a key event in the progression of metabolic syndrome. Recent evidence shows that insulin resistance and the incretin axis could be strongly related. Only a limited number of studies have been performed to evaluate the pathophysiology of incretin hormones in the metabolic syndrome as well as other conditions of reduced glucose tolerance and insulin resistance. So far, no differences have been observed in the secretion of GLP-1 after OGTT in patients with metabolic syndrome as compared with individuals without metabolic syndrome [1], while GIP plasma levels were increased in the metabolic syndrome.

It is well known that not all obese individuals have the same risk of developing cardiovascular disease or diabetes; risks differ as a function of insulin sensitivity, with insulin resistant, obese individuals at highest risk. Accordingly, reduced plasma levels of GLP-1, but elevated plasma levels of GIP, were found in obese subjects with high insulin resistance when compared with individuals with normal insulin sensitivity [2]. Another study evaluated secretion of incretin hormones and the incretin effect before and after induction of insulin resistance (using a combination of prednisolone administration, relative physical inactivity, and high-calorie diet), in perfectly healthy young males without a family disposition of type 2 diabetes [3]. Interestingly, these subjects demonstrated an increase in the secretion of GIP and an impaired incretin effect after the short period (12 days) of intervention, while no changes in GLP-1 response were observed (Fig. 12.1).

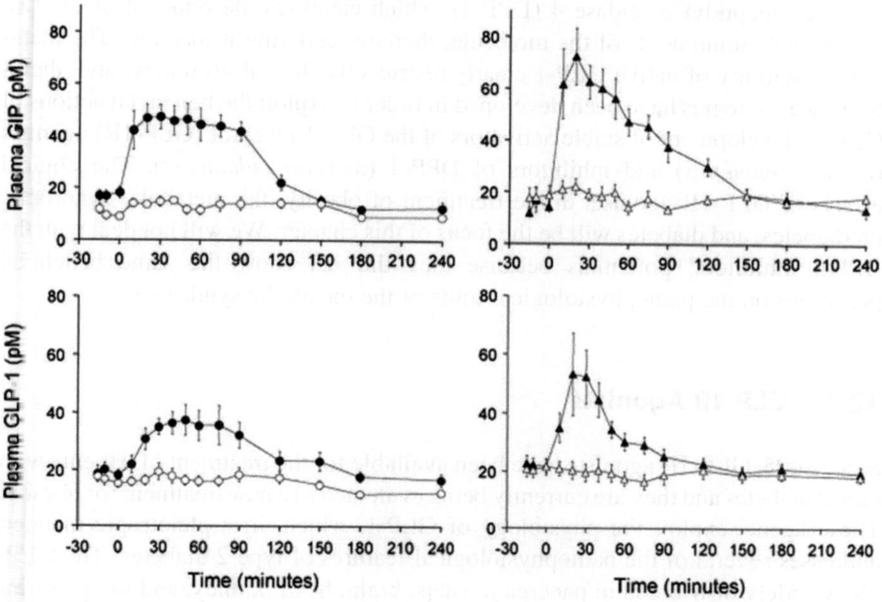

Fig. 12.1 Before intervention (*left, circles*) and after intervention (*right, triangles*) plasma glucose-dependent insulinotropic polypeptide (GIP) (*top*) and glucagon-like peptide-1 (GLP-1) (*bottom*) concentrations in healthy subjects during a 75-g oral glucose tolerance test (*black symbols*) and isoglycaemic glucose infusion IIGI (*white symbols*), respectively [3]

GLP-1 and GIP could play opposite roles in the metabolic syndrome and insulin resistance conditions. GIP, with its properties on lipid accumulation, glucagon stimulation, and pro-inflammatory effects on adipose tissue, could potentially be involved centrally in the pathogenesis of the metabolic syndrome, promoting or worsening insulin resistance and shortening the gap to developing diabetes. In contrast, GLP-1, with its favourable effects on body weight, lipid metabolism, blood pressure, and fasting glucose, presents an interesting potential for the use in the treatment of the metabolic syndrome. The rest of this chapter will focus on the beneficial actions of GLP-1 as a potential treatment of the metabolic syndrome.

12.2 GLP-1-Based Therapy

Patients with type 2 diabetes have preserved insulinotropic and glucagonostatic actions of GLP-1, and intravenous infusion of supraphysiological doses of GLP-1 is able to completely normalise plasma glucose in patients with long-standing and severe disease. However, a short duration of action of GLP-1 (minutes), due to an extremely rapid and extensive degradation, leaves the intact peptide with an apparent half-life in the body of 1–2 min and a plasma clearance amounting to 2–3 times the cardiac output. This degradation is due to the action of the ubiquitous enzyme dipeptidyl peptidase 4 (DPP-4), which catalyses the removal of the two N-terminal amino acids of the molecule, thereby rendering it inactive. The metabolic instability of native GLP-1 clearly restricts its clinical usefulness and, therefore, two strategies have been developed in order to exploit the beneficial actions of GLP-1: development of stable activators of the GLP-1 receptor (GLP-1R) agonists (*incretin mimetics*) and inhibitors of DPP-4 (*incretin enhancers*). The clinical effects of GLP-1R agonists in the treatment of obesity, the metabolic syndrome, prediabetes, and diabetes will be the focus of this chapter. We will not deal with the DPP-4 inhibitors' potentials because they did not show the same beneficial properties on the pathophysiological traits of the metabolic syndrome.

12.2.1 GLP-1R Agonists

Since 2005, GLP-1R agonists have been available for the treatment of patients with type 2 diabetes and they are currently being evaluated as a new treatment for obesity. These agents exploit the physiology of GLP-1, which, in a pleiotropic manner, addresses several of the pathophysiological features of type 2 diabetes. The GLP-1R is widely distributed in pancreatic islets, brain, heart, kidney, and the gastrointestinal tract including the stomach. Its function is not known for all these locations and numerous attempts have been made to identify alternative GLP-1Rs or subtypes, but at present only a single GLP-1R has been identified. Binding of GLP-1 to the GLP-1R on the beta-cell results in stimulation of insulin secretion in a strict glucose-dependent manner, but preclinical data have demonstrated that GLP-1 also has potential effects on beta-cell mass by stimulation of beta-cell proliferation, by differentiation of new beta-cells from progenitor cells, and by inhibition of beta-cell apoptosis. Furthermore, GLP-1R agonists robustly inhibit glucagon secretion, and the combined effects on insulin and glucagon secretion result in inhibition of hepatic glucose production, which contributes significantly to the overall glucose-lowering effect of GLP-1R agonists seen in patients with type 2 diabetes. Additionally, GLP-1 decreases gastrointestinal motility and promotes satiety, probably through activation of GLP-1Rs in the central nervous system in combination with GLP-1-induced decrease in gastric emptying. Clinical data have now demonstrated that chronic administration of GLP-1R agonists leads to weight loss.

12.3 Clinical Aspects of GLP-1R in the Treatment of Diabetes

Many meta-analyses, on data from randomised, controlled trials assessing GLP-1R agonists administered for longer periods, have been published. The results provide evidence that intervention with clinical relevant doses of currently available GLP-1R agonists (exenatide, exenatide once weekly, and liraglutide) facilitates reduction in body weight in obese patients both with and without diabetes. GLP-1R agonists also had beneficial effects on the systolic and diastolic blood pressure and cholesterol. For patients with type 2 diabetes, GLP-1R agonists improved glycaemic control (as assessed by HbA1c and fasting plasma glucose) and increased the proportion of patients who achieved their target HbA1c [4].

12.3.1 Specific GLP-1R Agonists

The development of the GLP-1R agonists is based on two different approaches. One strategy exploits the structure of native human GLP-1, modified in a way so that it is resistant to degradation by DPP-4, as the backbone for the compounds. The other approach uses a naturally occurring protein—exendin-4, originally isolated from the saliva of the lizard Heloderma suspectum—as the backbone of the compounds. Exendin-4 has a 53 % sequence homology with human GLP-1 in its first 30 amino acids and binds to and activates the GLP-1R with equal potency as human GLP-1. Today, three GLP-1R agonists have been approved for the treatment of type 2 diabetes, and all are injected subcutaneously: exenatide twice daily (Byetta®, Amylin/Lilly) and exenatide once weekly (Bydureon®, Amylin/Lilly), based on exendin-4, and liraglutide (Victoza®, Novo Nordisk), based on the structure of native human GLP-1, once daily (Fig. 12.2).

Exenatide was the first GLP-1R agonist to reach the market and was approved by the United States Food and Drug Administration in 2005 and by the European Medicines Agency (EMA) in 2007. Exenatide is a synthetic version of exendin-4 and is resistant to inactivation by DPP-4. Exenatide is primarily cleared by the kidneys by glomerular filtration, and the half-life after subcutaneous injection is approximately 2–3 h. Exenatide, therefore, has to be administered twice daily to achieve 24-h pharmacological plasma concentrations. In the early clinical AC2993: Diabetes Management for Improving Glucose Outcome (AMIGO) trials, the effects of exenatide were investigated in a total of 1,446 randomised patients. Exenatide was given as add-on therapy to metformin, sulphonylurea (SU), or both, and these studies reported statistically significant improvement of glycaemic control in the exenatide treatment groups (change of HbA1c of −1.0 % (baseline of 8.2 %) vs. an increase of approximately 0.2 % in the placebo groups) and change in fasting plasma glucose (−0.5 mM vs. an increase of nearly 1 mM in the placebo groups). On average, the weight loss in the three studies comparing exenatide with oral antidiabetics amounted to 1.6 kg (baseline of 95 kg) in the exenatide-treated patients. Additionally, a significant reduction in systolic blood pressure compared with placebo (difference of 2.8 mmHg) or insulin (difference of 3.7 mmHg) has been reported after 6 months of treatment with exenatide. In 2011, a large database analysis investigating the relative incidence of cardiovascular disease events in patients with type 2 diabetes either treated with exenatide twice daily ($n = 39{,}275$) or with other glucose-lowering agents ($n = 381{,}218$) was published. The study reported that treatment with exenatide twice daily was associated with a significantly lower risk of cardiovascular disease events than treatment with other glucose-lowering agents.

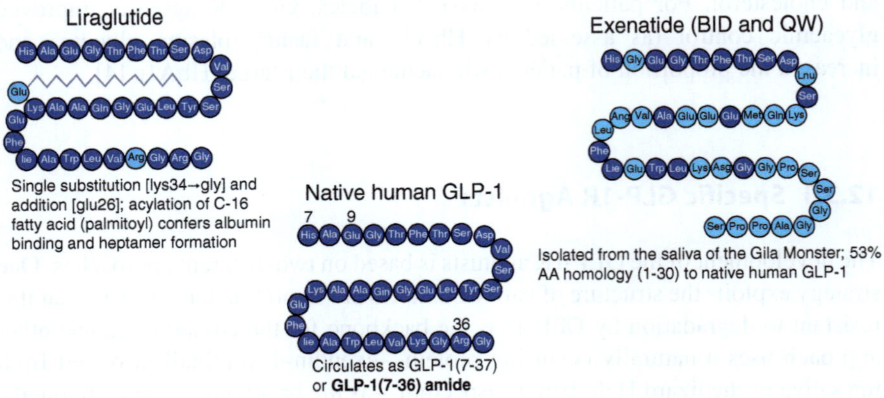

Fig. 12.2 Structure of glucagon-like peptide-1 (GLP-1) receptor agonists

12.3.2 Exenatide Once Weekly

Exenatide has been developed in a sustained-release formulation for once-weekly subcutaneous administration. The exenatide molecules are encapsulated in injectable microspheres, which consist of a biodegradable medical polymer also used in other extended-release pharmaceuticals. These microspheres allow gradual drug delivery at a controlled rate by diffusion and erosion of the microspheres. The clinical effects of exenatide once weekly have been examined in the Diabetes Therapy Utilisation: Researching changes in HbA1c, weight, and other factors Through Intervention with exenatide Once-weekly (DURATION) 1–6 trials. In all the DURATION trials, exenatide once weekly lowered HbA1c and body weight significantly. The HbA1c reduction by exenatide once weekly was up to 1.6 %, and in most cases this reduction was greater or similar to that of the comparator. Overall, a reduction in body weight by exenatide once weekly was seen in the range of 2.1–2.6 kg. The DURATION-6 study, comparing exenatide once weekly with liraglutide once daily, is a 26-week head-to-head, open-label study including approximately 900 patients with type 2 diabetes who were inadequately controlled with diet and exercise in conjunction with metformin, SU, metformin plus an SU or metformin plus a thiazolidinedione (TZD) [5]. The study revealed that patients receiving exenatide once weekly experienced a reduction in HbA1c of 1.3 % compared with 1.5 % for liraglutide. The mean change in weight from baseline to posttreatment assessment was −2.7 kg for exenatide and −3.6 kg for liraglutide, with a mean difference of 0.9 kg overall. Thus, exenatide once weekly therefore did not meet the pre-specified primary endpoint of non-inferiority to liraglutide with regard to HbA1c and body weight reductions. However, exenatide once weekly did appear to be slightly better tolerated than liraglutide with less gastrointestinal side effects (such as nausea and vomiting). Injection site reactions were observed more frequently in patients treated with exenatide once weekly vs. comparator-treated patients (16 % vs. range of 2–7 %) during the 6 months controlled phase of studies.

These injection site reactions were generally mild and usually did not lead to withdrawal from studies. Most individual nodules were asymptomatic, did not interfere with study participation, and resolved over 4–8 weeks.

Liraglutide is an acylated analogue of human GLP-1 (with 97 % homology with native GLP-1), which was approved for clinical use in Europe in 2009 and in the United States in 2010. In liraglutide, a C-16 acyl chain is linked to amino acid 20 via a γ-glutamic acid spacer, and the lysine in position 28 of native GLP-1 is exchanged with arginine. These changes result in a half-life after subcutaneous administration of approximately 11–15 h, making it suitable for once-daily dosing. The clinical effects of liraglutide treatment have been investigated in the Liraglutide Effect and Action in Diabetes (LEAD) series of phase III studies. These trials, lasting up to 52 weeks, showed that treatment with liraglutide both as monotherapy and in combination with metformin, SU, or TZD plus metformin lowered HbA1c and body weight. Liraglutide-induced change in HbA1c varied from −0.8 to −1.6 % (baseline HbA1c of 8.2–8.5 %), reductions that in most cases were similar or greater than compared with the oral comparator drug. Overall, a reduction in body weight was seen in all trials in the range of 2–3 kg, much like other phase III studies with liraglutide compared with placebo, and not different from exenatide. In the LEAD-6 study, liraglutide and exenatide were compared head to head. A significantly greater reduction in HbA1c with liraglutide than with exenatide treatment was observed (1.1 vs. 0.8 %), as well as greater reduction in fasting plasma glucose (1.6 vs. 0.6 mM, respectively). Furthermore, greater reductions in triglycerides (0.4 vs. 0.2 mM) and free fatty acids (FFA) (0.17 vs. 0.10 mM) in the liraglutide group were also observed. Both liraglutide and exenatide caused significant decreases in blood pressure. Newly published data from a 14 weeks extension of the LEAD-6 phase IIIb study, where subjects either continued with liraglutide or switched from exenatide to liraglutide, showed that switching from exenatide to liraglutide further and significantly reduced HbA1c (0.3 %), fasting plasma glucose (0.9 mM), and body weight (0.9 kg).

12.3.3 Safety of GLP-1R Agonists

GLP-1R agonists are associated with dose-dependent adverse events with gastrointestinal side effects (mild to moderate) including nausea, vomiting, and diarrhoea, which are the most common. These side effects often cease over time and do not seem to affect the number of losses to follow-up, which is in agreement with recent evidence showing that the overall patient satisfaction with GLP-1R agonists is relatively high. The incidence of treatment-associated hypoglycaemia is reported to be low. In fact, occurrence of hypoglycaemia during GLP-1R agonist treatment combined with metformin is similar to when metformin is used as monotherapy. However, combined with SU the risk of minor hypoglycaemic episodes is reported to be in the range of 15–36 % for exenatide and 8–25 % for liraglutide.

Antibody formation to therapeutic peptides is common. Recently, an analysis characterising the time course and cross-reactivity of anti-exenatide antibodies and potential effects on efficacy and safety has been published. No obvious correlation between change in HbA1c and titre was observed for exenatide twice daily, although mean reductions were attenuated in the small subset of patients (5 %) with higher titres. A significant correlation was observed for exenatide once weekly with no difference between antibody-negative and low-titre patients, but an attenuated mean reduction in the subset of patients (12 %) with higher titres. Thus, low-titre anti-exenatide antibodies were common with exenatide treatment (32 % exenatide twice daily, 45 % exenatide once weekly), but had no apparent effect on efficacy. Among liraglutide-treated patients only 4–10 % developed antibodies (low titres) and no correlation to impaired efficacy was observed. The exact impact of auto-antibodies on efficacy and safety in the longer term remains to be established.

After the approval of exenatide and liraglutide, post-marketing reports of several incidents of acute pancreatitis in patients treated with exenatide and liraglutide have been disclosed. However, it is not evident that the incidence of acute pancreatitis is higher in those receiving exenatide or liraglutide than in the background type 2 diabetic populations. Still, it is recommended that GLP-1R agonists are not used in subjects with a history of, or increased risk of, pancreatitis. Lately, the risk of pancreatic cancer has been discussed in patients treated with exenatide compared with other antidiabetic medications. However, EMA recently concluded that a correlation between GLP-1R agonists and pancreatic malignancies could not yet be confirmed nor excluded. In carcinogenicity studies with liraglutide, C cell tumours were observed in thyroid tissue of mice and rats. However, recent data identify key differences between rodent models, nonhuman primates, and humans with regard to this, and the long-term consequences of sustained GLP-1R activation in the human thyroid require further investigation, but so far no changes in thyroid function have been reported in clinical trials with GLP-1R agonists.

An increase in heart rate (by 2–4 beats per minute) has been reported during treatment with liraglutide and exenatide. Even a small increase in heart rate accompanying a decrease in blood pressure is, however, potentially troubling, as an increased heart rate is an independent risk factor for cardiac mortality. The mechanism behind the change in heart rate is not known, but may involve increased natriuresis and lowered blood pressure. In one study, patients with obesity, but without diabetes, were treated with liraglutide and an increase was detected in the heart rate for only the first 30 weeks of treatment. The patients' heart rates subsequently returned to basal levels. Whether the benefit of the decrease in blood pressure outweighs the harm of the temporary increase in heart rate remains to be determined. Several large cardiovascular outcome trials (liraglutide effect and action in diabetes: evaluation of cardiovascular outcome results—a long term evaluation (LEADER, liraglutid), exenatide study (EXSCEL, exenatide once weekly), evaluation of cardiovascular outcomes in patients with type 2 diabetes after acute coronary syndrome during treatment with lixisenatide (ELIXA, lixisenatide), and researching cardiovascular events with a weekly incretin in diabetes (REWIND, dulaglutide)) including up to 9,500 patients with type 2 diabetes are ongoing and are expected to be completed between 2016 and 2019.

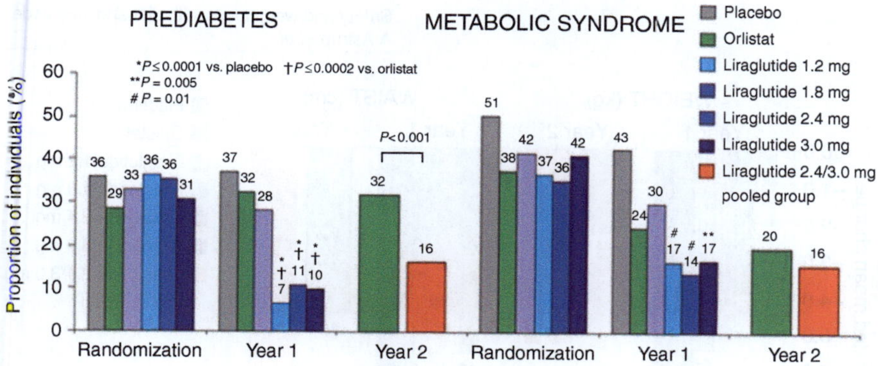

Fig. 12.3 The prevalence of prediabetes and the metabolic syndrome after one year of treatment with liraglutide 1.2–3.0 mg or placebo or orlistat and after two years with liraglutide 2.4–3.0 mg or orlistat. Prediabetes defined as either impaired fasting plasma glucose (FPG) (5.6–6.9 mM) or impaired glucose tolerance (7.8–11.0 mM) after two-hour oral glucose tolerance test (75 g glucose) [6]

12.4 Therapeutic and Pharmacological Potential in the Metabolic Syndrome

The fascinating extra-pancreatic properties of GLP-1R agonists, showed in type 2 diabetes patients, make these drugs potential candidates for the treatment of the metabolic syndrome. GLP-1R agonists have been shown to reduce the prevalence of the metabolic syndrome and prediabetes in obese adults subjects [6] (Fig. 12.3).

The separate impact of these drugs on lipid and glucose metabolism, as well as body weight and blood pressure, should be elucidated. Table 1.1 (Chap. 1) shows the newest criteria from the International Diabetes Federation (IDF) [7] for clinical diagnosis of the metabolic syndrome: Three or more components must be fulfilled to give the diagnosis. The effect of GLP-1R agonists on each target will be discussed separately.

12.4.1 GLP-1R Agonists and Waist Circumference

GLP-1R agonists have considerable effects on body weight. Increased body weight is a major risk factor for developing the metabolic syndrome. Obesity increases mortality and morbidity as well as the frequency of type 2 diabetes, hypertension, non-alcoholic fatty liver disease (NAFLD), and physical disability. It is associated with resistance to the effects of insulin on peripheral glucose and fatty acid utilisation. The metabolic syndrome criteria take into consideration the waist circumference as an indicator of the central, visceral fat. Visceral fat is considered an independent risk factor for cardiovascular disease, because it has a higher degree of lipolytic turnover and higher secretion of adipokines and inflammatory cytokines, in comparison to subcutaneous fat. Subcutaneous (extraperitoneal) fat, conversely,

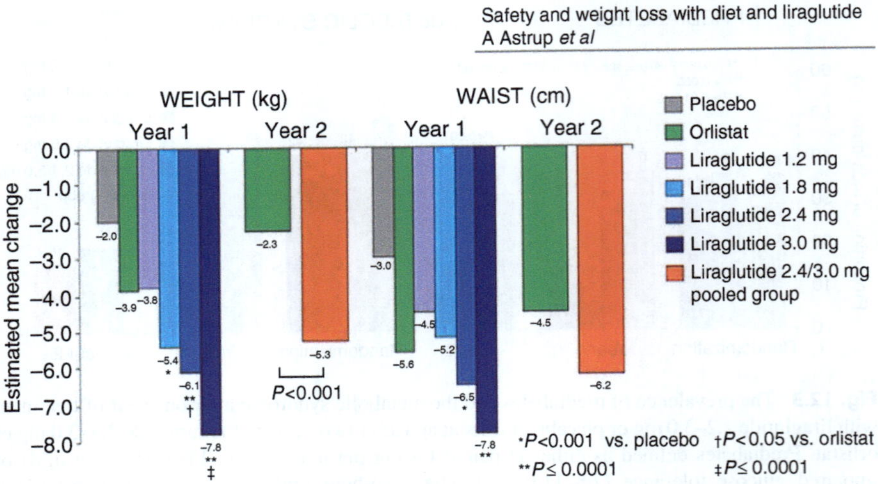

Fig. 12.4 Mean changes in body weight and waist circumference in obese non-diabetic adults after one year of treatment with liraglutide, 1.2–3.0 mg, placebo, or orlistat, and after 2 years with liraglutide, 2.4–3.0 mg, or orlistat [6]

functions as a neutral reservoir for the storage of excess lipids and, in patients with metabolic syndrome, is often lacking or dysfunctional. Indeed, enlarged fat cells are observed, resistant to the anti-lipolytic effects of insulin and incompetent to adequately store fat, which in turn leads to fat deposition ectopically in other organ systems. The change in percentage of visceral and subcutaneous adipose tissue, with consequent different pattern of pro-inflammatory cytokines and insulin resistance degree, could be the primary driver behind the cluster of pathophysiological traits in the metabolic syndrome. It may also be the basis for the existence of diverse subsets of patients, among obese patients characterised by a favourable metabolic profile (metabolically healthy but obese) or at-risk obese subjects.

In obese, non-diabetic adults, the estimated mean weight loss after 1 year of treatment with liraglutide (1.8–3.0 mg once daily) was significantly greater compared with placebo, and mean change in waist circumference was significantly greater both after 1 year vs. placebo and after 2 years with liraglutide, 2.4–3.0 mg, vs. orlistat (Fig. 12.4) [6].

In a recent meta-analysis [4], including data from 25 randomised, controlled trials, assessing clinically relevant doses of GLP-1R agonists given for at least 20 weeks, the treatment with GLP-1R agonists reduced body weight in patients, who were overweight or obese, compared with placebo, oral antidiabetic drugs, or insulin. Three of the included trials assessed the effect of GLP-1R agonists on patients without type 2 diabetes and 22 assessed patients with type 2 diabetes. The mean reduction in body weight achieved with the highest dose of GLP-1R agonists (20 μg/day for exenatide; 1.8 mg/day for liraglutide) ranged from −7.2 to −0.2 kg (Fig. 12.5).

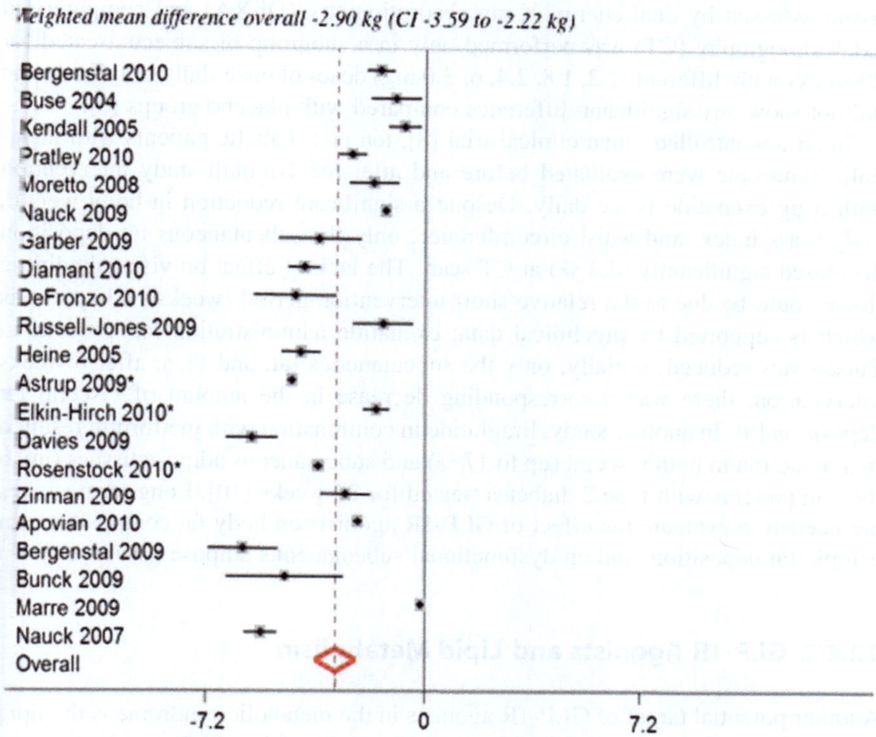

Fig. 12.5 Meta-analysis of change in body weight (kg), including data from 25 randomised, controlled trials included after at least 20 weeks of treatment with GLP-1R agonists, in comparison with placebo, no intervention, or other antidiabetic drugs [4]

Subgroup analyses showed a greater weight loss after treatment with the highest doses of GLP-1R agonists. Weight reduction was present both in patients without diabetes (−3.2 kg, −4.3 to −2.1) and in those with diabetes (−2.8 kg, −3.4 to −2.3). There was no difference in body weight changes for patients assigned to liraglutide or exenatide twice daily (−0.4 kg, 95 % confidence interval −1.3 to 0.6), or for those assigned exenatide as a long-acting release vs. exenatide twice daily (−0.6 kg, −1.5 to 0.3).

The favourable effect on body weight and waist circumference could give GLP-1R agonists a leading role in the treatment of the metabolic syndrome. However, body weight and waist circumference are only surrogate markers of high-risk conditions and not diseases per se. For this reason, before considering the clinical use of GLP-1R agonists in patients with metabolic syndrome, the effect of these drugs on the distribution of visceral and subcutaneous fat should be elucidated.

In the above-mentioned study by Astrup et al. [6], the changes in body weight and waist circumference occur simultaneously with the reduction of adipocytokines and inflammatory markers associated with visceral obesity, such as fibrinogen, PAI-1, and highly sensitive CRP. Nevertheless, the estimation of visceral adipose tissue assessed by dual-energy X-ray absorptiometry (DEXA) and computerised axial tomography (CT) was performed only in a subgroup of subjects treated for 20 weeks with different (1.2, 1.8, 2.4, or 3.0 mg) doses of once-daily liraglutide and did not show any significant difference compared with placebo groups [6].

In an uncontrolled, open clinical trial [8], ten non-diabetic patients with metabolic syndrome were evaluated before and after the 1-month study intervention with 5 μg exenatide twice daily. Despite a significant reduction in body weight, body mass index, and waist circumference, only the subcutaneous fat deposition decreased significantly (4.4 %) at CT scan. The lack of effect on visceral adipose tissue could be due to the relative short intervention period (weeks), a hypothesis which is supported by preclinical data; exenatide administration for 4 weeks in Zucker rats reduced, initially, only the subcutaneous fat, and then, after 8 weeks intervention, there was a corresponding decrease in the amount of visceral fat deposition [9]. In another study, liraglutide in combination with metformin resulted in a reduction in both visceral (up to 17 %) and subcutaneous adipose tissues (up to 9 %) in patients with type 2 diabetes treated for 26 weeks [10]. Long-term studies are needed to evaluate the effect of GLP-1R agonists on body fat composition, on ectopic fat deposition, and on dysfunctional subcutaneous adipose tissue.

12.4.2 GLP-1R Agonists and Lipid Metabolism

Another potential target of GLP-1R agonists in the metabolic syndrome is the lipid profile. Elevated plasma triglyceride concentrations and low high-density lipoprotein (HDL) cholesterol concentrations are associated with increased intima-media thickness and endothelial dysfunction and with high risk of macrovascular diseases, such as myocardial infarction or stroke.

Astrup et al. [6] showed that obese non-diabetic adults, after 2 years treatment with liraglutide (2.4–3.0 mg once daily) vs. orlistat, had increased HDL cholesterol and reduced plasma triglyceride levels (no effects of liraglutide vs. placebo or vs. orlistat on fasting lipids were apparent after 1 year of treatment).

Also, Meier et al. [11] showed that the administration of native GLP-1 during the ingestion of a mixed test meal is able to decrease postprandial triglycerides in healthy young men with normal triglycerides levels at baseline in comparison to placebo (Fig. 12.6).

This could be due to the effect of GLP-1 on the deceleration of gastric emptying or a possible inhibition of fat absorption from the gut. Moreover, the GLP-1 infusion markedly reduced the FFA levels that are chronically increased in individuals with dysfunctional adipose tissue. The elevated plasma FFA stimulate gluconeogenesis, induce hepatic and muscle insulin resistance, and impair insulin secretion in genetically predisposed individuals.

Exenatide treatment for 3.5 years, in 151 patients with type 2 diabetes, reduced serum triglyceride levels by 12 % (a reduction from baseline of 44 mg/dl), total cholesterol levels by 5 % (a reduction of 11 mg/dl), and low-density lipoprotein (LDL) cholesterol levels by 6 % (a reduction of 12 mg/dl) and increased HDL cholesterol levels by 24 % (a rise of 9 mg/dl) [12]. However, in 232 patients with

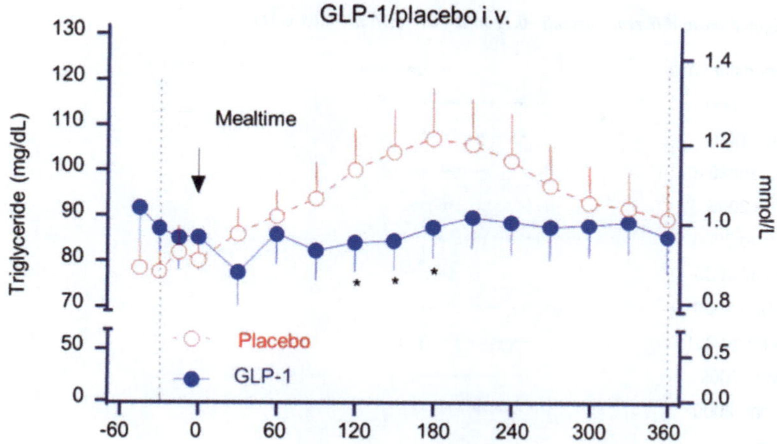

Fig. 12.6 Plasma concentrations of triglycerides during intravenous administration of glucagon-like peptide-1 (GLP-1) (1.2 pmol × kg^{-1} × min^{-1}, *filled circles*) or placebo (*open circles*) in 14 healthy male subjects. At $t = 0$ min, a mixed meal (1.05 MJ) meal was served (*arrows*). Data are mean ± SEM. *$p < 0.05$ for differences vs. placebo at individual time points [11]

type 2 diabetes (who had not previously taken any antidiabetic drugs), treated with exenatide in a double-blind, placebo-controlled study, no significant changes were found in total HDL cholesterol or LDL cholesterol levels [13].

In other papers, only modest reductions of fasting triglycerides have been reported after GLP-1R agonist treatment [14, 15]. Whether the changes in HDL cholesterol and triglyceride plasma levels associated with GLP-1 treatment have any clinical benefit is unknown. Moreover, whether these changes are a direct result of altered lipid metabolism or are an indirect effect of GLP-1-induced weight loss remains to be determined.

On the other hand, with regard to the reduction of total cholesterol [4] (Fig. 12.7) and LDL cholesterol [6, 14], GLP-1R agonists have shown fascinating properties.

Total cholesterol, and especially LDL cholesterol, plays a central role in the development of atherosclerosis and increased plasma levels are strongly associated with cardiovascular disease and mortality. Although it is not included in the main criteria of the metabolic syndrome, in people with this condition, LDL plasma levels of less than 80–100 mg/dl are recommended. Lipid-lowering therapy should be considered if diet and weight loss do not adequately reduce LDL levels. A drug with favourable effects on triglycerides, HDL cholesterol, and LDL cholesterol can be thought to reduce the number of drugs and increase compliance.

12.4.3 GLP-1R Agonists and Blood Pressure

Elevated blood pressure is an established risk factor for cardiovascular disease. GLP-1R agonists seem to reduce blood pressure independently of GLP-1R

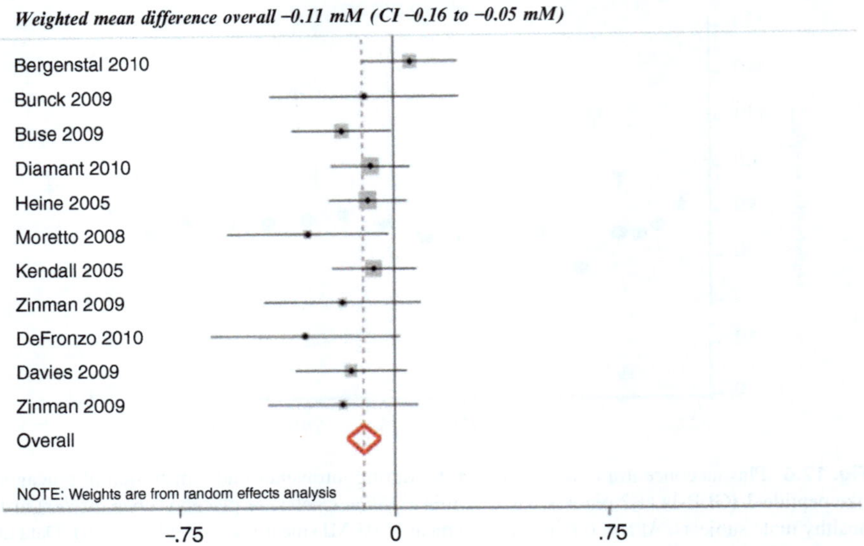

Fig. 12.7 Meta-analysis of change in concentration of total cholesterol (mM), including data from 25 randomised, controlled trials, after at least 20 weeks of treatment with glucagon-like peptide-1 receptor (GLP-1R) agonists, in comparison with placebo, no intervention, or other antidiabetic drugs [4]

agonist-induced weight loss. In the Liraglutide Effect and Action in Diabetes (LEAD) study that compared the effects of liraglutide with other antidiabetic drugs, it was shown that treatment with liraglutide reduced systolic blood pressure by 2–6 mmHg and diastolic blood pressure by 1–2 mmHg. These reductions were observed after 1–2 weeks of treatment and preceded any significant weight loss. The exact mechanisms behind these blood pressure-lowering effects could be several (Fig. 12.8) [16]: increased urine excretion and natriuresis; activation of neural pathways leading to decreased sympathetic nervous system activity; increased insulin production leading to vasodilatation; direct vasodilatory action through GLP-1R stimulation in blood vessels; and/or improved endothelial function owing to inhibition of the adverse effects of hyperglycaemia. In animals, GLP-1R agonists can also reach the area postrema in the brain (via leaks in the blood–brain barrier) and stimulate vagal afferent fibres (via GLP-1R in the gut and the hepatic portal vein). Signalling within the brainstem and hypothalamus may result in activation of vagal efferent fibres and sympathetic neurons. These events can be thought to affect pulse rate, contractions of the heart, vascular tone, catecholamine secretion from the adrenal medulla, and urine and sodium output in the kidney, thereby modulating blood pressure.

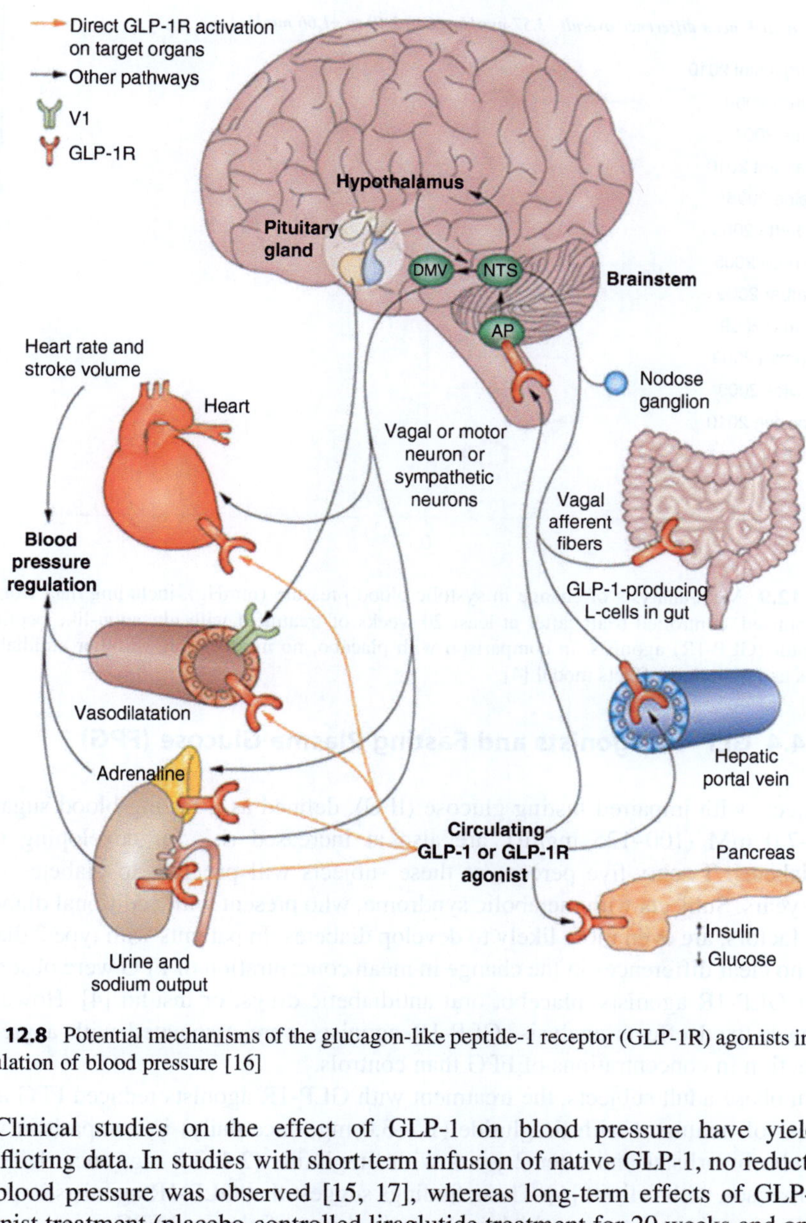

Fig. 12.8 Potential mechanisms of the glucagon-like peptide-1 receptor (GLP-1R) agonists in the regulation of blood pressure [16]

Clinical studies on the effect of GLP-1 on blood pressure have yielded conflicting data. In studies with short-term infusion of native GLP-1, no reduction of blood pressure was observed [15, 17], whereas long-term effects of GLP-1R agonist treatment (placebo-controlled liraglutide treatment for 20 weeks and open-label treatment for 2 years) in non-diabetic obese subjects resulted in significant reductions in systolic blood pressure (by up to 7.0 mmHg after 1 year and 4.6 mmHg after 2 years) [6]. Accordingly, our recent meta-analysis found that GLP-1R agonists reduced systolic blood pressure and diastolic blood pressure after long-term treatment (Fig. 12.9) [4].

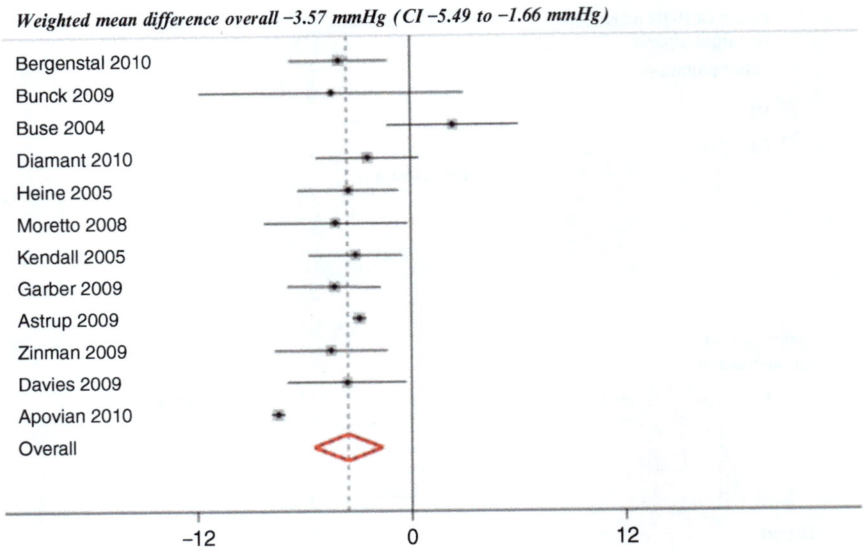

Fig. 12.9 Meta-analysis of change in systolic blood pressure (mmHg), including data from 25 randomised, controlled trials, after at least 20 weeks of treatment with glucagon-like peptide-1 receptor (GLP-1R) agonists, in comparison with placebo, no intervention, or other antidiabetic drugs using random effects model [4]

12.4.4 GLP-1R Agonists and Fasting Plasma Glucose (FPG)

Subjects with impaired fasting glucose (IFG), defined as a fasting blood sugar of 5.6–7.0 mM (100–125 mg/dl), are also at increased risk for developing type 2 diabetes. Twenty-five percent of these subjects will progress to diabetes over 3–5 years. Subjects with metabolic syndrome, who present with additional diabetes risk factors, are even more likely to develop diabetes. In patients with type 2 diabetes, no clear differences in the change in mean concentration of FPG were observed after GLP-1R agonists, placebo, oral antidiabetic drugs, or insulin [4]. However, using a fixed effects analysis, GLP-1R agonists were associated with a greater reduction in concentrations of FPG than controls.

In obese adult subjects, the treatment with GLP-1R agonists reduced FPG after 1 year of treatment with liraglutide (1.2–3.0 mg, once daily) in comparison with placebo or orlistat and after 2 years with liraglutide (2.4–3.0 mg, once daily) in comparison with orlistat [6]. These findings suggest that GLP-1R agonists improve hepatic insulin resistance, which is the main driver of elevated FPG.

12.5 Perspectives and Conclusion(s)

Overall, incretin-based therapy seems to target several of the metabolic derangements characterising the metabolic syndrome. First, these drugs provide significant improvements in glycaemic parameters by improving the function of both beta-cells and alpha-cells in the pancreatic islets. Second, the wide distribution and pleiotropic effects of GLP-1 signalling generally confer favourable effects on several of the co-morbidities of the metabolic syndrome and are expected to provide reductions in cardiovascular morbidity and mortality. Several large-scaled phase IV trials of incretin-based therapy with cardiovascular disease endpoints are ongoing and hold the promise to convey a cardiovascular risk reduction in type 2 diabetes. Third, the promising preclinical effects seen on beta-cell proliferation and preservation could hold true to some extent in humans too, thereby offering the potential to improve the natural history of type 2 diabetes. Nonetheless, we still need the clinical evidence that long-term treatment with incretin-based therapy will indeed attenuate the progressive nature of diabetes in humans.

The emerging GLP-1R agonists, to be introduced to the market in the next years, seem to be well tolerated (with some clinical relevant differences in head-to-head trials). Nevertheless, the general, and probably limiting, issue in regard to the treatment of patients with type 2 diabetes is the gastrointestinal side effects (nausea and diarrhoea). In spite of these side effects being mild to moderate, transient, and probably less frequent with the once-weekly GLP-1R agonists compared with the once-daily and twice-daily GLP-1R agonists currently on the market (likely because of reduced peak concentrations with the once-weekly compounds), the use will still be limited in some patients. Furthermore, the importance of antibody formation is not fully known. Although, so far, available data do not indicate that moderate antibody formation attenuates the clinical efficacy of the GLP-1R agonists. However, patients with high titres of antibodies seem to have less benefit of GLP-1R agonist treatment with regard to glycaemic control compared with patients who do not develop antibodies. It seems that compounds based on the exendin-4 backbone have a tendency to induce antibody formation at higher rates compared with the compounds built on the backbone of human GLP-1, plausible because of the closer resemblance to native GLP-1 of the latter. So far, no safety problems associated with the formation of antibodies against the GLP-1R agonists have been reported.

Within the next years, comparable efficacy and safety data, especially with regard to long-term safety and cardiovascular disease risk reduction of different GLP-1R agonists, are expected to be clarified further. The observations that GLP-1 might improve cardiovascular function and cardiovascular disease biomarkers in humans raise great expectations for the ongoing prospective trials. Furthermore, in coming years, other indications for incretin-based therapy may also be established. Importantly, an expansion of the indication to the treatment of obesity could be within reach, as exemplified by recent trials with GLP-1R agonists in obese non-diabetic subjects.

In patients identified as having the metabolic syndrome, aggressive lifestyle intervention (weight reduction and physical activity) is warranted to reduce the risks of type 2 diabetes and cardiovascular disease, but often this is not sufficient. The use of GLP-1R agonists could drastically modify or reverse the progression of the metabolic syndrome, through the fascinating effects on body weight and blood pressure, as well as on glucose and lipid metabolism. In several cohorts, the risk of diabetes increased with increasing number of components of the metabolic syndrome, and the pleiotropic effects of GLP-1R agonists may hold promise for the treatment of this multi-faceted condition.

Conflict of interest. The authors have no conflict of interests in relation to the present paper.

References

1. Calanna S, Urbano F, Piro S, Zagami RM, Di Pino A, Spadaro L, Purrello F, Rabuazzo AM (2012) Elevated plasma glucose-dependent insulinotropic polypeptide associates with hyperinsulinemia in metabolic syndrome. Eur J Endocrinol 166:917–922
2. Calanna S, Piro S, Pino A Di, Zagami RM, Urbano F, Purrello F, Rabuazzo AM (2012) Beta and alpha cell function in metabolically healthy but obese (MHO) subjects: relationship with entero-insular axis. Obesity in press (accepted 18-06-2012)
3. Hansen KB, Vilsbøll T, Bagger JI, Holst JJ, Knop FK (2010) Reduced glucose tolerance and insulin resistance induced by steroid treatment, relative physical inactivity, and high-calorie diet impairs the incretin effect in healthy subjects. J Clin Endocrinol Metab 95:3309–3317
4. Vilsbøll T, Christensen M, Junker AE, Knop FK, Gluud LL (2012) Effects of glucagon-like peptide-1 receptor agonists on weight loss: systematic review and meta-analyses of randomised controlled trials. BMJ 344:d7771
5. Buse JB et al. (2012) Exenatide once weekly versus liraglutide once daily in patients with type 2 diabetes (DURATION-6): a randomised,open-label study. Lancet. Published online 7 Nov 2012
6. Astrup A, Carraro R, Finer N, Harper A, Kunesova M, Lean MEJ, Niskanen L, Rasmussen MF, Rissanen A, Rössner S, Savolainen MJ, Van Gaal L (2012) Safety, tolerability and sustained weight loss over 2 years with the once-daily human GLP-1 analog, liraglutide. Int J Obes (Lond) 36:843–854
7. Alberti KGMM, Eckel RH, Grundy SM, Zimmet PZ, Cleeman JI, Donato KA, Fruchart J-C, James WPT, Loria CM, Smith SC Jr (2009) Harmonizing the metabolic syndrome: a joint interim statement of the International Diabetes Federation Task Force on Epidemiology and Prevention; National Heart, Lung, and Blood Institute; American Heart Association; World Heart Federation; International Atherosclerosis Society; and International Association for the Study of Obesity. Circulation 120:1640–1645
8. González-Ortiz M, Martínez-Abundis E, Robles-Cervantes JA, Ramos-Zavala MG (2011) Effect of exenatide on fat deposition and a metabolic profile in patients with metabolic syndrome. Metab Syndr Relat Disord 9:31–34
9. Szayna M, Doyle ME, Betkey JA, Holloway HW, Spencer RG, Greig NH, Egan JM (2000) Exendin-4 decelerates food intake, weight gain, and fat deposition in Zucker rats. Endocrinology 141:1936–1941
10. Jendle J, Nauck MA, Matthews DR, Frid A, Hermansen K, Düring M, Zdravkovic M, Strauss BJ, Garber AJ (2009) Weight loss with liraglutide, a once-daily human glucagon-like peptide-1 analogue for type 2 diabetes treatment as monotherapy or added to metformin, is primarily as a result of a reduction in fat tissue. Diabetes Obes Metab 11:1163–1172
11. Meier JJ, Gethmann A, Götze O, Gallwitz B, Holst JJ, Schmidt WE, Nauck MA (2006) Glucagon-like peptide 1 abolishes the postprandial rise in triglyceride concentrations and lowers levels of non-esterified fatty acids in humans. Diabetologia 49:452–458
12. Klonoff DC, Buse JB, Nielsen LL, Guan X, Bowlus CL, Holcombe JH, Wintle ME, Maggs DG (2008) Exenatide effects on diabetes, obesity, cardiovascular risk factors and hepatic biomarkers in patients with type 2 diabetes treated for at least 3 years. Curr Med Res Opin 24:275–286

13. Moretto TJ, Milton DR, Ridge TD, Macconell LA, Okerson T, Wolka AM, Brodows RG (2008) Efficacy and tolerability of exenatide monotherapy over 24 weeks in antidiabetic drug-naive patients with type 2 diabetes: a randomized, double-blind, placebo-controlled, parallel-group study. Clin Ther 30:1448–1460
14. Buse JB, Henry RR, Han J, Kim DD, Fineman MS, Baron AD (2004) Effects of exenatide (exendin-4) on glycemic control over 30 weeks in sulfonylurea-treated patients with type 2 diabetes. Diabetes Care 27:2628–2635
15. Toft-Nielsen MB, Madsbad S, Holst JJ (1999) Continuous subcutaneous infusion of glucagon-like peptide 1 lowers plasma glucose and reduces appetite in type 2 diabetic patients. Diabetes Care 22:1137–1143
16. Sivertsen J, Rosenmeier J, Holst JJ, Vilsbøll T (2012) The effect of glucagon-like peptide 1 on cardiovascular risk. Nat Rev Cardiol 9:209–222
17. Halbirk M, Nørrelund H, Møller N, Holst JJ, Schmitz O, Nielsen R, Nielsen-Kudsk JE, Nielsen SS, Nielsen TT, Eiskjaer H, Bøtker HE, Wiggers H (2010) Cardiovascular and metabolic effects of 48-h glucagon-like peptide-1 infusion in compensated chronic patients with heart failure. Am J Physiol Heart Circ Physiol 298:H1096–1102

13 Treatment of Hypertension in the Metabolic Syndrome

Michael Hecht Olsen

13.1 Introduction

In subjects with metabolic syndrome, intense lifestyle measures should be adopted and antihypertensive drug treatment instituted whenever blood pressure is ≥140/90 mmHg because subjects with metabolic syndrome have higher prevalence of multiple target organ damage (TOD) and increased levels of inflammatory markers, which are associated with higher cardiovascular risk. The antihypertensive treatment should preferably consist of blockers of the renin–angiotensin system with the addition, when needed, of a calcium antagonist and/or a low-dose thiazide diuretic. As the other cardiovascular risk factors like for example the other elements of the metabolic syndrome broaden the blood pressure ranges associated with increased cardiovascular risk, the blood pressure goal in subjects with metabolic syndrome is suggested to be 130/85 mmHg even in the absence of diabetes. Hypertensive patients with metabolic syndrome should receive hypertensive drugs according to the 2007 European Society of Hypertension/European Society of Cardiology guidelines on hypertension diagnosis and treatment [1]; that is, in addition to recommendations to undergo intense lifestyle modifications, antihypertensive drugs should be given whenever blood pressure is persistently 140 mmHg systolic at least or 90 mmHg diastolic at least. In the presence of diabetes, the threshold for drug intervention should be lower with a blood pressure goal just below 130/85 mmHg in line with the goal that is recommended whenever total cardiovascular risk is high [1–4]. Administration of a renin–angiotensin system blocker in subjects with metabolic syndrome and high normal blood pressure, in order to protect against organ damage and prevent new onset diabetes or hypertension may be reasonable, but cannot be generally recommended at present due to the lack of

M.H. Olsen (✉)
Department of Endocrinology, Odense University Hospital, Kloevervaenget 6, 5th floor, 5000 Odense C, Denmark
e-mail: Michael.olsen@dadlnet.dk

H. Beck-Nielsen (ed.), *The Metabolic Syndrome*,
DOI 10.1007/978-3-7091-1331-8_13, © Springer-Verlag Wien 2013

clinical evidence. Treatment should aim at preventing progression or causing regression of the existing organ damage as well as at reducing the much greater chance an individual with metabolic syndrome has to develop new onset diabetes or hypertension. This calls for avoidance of some antihypertensive agents and elective use of some others, as outlined in the following section.

13.2 Treatments

Ideally, treatment of high blood pressure in the metabolic syndrome should be based on lifestyle changes, diet and physical exercise, which allow for weight reduction and improve muscular blood flow.

Concerning antihypertensive drugs, whether or not a particular antihypertensive agent is superior to others has not been tested in trials including individuals specifically with metabolic syndrome. A large body of information is, however, available from both long-term antihypertensive trials with major outcomes and from a myriad of shorter studies.

After changes in lifestyle are introduced, the drugs to be preferred should be those that may induce reduction of insulin resistance and subsequent changes in the lipid profile and in glucose levels. Therefore, angiotensin-converting enzyme inhibitors (ACEi), angiotensin II-AT1 receptor blockers (ARB) or even calcium channel blockers are preferable over diuretics and beta-blockers in monotherapy, if no compelling indications are present for its use. If a combination of drugs is required, low-dose diuretics can be used. A combination of thiazide diuretics and beta-blockers should be avoided.

13.3 Impact on Other Metabolic Syndrome Components

The impact of particular antihypertensive drugs on other components of the metabolic syndrome is an important clinical issue with consequences for the success of the treatment. Changes in metabolic components, mainly in the lipid profile and insulin resistance, during antihypertensive treatment with diuretics and beta-blockers have been claimed as the culprit of lower reductions than expected in coronary heart disease morbidity and mortality [5]. On the contrary, reductions in the rates of new onset diabetes have been observed during treatment with ACEi, ARB or even calcium channel blockers as compared with diuretics and beta-blockers [6, 7].

The recently published STAR study (The Study of Trandolapril/Verapamil SR and Insulin Resistance) reduced the risk of new onset diabetes in obese patients with impaired glucose tolerance, normal kidney function and hypertension treated with the fixed-dose combination of trandolapril/verapamil as compared with losartan/hydrochlorothiazide-based therapy [8].

For many years, metabolic changes associated with the use of antihypertensive drugs have received attention, looking at both worsening and improvement in the metabolic profile. However, not all the studies report the same conclusions, in part, due to the different dose of the drugs used, particularities of drug mechanisms of action even within the same therapeutic group, duration of treatment and, mainly, because of the different characteristics of the individuals included. Age and hormonal status have been recognized as important modulators of drug impact but, besides these, personal or family histories of metabolic disorders were among the most important factors.

The most recognized metabolic change associated with the antihypertensive drug classes is insulin resistance: it is induced by a combination of different mechanisms including a reduction of the microcirculatory flow in the muscle and a reduction in the rate of intracellular glucose disposal. The former is a consequence of the use of beta-blockers, as beta-blockade activity goes unopposed by the alpha-receptors. The latter is not well understood. Beta-blocker agents with additional properties can reduce the impact of the pure beta-blockade and even exert partially beneficial effects. The simultaneous alpha-blockade of carvedilol [9] or the increment in the nitric oxide bioavailability of nebivolol [10] has shown a neutral effect on glucose metabolism indexes and a trend towards a favorable lipid profile [11, 12].

The potential effect of beta-blockers in favoring gaining weight needs to be mentioned. A large review concerning weight changes in studies using beta-blockers showed that they tend to increase body weight as a consequence of reducing fuel expenditure [13]. The clinical consequences of the gain of weight during beta-blocker treatment, however, seem to be negligible.

The reduction of glucose disposal is worse when insulin secretion decreases. This can occur as a direct consequence of the beta-blockade, reducing the response of the pancreatic beta-cell, and by hypokalemia induced by thiazide-like diuretics. Reductions in glucose disposal and in the compensatory insulin secretion lead to metabolic abnormalities of the glucose homeostasis and dyslipidaemia, as previously described and, in the English Longitudinal Study of Ageing (ELSA), the incidence of new metabolic syndrome was significantly greater in patients under atenolol than lacidipine [14].

Nevertheless, a beneficial impact of decreasing the risk of the development of diabetes with ACEi-based or ARB-based treatments has been described. Detailed systematic reviews of the potential beneficial effects have been published recently. In general, treatment with these classes of drugs reduces the rate of new onset diabetes as compared with the use of diuretic and/or beta-blockers [5, 6]. Inhibiting the renin–angiotensin system may improve blood flow to muscles, decrease the activity of the sympathetic nervous system, enhance insulin signaling, lower free fatty acid levels, increase plasma adiponectin levels and improve glucose disposal. Another putative mechanism by which the inhibition of the renin–angiotensin system may improve insulin sensitivity is through effects on peroxisome proliferator-activated receptor (PPAR)-gamma, which is inhibited by angiotensin II [15].

The controversy over whether this effect is a consequence of the risk induced by diuretics or beta-blockers and not a real beneficial effect was, in part, resolved by the observation that the reduction in new onset diabetes was also observed in a trial against placebo [16] and by data furnished by the Valsartan Antihypertensive Long-Term Use Evaluation (VALUE) study [17, 18]. In this study, valsartan-based treatment significantly reduced the rate of new onset diabetes as compared with amlodipine, a calcium channel blocker. Mechanisms that led to improved glucose metabolism were increment in the microcirculatory flow and in the bioavailability of the glucose transporter 4 (Glut4). The results of the Diabetes Reduction Assessment with ramipril and rosiglitazone Medication Study (DREAM) [19] challenge the concept of protection against development of new onset diabetes by using drugs blocking the renin–angiotensin system. The study reports the effects of ramipril on the risk of diabetes in a randomised trial designed with diabetes as a primary outcome in subjects who had impaired plasma glucose levels after an overnight fast or impaired glucose tolerance. Rates of the primary endpoint, mainly diabetes, were not significantly lower in the ramipril group. However, regression to normoglycemia, a secondary outcome, was significantly more frequent in the ramipril group than in the placebo group, although the absolute difference between the groups was small. Several reasons may explain the negative result in the impact of ACEi to reduce the risk of developing diabetes: there was only 43 % of hypertensive patients in the study; these hypertensive patients were under multiple treatments including diuretics and beta-blockers; some of the effect can be masked by the treatment with rosiglitazone; and the follow-up of the study was only three years, a short period for the risk of developing diabetes.

An additional mechanism for some ARB that has been tested in experimental models is the partial PPAR-gamma agonism of telmisartan [20] and even irbesartan [21], with further improvement of insulin resistance. The significance and clinical impact of this additional mechanism, however, need to be tested in appropriately designed studies.

The impact of other antihypertensive drug classes demonstrated the neutral effect of both long-acting calcium channel blockers as well as other sympatholytic drugs with central action, such as reserpine, a-methyl-dopa or moxonidine. The pure peripheral alpha-blocker, doxazosin, improves the lipid profile, reducing insulin resistance and consequently increasing high-density lipoprotein (HDL) cholesterol and reducing triglycerides [5]. A trend to reduce total cholesterol has also been described. The main mechanism implicated in the positive changes of alpha-blockers seems to be mediated by increasing microcirculation flow. Additional effects of alpha-blockade on the activity of key enzymes of lipid metabolism are less well known.

A final question is the net effect of the interaction when two different kinds of drugs, with opposite effects, are combined. This is the case of combination treatments with diuretics. Simultaneous administration of a thiazide diuretic with ACEi or ARB reduces hypokalemia and does not significantly modify the lipid and glucose profiles. Whether or not this combination reduces at large the beneficial effects in cardiovascular risk needs to be assessed. A recent publication points out that valsartan alone reduced the levels of high sensitivity C-reactive protein (CRP) [22]. In contrast, a combination of valsartan plus hydrochlorothiazide, despite a significantly larger blood pressure reduction, was unable to reduce high-sensitivity CRP values. No interaction with statins was demonstrated.

13.4 Conclusion

The metabolic syndrome is a highly prevalent condition currently considered to be a cluster of metabolic and cardiovascular risk factors, including blood pressure elevation. A higher risk for progression in metabolic syndrome individuals with high normal blood pressure has been observed and, when hypertension is established, this seems to confer a higher cardiovascular risk on top of the risk induced by blood pressure elevation. Therefore, assessment of metabolic syndrome components can result in a clinical utility strategy to manage hypertension based on individual risk.

References

1. Mancia G, De Backer G, Dominiczak A, Cifkova R, Fagard R, Germano G et al (2007) Management of Arterial Hypertension of the European Society of Hypertension; European Society of Cardiology. 2007 Guidelines for the Management of Arterial Hypertension: The Task Force for the Management of Arterial Hypertension of the European Society of Hypertension (ESH) and of the European Society of Cardiology (ESC). J Hypertens 25:1105–1187
2. Rizzoni D, Porteri E, Guelfi D, Muiesan ML, Valentini U, Cimino A et al (2001) Structural alterations in subcutaneous small arteries of normotensive and hypertensive patients with noninsulin-dependent diabetes mellitus. Circulation 103:1238–1244
3. Chobanian AV, Bakris GL, Black HR, Cushman WC, Green LA, Izzo JL Jr et al (2003) National Heart, Lung, and Blood Institute Joint National Committee on Prevention, Detection, Evaluation, and Treatment of High Blood Pressure; National High Blood Pressure Education Program Coordinating Committee. The Seventh Report of the Joint National Committee on Prevention, Detection, Evaluation, and Treatment of High Blood Pressure: the JNC 7 report. JAMA 289:2560–2572
4. American Diabetes Association (2005) Clinical practice recommendations 2005. Diabetes Care 28(Suppl 1):S1–S79
5. Lithell H (1993) Hypertension and hyperlipidemia. A review. Am J Hypertens 6:303S–308S
6. Messerli FH, Grossman E, Leonetti G (2004) Antihypertensive therapy and new onset diabetes. J Hypertens 22:1845–1847
7. Mancia G, Grassi G, Zanchetti A (2006) New-onset diabetes and antihypertensive drugs. J Hypertens 24:3–10
8. Bakris G, Molitch M, Hewkin A, Kipnes M, Sarafidis P, Fakouhi K et al (2006) On behalf of the STAR Investigators. Differences in glucose tolerance between fixed-dose antihypertensive drug combinations in people with metabolic syndrome. Diabetes Care 29:2592–2597
9. McTavish D, Campoli-Richards D, Sorkin EM (1993) Carvedilol: a review of its pharmacodynamic and pharmacokinetic properties, and therapeutic efficacy. Drugs 45:232–258
10. Tzemos N, Lim PO, MacDonald TM (2001) Nebivolol reverses endothelial dysfunction in essential hypertension: a randomized, double-blind, crossover study. Circulation 104:511–514
11. Bakris GL, Fonseca V, Katholi RE, McGill JB, Messerli FH, Phillips RA et al (2004) GEMINI Investigators. Metabolic effects of carvedilol vs metoprolol in patients with type 2 diabetes mellitus and hypertension: a randomized controlled trial. JAMA 292:2227–2236

12. Kaiser T, Heise T, Nosek L, Eckers U, Sawicki PT (2006) Influence of nevibolol and enalapril on metabolic parameters an arterial stiffness in hypertensive type 2 diabetic patients. J Hypertens 24:1397–1403
13. Zanchetti A, Hennig M, Baurecht H, Tang R, Cuspidi C, Carugo S, Mancia G (2007) Prevalence and incidence of the metabolic syndrome in the European Lacidipine Study on Atherosclerosis (ELSA) and its relation with carotid intima-media thickness. J Hypertens 25: 2463–2470
14. Sharma AM, Pischon T, Hardt S, Kunz I, Luft FC (2001) Hypothesis: betaadrenergic receptor blockers and weight gain: a systematic analysis. Hypertension 37:250–254
15. Horiuchi M, Mogi M, Iwai M (2006) Signaling crosstalk angiotensin II receptor subtypes and insulin. Endocr J 53:1–5
16. Yusuf S, Sleight P, Pogue J, Bosch J, Davies R, Dagenais G (2000) Effects of an angiotensin-converting-enzyme inhibitor, ramipril, on cardiovascular events in high-risk patients. The Heart Outcomes Prevention Evaluation Study Investigators. N Engl J Med 342:145–153
17. Julius S, Kjeldsen SE, Weber M, Brunner HR, Ekman S, Hansson L et al (2004) VALUE trial group Outcomes in hypertensive patients at high cardiovascular risk treated with regimens based on valsartan or amlodipine: the VALUE randomised trial. Lancet 363:2022–2031
18. Kjeldsen SE, Julius S, Mancia G, McInnes GT, Hua T, Weber MA et al (2006) VALUE Trial Investigators. Effects of valsartan compared to amlodipine on preventing type 2 diabetes in high-risk hypertensive patients: the VALUE trial. J Hypertens 24:1405–1412
19. Bosch J, Yusuf S, Gerstein HC, Pogue J, Sheridan P, Dagenais G et al (2006) DREAM Trial Investigators Effect of ramipril on the incidence of diabetes. N Engl J Med 355:1551–1562
20. Benson SC, Pershadsingh HA, Ho CI, Chittiboyina A, Desai P, Pravenec M et al (2004) Identification of telmisartan as a unique angiotensin II receptor antagonist with selective PPARgamma-modulating activity. Hypertension 43:993–1002
21. Di Filippo C, Lampa E, Tufariello E, Petronella P, Freda F, Capuano A, D'Amico M (2005) Effects of irbesartan on the growth and differentiation of adipocytes in obese zucker rats. Obes Res 13:1909–1914
22. Ridker PM, Danielson E, Rifai N, Glynn RJ (2006) Val-MARC Investigators. Valsartan, blood pressure reduction, and C-reactive protein: primary report of the Val-MARC trial. Hypertension 48:73–79

Treatment of the Metabolic Syndrome by Bariatric Surgery

14

Sten Madsbad

14.1 Introduction

The increase in obesity has generated a secondary epidemic of the metabolic syndrome with hypertension, dyslipidaemia, abdominal obesity and increased risk of type 2 diabetes and cardiovascular diseases [1–5]. The aetiological connections between obesity and the metabolic syndrome seem to be multiple. Insulin resistance, abdominal obesity and an excess of visceral adipose tissue are key abnormalities in people with metabolic syndrome [3–5]. The aetiology includes elevated levels of free fatty acids (FFA), suppressed adiponectin, elevated levels of cytokines, i.e. tumour necrosis factor (TNF) α, interleukin (IL) 6 and fibrinogen [3, 6]. The cytokines and FFA induce insulin resistance, beta-cell dysfunction and "low-grade" inflammation in the vascular system and increase triglyceride content in the liver, pancreas, and skeletal and heart muscles [3–5, 7]. The metabolic syndrome also includes a prothrombotic state with, i.e., elevation of C-reactive protein and plasma activator inhibitor (PAI)-1 [3, 6].

Patients with metabolic syndrome have an increased risk of cardiovascular diseases and of developing type 2 diabetes [1–3, 5, 6]. Additional metabolic comorbidities include polycystic ovary syndrome (PCOS) and non-alcoholic steatohepatitis (NASH) [8, 9]. Morbid obesity is also related to obstructive sleep apnoea and several forms of cancers [10].

The treatment of the metabolic syndrome is lifestyle changes focusing on weight loss and increased physical activity. It is possible to lose 5–10 % in weight by lifestyle changes, but most patients will start to gain weight after 3–6 months, and after 1–5 years about 90 % will have relapse to the weight or a higher weight than before the start of lifestyle treatment, indicating that obesity in most cases is

S. Madsbad (✉)
Department of Endocrinology, Hvidovre University Hospital, University of Copenhagen, Kettegaard Allé 30, 2650 Hvidovre, Denmark
e-mail: sten.madsbad@regionh.dk

H. Beck-Nielsen (ed.), *The Metabolic Syndrome*,
DOI 10.1007/978-3-7091-1331-8_14, © Springer-Verlag Wien 2013

Table 14.1 Effects of bariatric surgery on the metabolic syndrome and cardiovascular risk factors

Obesity	Weight loss
	Reduction in abdominal obesity
	Reduction on waist
Hypertension	Lowering of systolic and diastolic blood pressure
Dyslipidaemia	Lowering of low-density lipoprotein cholesterol
	Lowering of triglycerides
	Lowering of total cholesterol
	Increase in high-density lipoprotein cholesterol
Type 2 diabetes	Prevention of type 2 diabetes
	Remission of prediabetes
	Improvement in HbA1c
	Remission of type 2 diabetes
	Improvement in insulin sensitivity and insulin secretion
Metabolic syndrome	Resolution of metabolic syndrome
Cardiovascular diseases	Reduction in cardiovascular risk factors
	Reduction in cardiovascular events
	Reduction in cardiovascular mortality

refractory to lifestyle therapy. By use of anti-obesity agents 2–8 kg further weight loss can be added, but with the agents at present on the market or in the phase of development, a mean weight loss of more than 10 kg has not been possible to obtain in clinical trials [11].

Bariatric surgery is regarded as "metabolic" surgery due to its effects on the metabolic syndrome and type 2 diabetes (Table 14.1). At present an estimated 350,000 bariatric operations are performed worldwide per year [12]. Obesity responds well to bariatric surgery with major weight loss [13–19]. Laparoscopic adjustable gastric banding (LAGB) and laparoscopic Roux-en-Y gastric bypass (RYGB) are the two more commonly performed bariatric procedures [13, 19].

The present chapter reviews the metabolic mechanisms behind bariatric surgery, the effects of bariatric surgery on the metabolic syndrome, its individual components and the impact on cardiovascular diseases, type 2 diabetes, cancers and mortality. The risks and adverse effects of LAGB and laparoscopic RYGB will also be discussed.

14.2 The Bariatric Operations

The major breakthrough in bariatric surgery came with Dr. Edward Mason from Minnesota, who documented that major weight loss could be achieved through the gastric banding procedure and the gastric bypass operation [20, 21]. The gastric bypass operation has been modified with the biliopancreatic bypass with the addition of a duodenal switch and more recently with the gastric sleeve procedure [21].

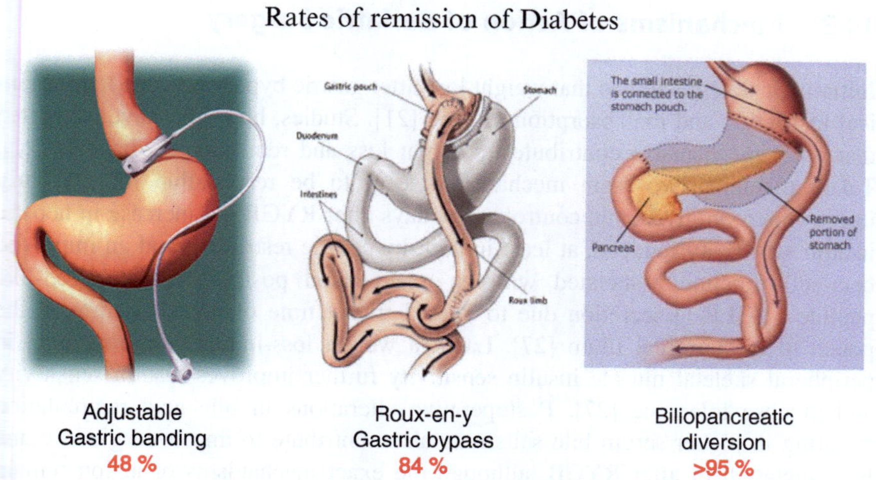

Fig. 14.1 Illustrates to the left the gastric banding, in the middle the Roux-en-Y gastric bypass and to the right the biliopancreatic diversion operation. The remission rates of type 2 diabetes for the different procedures are also depicted. Adopted from [13]

Other operations are duodenal–jejunal bypass and ileal transposition, i.e. translocation of a segment of ilium including vessels and nerves close to the Ligament of Treitz [22–26].

The adjustable gastric banding is a restrictive procedure that produces weight loss by limiting food intake (Fig. 14.1). A small bracelet silicone band is placed high around the stomach to produce a pouch of about 30 ml. The band is lined by an inflatable cuff that is joined to a subcutaneous abdominal reservoir allowing adjustment of the pouch outflow [21].

The laparoscopic RYGB procedure creates a gastric pouch of about 30 ml [21]. The pouch is drained with an Roux-an-Y by dividing the proximal jejunum 30 ml below the Ligament of Treitz, bringing the distal segment (the alimentary limb) up to form a gastroenterostomy, and joining the proximal segment (the secretory limb) to the small bowel about 100 cm below the point of division (Fig. 14.1). Thus, nutrients bypass the major part of the stomach, the duodenum and the upper part of the jejunum.

The biliopancreatic bypass with duodenal switch reduces the gastric pouch leaving only a gastric sleeve [21]. The duodenum is divided about 2 cm below the pylorus and is reconstituted by a Roux-en-Y anastomosis to the distal jejunum and excludes more small bowel than a gastric bypass operation (Fig. 14.1).

The gastric sleeve operation creates a narrow tube through the excision of most of the stomach and is used as a bridge to a gastric bypass in severely obese patients with a body mass index (BMI) >55 kg/m^2 [21]. Lastly, the ileal transposition is an experimental procedure and has shown to induce remission of diabetes without major weight loss [21, 23–26].

14.3 Mechanisms of Action of Bariatric Surgery

Initially, it was speculated that weight loss after gastric bypass was due to mechanical restriction and malabsorption of food [21]. Studies, however, have suggested that other mechanisms contribute to weight loss and remission of diabetes [21]. Taken together, two main mechanisms seem to be responsible for the early improvement in glycaemic control a few days after RYGB: an increase in hepatic insulin sensitivity induced, at least in part, by calorie restriction and an improved beta-cell function associated with an exaggerated postprandial glucagon-like peptide-1 (GLP-1) secretion due to altered transit time of nutrients through the pouch to the terminal ilium [27]. Later, a weight loss-induced improvement in peripheral skeletal muscle insulin sensitivity further improves insulin sensitivity and glucose tolerance [27]. Postoperative alterations in bile acid recirculation resulting in higher serum bile salts may also contribute to improved glucose and lipid metabolism after RYGB, although the exact mechanisms of action remain poorly understood [28, 29]. Bariatric surgery has been shown to have beneficial effects on the levels of adiponectin, resistin, visfatin and other adipokines, which may contribute to the reduction in type 2 diabetes and cardiovascular diseases after surgery [3, 27].

RYGB alters the physiology of weight regulation and eating behaviours. It has been realised that the gastrointestinal tract exerts significant neuroendocrine control over appetite, food intake and energy expenditure [17, 27, 30–32] via postprandial release of gut hormones like GLP-1, peptide YY (PYY), oxyntomodulin and cholecystokinin (CCK) as well as the preprandial increase in ghrelin levels, the only orexigenic hormone. PYY and GLP-1 are released from the intestinal L-cells [27, 30–39]. Oxyntomodulin, another L-cell product, has been reported to be elevated postoperatively by Laferrere et al. [40]. These hormones from the L-cell stimulate anorectic pathways in the hypothalamus and brain stem leading to reduced food intake and may also influence energy expenditure [30, 41, 42].

In rats, RYGB has been shown to increase energy expenditure after weight loss compared with after a food restriction-induced weight loss, where compensatory mechanisms decrease energy expenditure and thereby combat the weight loss [11, 43, 44]. Two small human studies have also suggested that RYGB may be associated with increased energy expenditure, while other studies have failed to find such an association [45–47]. Human studies have suggested that RYGB decreases non-hunger-related hedonic driven and reward-based desire to eat [48, 49].

Taken all together, the altered gastrointestinal anatomy after RYGB and consequently the very rapid delivery of nutrients to the distal part of the small intestine provoke an exaggerated release of GLP-1-potentiating postprandial insulin secretion. Furthermore, the increased release of GLP-1, PYY and other anorexigenic hormones like oxyntomodulin and CCK may contribute to the postoperative weight loss and thereby indirectly to improved insulin sensitivity. Hence, RYGB is a unique opportunity to explore the mechanism of energy homeostasis and pathophysiology of type 2 diabetes and thereby to identify novel therapies for obesity and related metabolic diseases as diabetes.

14.4 Effect of Bariatric Surgery on Weight

Bariatric surgery is the most effective treatment for obesity and produces major and durable weight loss. The mean weight loss is about 40–50 kg or about 15 BMI units [13, 50]. An additional method to express the weight loss is to relate it to "excess weight", which is actual weight minus ideal body weight. In the meta-analysis of Buchwald et al. [13] the weight loss, expressed as percent of excess weight, was after gastric banding 47 %, after RYGB 61.6 % and after biliopancreatic bypass with duodenal switch 79 %, respectively. After RYGB the maximal weight loss was obtained after 1.5–2.0 years in most patients [13]. Thereafter, 10–20 % of the patients will gain weight [13].

The Swedish Obesity Study (SOS), a landmark study, was initiated to ascertain the effects of intentional weight loss induced by bariatric surgery on mortality [51]. The intervention group consists of one surgical group ($n = 2{,}010$) and one obese control group ($n = 2{,}037$). The matching programme between the groups used 18 matching variables, and the matching could not be influenced by the investigators [51]. Inclusion criteria were age 37–60 years and BMI of 34 or more for men and 38 or more for women. The surgically treated patients underwent adjustable or nonadjustable gastric banding ($n = 376$), vertical banding gastroplasty ($n = 1{,}369$) or gastric bypass ($n = 265$). The control group received the customary non-surgical obesity treatment for their given centre of registration, which ranged form sophisticated lifestyle treatment to no treatment. The surgically treated patients were on average 2.3 kg heavier (119.2 vs. 116.9 kg), 1.3 years younger (46.1 vs. 47.4 years) and were smoking more frequently (27.9 vs. 20.2 %) [51]. The weight changes in the control group were during follow-up ±2.0 % of basal weight, while the weight loss after surgery was maximal after 1–2 years (RYGB 32 %, vertical banding 25 % and banding 20 %, Fig. 14.2) in the surgical groups [52–54].

The weight loss after gastric banding is slower and less compared with RYGB [52–54]. Weight increase was seen in all surgical subgroups in the following years, but the relapse levelled off after 8–10 years, and after 10 years the weight loss was 25, 16 and 14 % in the three groups, respectively (Fig. 14.2). After 15 years the weight loss was 27, 18 and 13 %, respectively [52–54]. About 5–10 % of the patients will regain the weight lost after gastric bypass and even a higher number of patients after gastric banding, and on average it is expected that 20–25 % of the weight lost will be regained over a period of 10 years after bariatric surgery [52–54]. The explanation of the weight gain is non-compliance with dietary and lifestyle recommendations, variations in response to surgery and surgical failure [55].

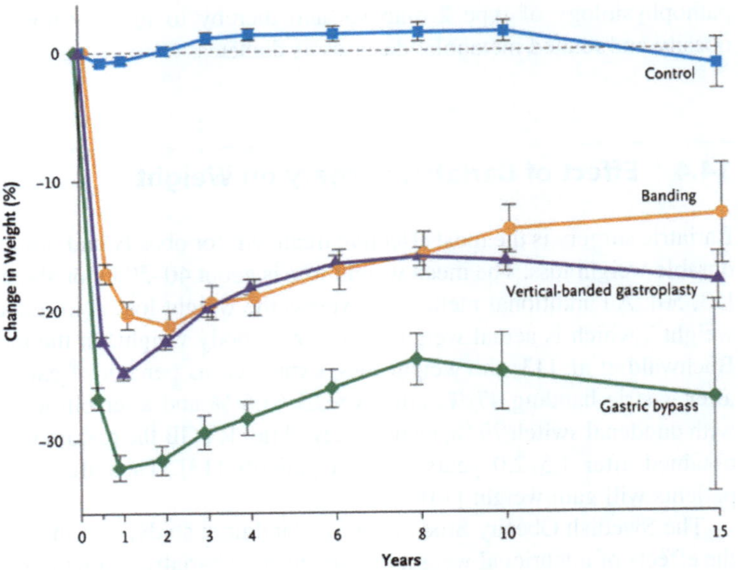

No. Examined	0	1	2	3	4	6	8	10	15
Control	2037	1768	1660	1553	1490	1281	982	886	190
Banding	376	363	357	328	333	298	267	237	52
Vertical-banded gastroplasty	1369	1298	1244	1121	1086	1004	899	746	108
Gastric bypass	265	245	245	211	209	166	92	58	10

Fig. 14.2 Mean percent weight change during a 15-year period in the control group and the surgery group according to the method of bariatric surgery. Adapted from [53]

14.5 Effects of Bariatric Surgery on Comorbidities

14.5.1 Effect on Blood Pressure

Bariatric surgery has a significant effect on hypertension, with a resolution in about 30–50 % of the patients and a reduced need for antihypertensive treatment in further 20–30 % of the patients [56, 57]. An interesting observation is that a rebound in hypertension was observed after 5–8 years follow-up in the SOS study, where most patients were treated with gastric banding [52, 58]. Whether the same phenomenon will be observed after gastric bypass is unknown.

14.5.2 Effect on Lipids

RYGB surgery improved lipid profile with a 30 % decrease in low-density lipoprotein (LDL) cholesterol and an increase in high-density lipoprotein (HDL) cholesterol of 39 % combined with a 63 % decrease in triglycerides 12 months after gastric banding surgery [59]. Similar results have been described by Segal JB et al. [60]. In the last study, the medications used for treatment of type 2 diabetes, hypertension and dyslipidaemia were reduced from 76 to 51 %, respectively [60]. In the SOS study, the triglycerides did not differ between the surgery and control group after 2 and 10 years follow-up, although the reduction in triglycerides was greater in the subgroup treated with gastric bypass [52]. The lipid changes in people with type 2 diabetes after bariatric surgery are discussed below.

14.5.3 Effect on NAFLD

NAFLD is an independent risk factor for type 2 diabetes, cardiovascular disease and liver cirrhosis, and patients with NAFLD had much higher mortality rates than the background population [8, 61, 62]. After bariatric surgery a reduction in liver steatosis (from 88 to 8 %), inflammation (from 23 to 2 %) and fibrosis (from 31 to 13 %) was observed 15 months after surgery [63]. Inflammation and fibrosis resolved in 37 % and 20 % of the patients. In another study NASH resolved in 89 % of the patients [64]. Other studies have found similar results [65, 66].

A significant removal of fat from the liver is probably evident already a few days after bariatric surgery and may be one of the main explanations of the improved glucose tolerance observed in patients with type 2 diabetes already a few days after operation [27].

14.5.4 Effect on Obstructive Sleep Apnoea

Obesity is a major risk factor for obstructive sleep apnoea [67–69] and is very frequent in morbid obese people (approximately 70 %). A meta-analysis indicated that after bariatric surgery obstructive sleep apnoea is resolved in 86 % of the patients and improved in 95 % [13]. Other investigators have presented similar beneficial effects of bariatric surgery on obstructive sleep apnoea [67, 68].

14.5.5 Effect on Type 2 Diabetes

Type 2 diabetes is a major cause of premature illness and death. The key goal in treating type 2 diabetes is to keep blood glucose levels as close to normal as possible. However, therapies must also include active treatment of all cardiovascular risk factors (hypertension, dyslipidaemia, smoking, abdominal obesity and sedentary lifestyle) [70]. Type 2 diabetes is a progressive disease characterised by increasing insulin secretory impairment with duration of disease. Obesity is considered the primary risk factor for development of type 2 diabetes [71], and weight loss should be the most logical means of controlling the disease [72].

The most fascinating effect of bariatric surgery is the effect on type 2 diabetes. In 1995 Pories et al. reported that among 146 morbidly obese patients with type 2 diabetes, who underwent gastric bypass, 121 (83 %) experienced a rapid and prolonged postoperative normalisation of plasma glucose levels without the need for antidiabetic medication [73]. This remarkable observation has later been reported in several other studies and confirmed in a large meta-analysis of 621 studies, including nearly 5,000 patients with type 2 diabetes, where diabetes remission was seen in 80.3 % after RYGB [13]. After gastric banding the rate of remission was lower and about 50–60 % [13]. In patients with prediabetes the remission was about 85–100 % [13, 52].

In the SOS study using primarily the banding procedures the remission of diabetes dropped from 72 % at 2 years to 36 % at 10 years following surgery (Fig. 14.5) [52]. In the surgical and control groups 1,658 and 1,771 participants, respectively, had normal glucose tolerance at baseline [74]. After up to 15 years follow-up (mean 10 years) 392 participants in the control group and 110 in the bariatric group (adjusted hazard ratio (HR) 0.17) had developed diabetes, indicating that bariatric surgery is efficient in the prevention of diabetes (Fig. 14.6) [74]. The average weight loss in the surgical group was approximately 20 kg during follow-up compared with no significant weight change in the control group. The number needed to treat was 1.3 to prevent one case of diabetes. In patients with impaired glucose tolerance bariatric surgery reduced the risk of developing diabetes with 87 % [74]. The risk reduction did not differ among participants with a BMI below or above the median BMI of 40.8 kg/m^2 at baseline.

In another randomised, controlled trial patients with type 2 diabetes, who underwent laparoscopic adjustable gastric banding, had a higher remission rate than patients, who were treated with intensive pharmacological and lifestyle intervention [75]. Remission of type 2 diabetes was achieved in 73 % in the surgical group and 13 % in the conventionally treated group after 2 years. The weight loss was 20.5 % and 1.7 % of baseline weight. Remission of diabetes was related to weight loss and lower baseline HbA1c levels [75].

In a recent study, 60 patients with type 2 diabetes were randomised to receive conventional, medical therapy or undergo either gastric bypass or biliopancreatic diversion surgery [76]. At 2 years follow-up diabetes remission (fasting glucose below 5.6 mmol/l and HbA1c $<$ 6.5 % in the absence of pharmacological therapy) occurred in no patients in the medical group compared with 75 % in the gastric bypass group and 95 % in the biliopancreatic diversion group. The baseline HbA1c decreased from 8.65 to 7.69 % in the medical group to 6.35 % in the gastric bypass group and to 4.95 % in the biliopancreatic group, respectively (Fig. 14.3).

All lipid profile measures were significantly lower (except HDL cholesterol) among patients undergoing biliopancreatic diversion compared with the medically treated group. After 2 years the different lipid profile measurements were normal for 0–27 % in the medical group compared with 72–100 % in the two surgical groups. The weight loss was 4.7, 33.3 and 33. 8 % for the three groups, respectively.

In another randomised study the efficacy of intensive medical therapy alone versus RYGB or gastric sleeve gastrectomy was investigated in 150 obese patients with type 2 diabetes with an average HbA1c of 9.2 % and diabetes duration of 8 years [77]. Forty-four percent of the patients were treated with insulin. The primary endpoint was a HbA1c below 6.0 % with or without antidiabetic treatment, and in the medically treated group 12 % compared with 42 % and 37 % in the two

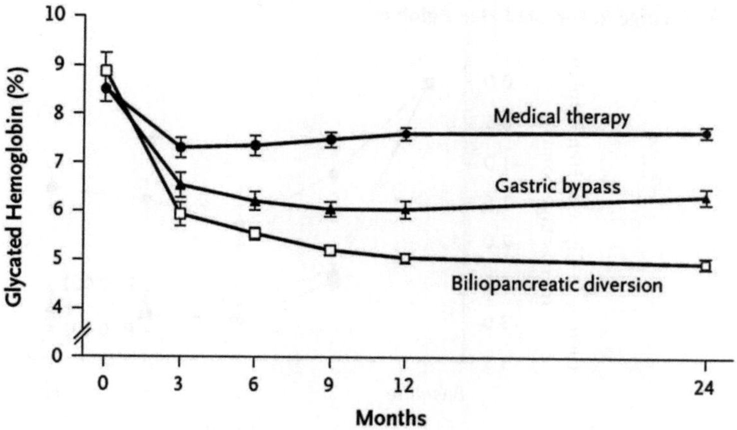

Fig. 14.3 Changes in HbA1c levels during 2 years of follow-up in patients treated with medical therapy compared with patients treated with gastric bypass or biliopancreatic diversion. Adapted from [76]

surgery groups obtained the endpoint after 12 months. The mean HbA1c was 7.5 %, 6.4 % and 6.0 % in the three groups (Fig. 14.4).

Particularly those in the gastric bypass group obtained remission without use of medications. The weight loss was greater in the two surgery groups (−29 % and −25 %) compared with −5.4 % in the medically treated group. The use of drugs for treatment of hypertension, lipids and glucose decreased significantly in the two surgical groups, but increased in patients receiving medical treatment alone (Fig. 14.4).

Accordingly, the remission rate of diabetes is higher after gastric bypass than after gastric banding, and after gastric banding the remission follows the weight loss, while after gastric bypass the remission is observed already a few days after the operation before any significant weight loss [27]. In persistent cases of type 2 diabetes after bariatric surgery glycaemic control often improves in parallel with weight loss despite the use of fewer antidiabetic drugs [75]. For that reason, the explanations of the remission of diabetes differ after the two types of operations. Both after banding and gastric bypass the very low caloric intake will improve glycaemic control directly, but also indirectly via improved hepatic insulin sensitivity following the reduction in hepatic fat content [27]. After gastric bypass, improved insulin secretion is associated with the exaggerated GLP-1 response during meals [27]. Later, after major weight loss the insulin sensitivity in the skeletal muscles also improved significantly [27].

In a recent consensus report, remission was defined as HbA1c < 6 % without the need for diabetic medications, and partial remission as HbA1c < 6.5 % without the need for diabetic agents [78]. Applying this definition the complete remission seems to be 30–50 % after different procedures of bariatric surgery, and in 209 patients with type 2 diabetes undergoing gastric bypass, sleeve gastrectomy and gastric banding the remission rates were 41, 26 and 7 % in the three groups, and in

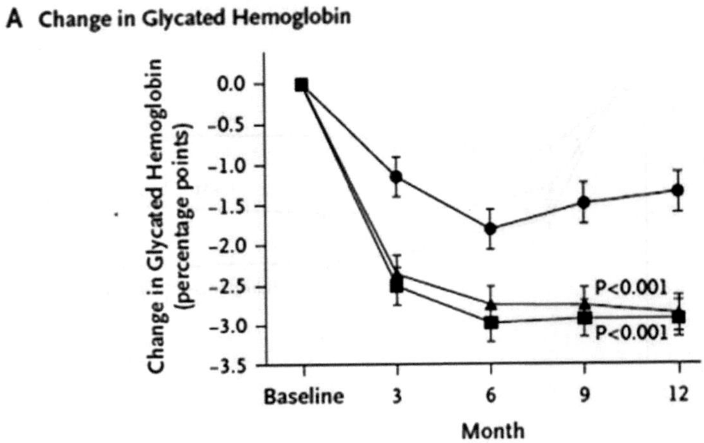

Value at Visit

	Baseline	3	6	9	12
Intensive medical therapy	8.9	7.7	7.1	7.4	7.5
Roux-en-Y gastric bypass	9.3	6.8	6.3	6.4	6.4
Sleeve gastrectomy	9.5	7.1	6.7	6.7	6.6

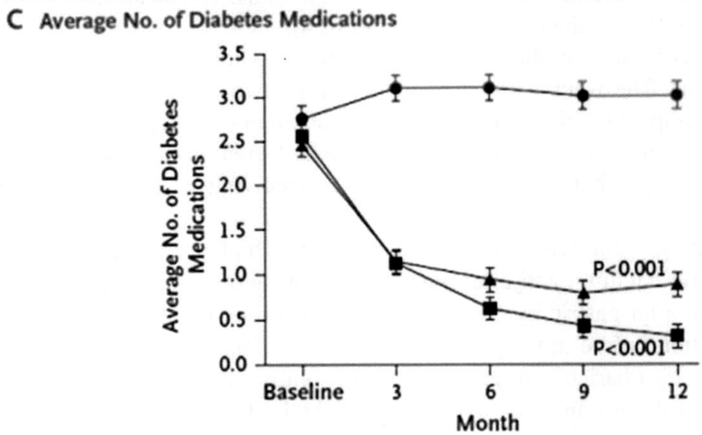

Value at Visit

	Baseline	3	6	9	12
Intensive medical therapy	2.8	3.1	3.1	3.0	3.0
Roux-en-Y gastric bypass	2.6	1.1	0.6	0.4	0.3
Sleeve gastrectomy	2.4	1.1	0.9	0.8	0.9

Fig. 14.4 Change in HbA1c and number of diabetes medication after 3, 6, 9 and 12 months in a medically treated group and patients treated with gastric bypass or sleeve gastrectomy. Adapted from [77]

another study remission rate was 43 % after gastric bypass [79, 80]. Therefore, the rate of diabetes remission after RYGB strongly depends on the definition of remission and the type of bariatric procedure. Low remission rates are associated with advanced stages of diabetes, long diabetes duration, poorly glycaemic control before operation despite treatment with insulin, inadequate weight loss or weight regain [81]. The primary physiological explanation of the relapse seems to be failing beta-cell function, which explains that remission rates are higher in patients with short duration of type 2 diabetes compared with patients with long duration of diabetes [78, 82]. On this background RYGB should also be considered as a tool to improve glycaemic control in many patients rather than to obtain a complete diabetes remission. Even in patients with type 1 diabetes without endogenous insulin secretion a 50 % reduction in insulin dose is observed the first 1–2 years after gastric bypass.

Which patients with type 2 diabetes should be offered bariatric surgery? The position statement of the International Diabetes Federation (IDF) considers bariatric surgery an appropriate treatment for patients with type 2 diabetes and obesity not achieving treatment targets with medical therapies, especially in the presence of other comorbidities, and even in patients with a BMI of 30–35 kg/m^2 [83]. Furthermore, bariatric surgery should be considered early rather than being a last resort, since early intervention increases the likelihood of diabetes remission [83]. A few studies indicate that, at least in patients with short duration and a reliable beta-cell function evaluated from C-peptide values, gastric bypass surgery induces remission of diabetes in most patients with a BMI of 25–35 kg/m^2 [22, 84, 85].

Notably, studies in high-income countries indicate that bariatric surgery is a cost-effective treatment for type 2 diabetes, or even generating cost savings already a few years after surgery [86–90].

14.5.6 Effect on Other Cardiovascular Risk Factors

Bariatric surgery reduced highly sensitive C-reactive protein to the normal range in more than 90 % of the patients [91]. Markers of thrombosis and fibrinolysis including PAI-1 also improved after bariatric surgery [92].

Two years after bariatric surgery mean carotid intima thickness was reduced from 0.84 to 0.50 mm [93]. Also, flow-mediated vessel dilatation improved.

Obesity is associated with left ventricular hypertrophy [94]. Some studies have indicated a decrease in left ventricular hypertrophy after bariatric surgery, and with the greatest reduction in patients with the most pronounced weight loss [94, 95].

In one study the estimated cardiovascular risk evaluated by the Framingham risk score declined from 11 to 5 % in men and from 6 to 3 % in women [96]. Similar results have been presented in other studies [96–98].

In the SOS study the 2 and 10 years recovery rates from diabetes, hypertriglyceridaemia, hypertension and hyperuricaemia were more favourable in the surgery group (Fig. 14.5), whereas the recovery of hypercholesterolaemia did not differ between the groups [52]. The surgery group had lower 2 and 10 years incidence rates of diabetes, hypertriglyceridaemia and hyperuricaemia than the control group, whereas the differences between the groups in the incidence of hypercholesterolaemia and hypertension did not differ between the groups (Fig. 14.6) [52].

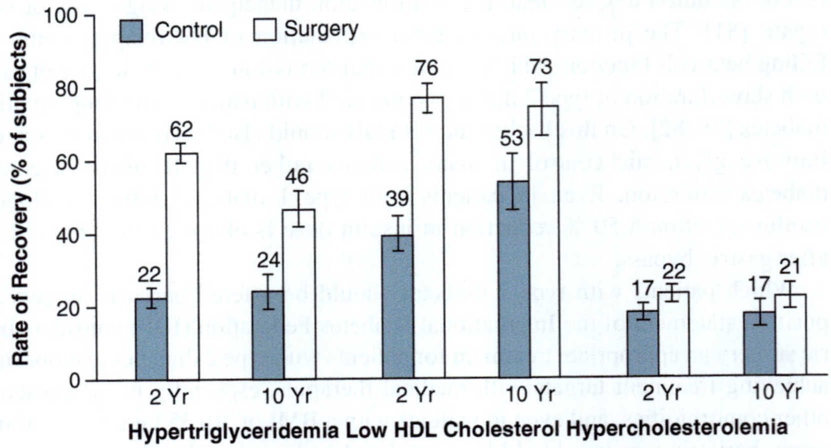

	2 Yr	10 Yr	2 Yr	10 Yr	2 Yr	10 Yr
No. of subjects	850 1102	331 402	1396 445	166 169	1048 1327	435 498
Odds ratio	5.28	2.57	5.28	2.35	1.22	1.30
95% CI	4.29-6.49	1.85-3.57	3.85-7.23	1.44-3.84	0.98-1.51	0.92-1.83
P value	<0.001	<0.001	<0.001	0.001	0.07	0.14

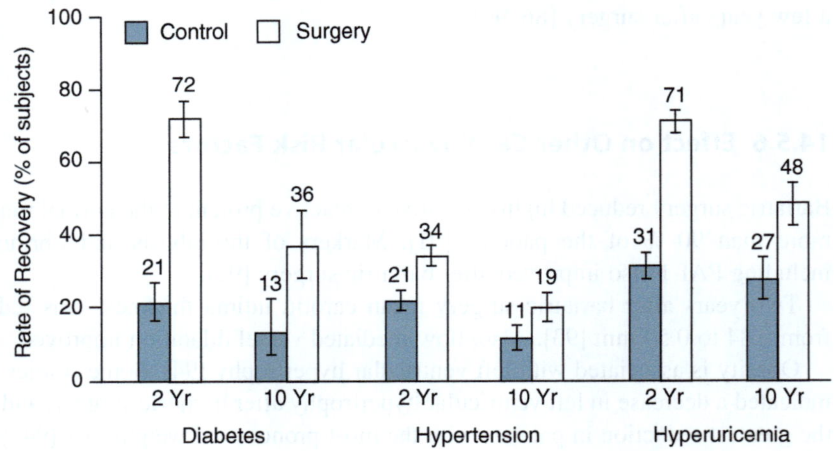

	2 Yr	10 Yr	2 Yr	10 Yr	2 Yr	10 Yr
No. of subjects	248 342	84 118	880 1204	342 424	637 792	243 292
Odds ratio	8.42	3.45	1.72	1.68	5.36	2.37
95% CI	5.68-12.5	1.64-7.28	1.40-2.12	1.09-2.58	4.23-6.78	1.61-3.47
P value	<0.001	0.001	<0.001	0.02	<0.001	<0.001

Fig. 14.5 Recovery from diabetes, lipid disturbances, hypertension and hyperuricemia over 2- and 10-year period among surgically treated subjects and their obese controls in the SOS intervention study. Adapted from [52]

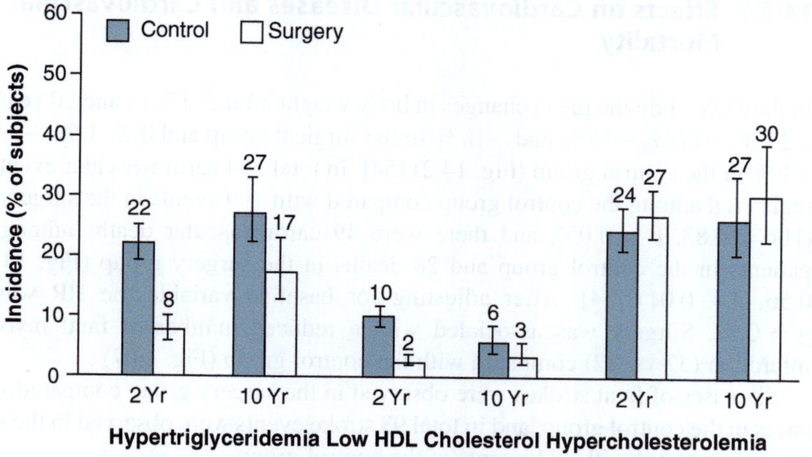

	Hypertriglyceridemia 2 Yr	Hypertriglyceridemia 10 Yr	Low HDL Cholesterol 2 Yr	Low HDL Cholesterol 10 Yr	Hypercholesterolemia 2 Yr	Hypercholesterolemia 10 Yr
No. of subjects	801 731	281 225	1174 1293	440 431	596 504	188 135
Odds ratio	0.29	0.61	0.21	0.57	1.27	1.16
P value	<0.001	0.03	<0.001	0.12	0.11	0.57

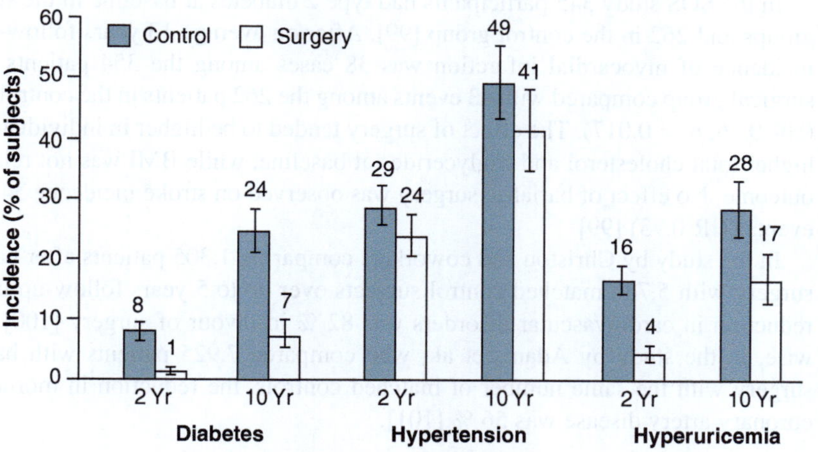

	Diabetes 2 Yr	Diabetes 10 Yr	Hypertension 2 Yr	Hypertension 10 Yr	Hyperuricemia 2 Yr	Hyperuricemia 10 Yr
No. of subjects	1402 1489	539 517	770 623	279 215	1017 1044	382 342
Odds ratio	0.14	0.25	0.78	0.75	0.22	0.49
95% CI	0.08-0.24	0.17-0.38	0.60-1.01	0.52-1.08	0.15-0.31	0.34-0.71
P value	<0.001	<0.001	0.06	0.13	<0.001	<0.001

Fig. 14.6 Incidence of diabetes, lipid disturbances and hyperuricemia over 2- and 10-year period among surgically treated subjects and their obese controls in the SOS intervention study. Adapted from [52]

14.5.7 Effects on Cardiovascular Diseases and Cardiovascular Mortality

In the SOS study the mean changes in body weight after 2, 10, 15 and 20 years were −23 %, −17 %, −16 % and −18 % in the surgical group and 0 %, 1 %, −1 %, and −1 % in the control group (Fig. 14.2) [54]. In total 234 cardiovascular events were registered among the control group compared with 199 events in the surgery group (HR = 0.83, $p = 0.05$), and there were 49 cardiovascular deaths among 2,037 patients in the control group and 28 deaths in the surgery group (Fig. 14.7, HR 0.56, $p < 0.01$) [54]. After adjusting for baseline variable the HR was 0.47, $p = 0.02$. Surgery was associated with a reduced number of fatal myocardial infarction (37 vs. 22) compared with the control group (Fig. 14.7).

Six cases of fatal strokes were observed in the surgery group compared with 12 cases in the control group, and in total 93 stroke events were observed in the surgery group compared with 111 events in the control group.

The benefits of surgery were associated with fasting plasma insulin at baseline, with greatest benefit in participants with higher insulin (insulin resistance), but not with BMI or waist-to-hip ratio [54]. The reduction in cardiovascular diseases was primarily seen in patients with type 2 diabetes, while mortality did not differ in the nondiabetic groups.

In the SOS study 345 participants had type 2 diabetes at baseline in the surgical groups and 262 in the control group [99]. After on average 13 years follow-up the incidence of myocardial infarction was 38 cases among the 354 patients in the surgical group compared with 43 events among the 262 patients in the control group (HR 0.56, $p = 0.017$). The effect of surgery tended to be higher in individuals with higher total cholesterol and triglycerides at baseline, while BMI was not related to outcome. No effect of bariatric surgery was observed on stroke incidence 34 vs. 24 events (HR 0.73) [99].

In the study by Christou and coworkers comparing 1,305 patients after bariatric surgery with 5,746 matched control subjects over up to 5 years follow-up the risk reduction in cardiovascular disorders was 82 % in favour of surgery [100]. Likewise, in the study by Adams et al., who compared 7,925 patients with bariatric surgery with the same number of matched controls, the reduction in mortality of coronary artery disease was 56 % [101].

14.5.8 Effects on Cancers

Obesity is a risk factor for cancer and one meta-analysis of prospective, observational studies estimated that overweight or obesity accounts for 14 % of cancer deaths in men and 20 % in women [102].

After 10.9 years follow-up in the SOS study and a weight loss of approximately 20 kg in the bariatric groups and a weight gain of 1.3 kg in the control group the number of first-time cancers in the bariatrically treated group ($n = 117$ in 2,010 patients) was reduced compared with the control group ($n = 169$ in 2,037 patients,

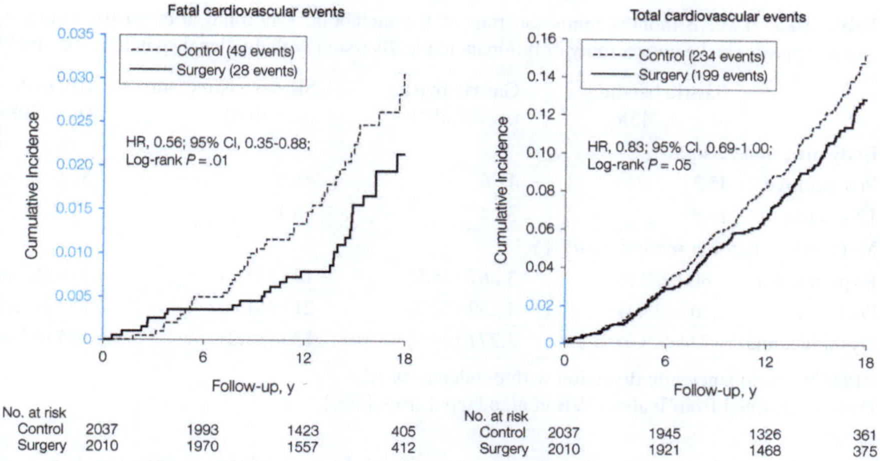

Fig. 14.7 Cumulative incidence of fatal and total cardiovascular events in control and surgical groups in the SOS intervention study. Adapted from [54]

HR 0.67) [103]. In women the number was 79 vs. 130 patients (HR 0.58), whereas there was no effect of surgery in men (38 vs. 39 patients).

Christou et al. reported after a maximum follow-up of 5 years 21 cancers in the surgery group ($n = 1{,}035$) compared with 487 cancers in the control group ($n = 5.746$, HR 0.22) [104, 105]. For breast cancer the relative risk ratio was 0.17 in favour of surgery.

Adams et al. found after a mean follow-up of 7.1 years that the reduction in cancer-caused mortality was 60 % [101]. In a later follow-up after a mean of 12.5 years a 24 % reduction in cancers was found in the surgical group compared with the control group [106]. The reduction was only observed in women. Especially the incidence of uterine cancer was significantly lower among surgical patients.

The quality of the studies, except for the SOS studies, is poor, and the results can at best be viewed as hypothesis-generating and inspire to new randomised, controlled studies with long-term follow-up. Experiments exploring the possible mechanisms of reduction in cancer incidence after bariatric surgery are also needed, especially to explain that the reduction in cancers is mainly observed in women.

14.5.9 Effects on Metabolic Syndrome

Before surgery most of the patients will display the metabolic syndrome, and in one study the resolution of the syndrome was 84 % after 2 years [107]. In another study the prevalence of the metabolic syndrome decreased after 3.4 years follow-up from 87 to 29 % after gastric bypass surgery compared with a decrease from 85 to 75 % in a control group treated with conventional lifestyle intervention [108]. The number needed to treat to obtain a resolution of the metabolic syndrome was about two patients after surgery. The strongest predictor for reversibility of the

Table 14.2 Twelve months remission rate of the metabolic syndrome after gastric banding, gastric bypass, sleeve gastrectomy or biliopancreatic diversion with duodenal switch, respectively

	Gastric banding (n = 4,245)	Gastric bypass (n = 7,285)	Sleeve gastrectomy (n = 406)	BPD/DS (n = 208)
Body mass index (kg/m^2)				
Preoperative	45.5	47.6	48.6	51.0
12 months	38.5	32.4	36.1	31.8
Metabolic syndrome remission, n (%)				
Hypertension	800 (18.8)	3,267 (44.8)	143 (35.2)	110 (52.9)
Diabetes	1,206 (28.4)	4,532 (62.2)	211 (51.0)	154 (74.0)
Dyslipidaemia	734 (17.3)	3,271 (44.9)	139 (34.2)	135 (64.9)

BPD/DS: Biliopancreatic diversion with duodenal switch
Data are adapted from Inabnet WB et al. adapted from [109]

metabolic syndrome was the percentage of weight lost of the excess weight. In a recent study using the Bariatric Outcome Longitudinal Database for the American Society for Metabolic Surgery 23,106 patients were identified with the metabolic syndrome before surgery [109]. Of the patients 62 % underwent RYGB, 32 % gastric banding, 4.5 % sleeve gastrectomy, and biliopancreatic diversion with duodenal switch was performed in 1.5 %. BMIs are given in Table 14.2. The patients with metabolic syndrome had an increased mortality compared with patients without metabolic syndrome (0.3 % vs. 0.1 %) the first 90 days after operation. Biliopancreatic diversion with duodenal switch had the highest rate of complications while gastric banding had the lowest rate of adverse events, but on the cost of decreased remission of the metabolic syndrome. The 12 months remission rate of the metabolic syndrome is illustrated in Table 14.2. The resolution of hypertension, diabetes and dyslipidaemia after gastric banding was 18.8, 28.4 and 17.3 %, and after gastric bypass 44.8, 62.2 and 44.9 %, respectively. Other investigators have presented similar results [63, 108, 110–115]. Thus bariatric surgery induces consistent and durable improvement in the prevalence of the metabolic syndrome. The study by Batsis et al. estimated that four deaths and 16 cardiovascular events would be prevented by bariatric surgery per 100 patients over a 10-year period [108].

14.5.10 Effects on Mortality

The majority of long-term epidemiological studies have indicated that obesity is associated with increased mortality [116–118]. Interestingly, several observational, epidemiological studies have indicated that overall mortality and cardiovascular mortality are increased with weight loss [119, 120]. The discrepancy between the beneficial effects of weight loss on cardiovascular risk factors as compared with mortality has been related to inability of such studies to distinguish between unintentional and intentional weight loss. The observed weight loss might be a consequence of conditions that lead to death rather than the course of increased mortality.

In the SOS study after an average of 11 years follow-up the cumulative overall mortality was 129 subjects (6.3 %) in the control group compared with 101 (5.0 %) in the surgery group, indicating a relative risk reduction of 24 % (HR 0.76, $p = 0.04$) [53]. The reduction in mortality in the surgical group was about 30 % in subjects with a BMI above the median BMI of 40.8 kg/m^2 and about 20 % in subjects below the median [53]. There were 53 cardiovascular deaths in the control group and 43 in the surgery group.

In the study by Adams et al. during the 7 years follow-up of 7,925 people, who underwent gastric bypass, and 7,925 severely obese persons matched for age, sex and BMI, total mortality was reduced with 40 % in the surgical group [101]. The mortality of coronary heart disease, type 2 diabetes and cancer was reduced by 56 %, 92 % and 60 %, respectively, in the surgical group. Mortality because of cancer was reduced more in men than in women [101].

In a third study the reduction in all-cause mortality was 89 % in the surgical group compared with a control group after at least 5 years follow-up [104]. A limitation of all three studies is that the design is not randomised and controlled.

14.5.11 Effects on Quality of Life

Obesity is associated with social discrimination and low self-esteem [10, 121–123]. The substantial and long-term weight loss has been shown to have a beneficial effect on quality of life in most patients [10, 121–123]. In the SOS study health-related quality of life followed phases of weight loss, weight gain and weight stability, and was related to the magnitude of weight loss and weight regain [123]. Peak improvements in the surgical group were observed during the first year, whereas the weight gain phase was accompanied by a gradual decline in quality of life. At 10 years follow-up a net gain was noted in quality of life compared with baseline and compared with the control group [123]. No significant differences were found for overall mood and anxiety [123]. The study also indicated that a maintained weight loss of about 10 % is sufficient for positive long-term effects on quality of life [123]. On the other hand in the study from Adams and coworkers mood disorders showed to be higher after bariatric surgery compared with an obese control group [101]. Suicide rates did not differ between the groups. In the SOS study bariatric surgery was associated with favourable effects on disability pension in men, whereas no effects could be detected in women [122].

14.6 Indications and Contraindications to Bariatric Surgery

In practical terms patients are eligible for bariatric surgery if BMI > 35 kg/m^2 and comorbidities as diabetes, hypertension, arthritis limiting daily function, cardiopulmonary failure and sleep apnoea. For patients without comorbidities the BMI limit is > 40 kg/m^2. The age limit is in most countries from 18 to 65 years. These criteria were established in recognition of the relationship between obesity and the risk of coronary artery disease, type 2 diabetes and sleep apnoea among other risks factors.

14.7 Risks of Bariatric Surgery

At the best centres the 30 days mortality is about 0.3–0.5 % after gastric bypass and about 0.1 % after gastric banding [13]. The acute complications are bleeding, infections, anastomotic leak, arrhythmias and pulmonary emboli [55]. Long-term complications are nutritional deficiencies, internal hernias and anastomotic stenosis with vomiting, stoma ulceration and erosions [55]. In the SOS study, where most patients were treated with banding, the 90 days mortality was 0.25 % [53, 58]. In 151 individuals 193 complications (bleeding 0.5 %, thrombosis and embolism 0.8 %, wound complication and infections 4.8 %) were registered. In 26 patients (2.2 %) the complications required reoperation. The frequencies of reoperation and/or conversions among 1,338 patients followed for at least 10 years were 31 %, 21 % and 17 % for those obtaining banding, vertical banding and gastric bypass [53, 58].

The risk of nutritional deficiencies includes thiamine, vitamins B6, B12 and D, calcium, iron, copper and zinc [55, 124, 125]. After gastric bypass the patients need to take lifelong calcium, D-vitamin, A-vitamin, iron, folate, and thiamine and to receive B12 injections [55, 124, 125]. It is also recommended that nutritional management includes an average 60–120 g protein daily to maintain lean body mass [55, 124, 125]. Periodical biochemical monitoring for micro- and macronutriotinal deficiencies is recommended [55].

Some patients will have dumping 15 min to 1 h after the meal with symptoms such as abdominal pain and cramping, sweating, dizziness, nausea, tachycardia and diarrhoea explained by the rapid entry of hyperosmotic food into the small intestine [55], which draws fluid from plasma into the intestinal lumen with a decrease in blood volume and sympathetic nervous stimulation [55, 126]. Dumping symptoms become less prominent with time. The treatment is to eat small, frequent meals, avoiding ingestion of liquid meals and avoiding simple sugars [55].

Few patients will develop postprandial hypoglycaemia because of an excessive insulin response in relation to the ambient insulin sensitivity [127, 128]. The pathogenesis of this syndrome is not clarified, but an imbalance between improved insulin sensitivity and exaggerated GLP-1 responses resulting in an excessive postprandial insulin secretion may be part of the explanation [127]. Indeed, in a patient with severe postoperative hypoglycaemia it has been possible to prevent the exaggerated release of GLP-1 and insulin and to avoid hypoglycaemia by feeding through a gastrostomy catheter inserted in the gastric remnant [129]. In some patients islet expansion (nesidioblastosis) has been described, while other studies have not found increased beta-cell mass in patients with hypoglycaemia [130, 131]. In a study using nationwide registries in Sweden the incidence of postprandial hypoglycaemia was about 0.2 % of gastric bypass patients, but was not observed after gastric banding [132]. The postprandial hypoglycaemia is typically observed

2–3 years after gastric bypass surgery. The most drastic intervention for this complication is pancreatic resection.

14.8 Final Comments

Many areas of the world are in the midst of an obesity epidemic, and one concern is that increasing rates of obesity will be associated with increasing mortality. However, risk estimates have been downgraded, most likely due to improved control of comorbidities of obesity by intensive pharmacological treatment [133].

Diet and exercise and use of medications usually only lead to a modest and transient degree of weight loss [11, 134, 135]. Bariatric surgery is the most effective therapy to obtain substantial, long-lasting weight loss and improvement or complete resolution of obesity comorbidities [13]. Bariatric surgery reduces mortality because of diabetes, cardiovascular diseases and cancers and also improves quality of life.

Body weight is centrally regulated, via peripheral hormonal signals released from the gastrointestinal tract, pancreas and adipose tissue, which is integrated primarily in the hypothalamus to regulate food intake and appetite [30, 36, 39, 41, 42, 48]. The modulators of appetite include leptin, ghrelin, cholecystokinin, PYY, insulin, pancreatic polypeptide, GLP-1 and glucose-dependent insulinotropic polypeptide, which except for ghrelin all inhibit hunger. Ghrelin stimulates hunger and is found in highest concentration preprandially. RYGB diminishes hunger and increases the experience of satiety after meals by generating a neuroendocrine response that is consistent with reduced appetite and energy intake [36, 136]. In obese people a 10 % weight loss induces a 10–20 % reduction in energy expenditure beyond what can be accounted for by the reduced body weight [137]. In addition, after weight loss hunger will increase consistently for defence of body fat stores [137, 138]. The combination of reduced energy expenditure and increased hunger may account for the recidivism to previous weight after weight loss [137–139]. In rats gastric bypass prevents the expected decrease in energy expenditure to weight loss, indicating that a "set point" for body weight has been interrupted by surgery [137]. In humans the results have not been so conclusive in relation to effect on energy expenditure after gastric bypass [45–47].

Many short-term studies have indicated that a 5 % weight loss in obese people is enough to induce significant improvements in cardiovascular risk factors [72, 140–142]. It has also been suggested that a 10 kg weight loss is associated with reduction of 10 mm Hg and 20 mm Hg reduction in systolic and diastolic blood pressure, 10–15 % reduction in total and LDL cholesterol, 30 % reduction in triglycerides and 8 % increase in HDL cholesterol [72, 140–142]. However, the estimates are often based on studies shorter than 2 years. Analysis of studies with at least 2 years follow-up has resulted in more modest expectations [143, 144]. In the 10-year follow-up of the SOS study the necessary weight loss for a significant alteration of a risk factor was estimated [145]. A 5 kg weight loss was not associated with any significant risk factor reduction over a 10-year period, while a 10 kg weight loss was associated with a 6 mm Hg improvement in systolic blood pressure and in fasting insulin. A 15 kg weight loss increased HDL cholesterol significantly and reduced fasting glucose with 0.75 mmol/l. Improvement in diastolic blood pressure and triglycerides was only seen in the patients with the largest weight loss of 44 kg. Total cholesterol was not significantly improved in even the group of patients with the greatest weight loss. Hypertension was unaffected by gastric banding surgery after 10 years follow-up. The analysis illustrates that large weight loss is needed to achieve effects on risk factors during a 10-year period. This conclusion may be considered in the light that 10 years of ageing in an obese person will per se deteriorate the status of the risk factors resulting in a neutralising effect of weight loss on the risk factors. Therefore, effects of bariatric surgery are influenced by non-weight change-dependent shifts in risk factor levels [145].

Although lifestyle, including weight loss and physical activities, should be first-line treatment in addition to pharmacological treatment of patients with type 2 diabetes other approaches are needed, since less than 50 % of the patients reach the target for glycaemic control [146]. Management of type 2 diabetes is challenging, since with the exception of incretin-based therapy and metformin, oral hypoglycaemic agents and insulin therapy induce weight gain, which may further impair glycaemic control [146]. On this background, a consensus meeting on bariatric surgery and the IDF have recommended consideration of bariatric surgery for control of type 2 diabetes in whom recommended glycaemic targets are not reached with available medical therapies, especially when the patient has major coexisting illnesses, such as hypertension and dyslipidaemia [83, 147].

In the meta-analysis of Buchwald et al. the resolution rates of diabetes, hyperlipidaemia, hypertension and sleep apnoea were 77, 79, 62 and 80 %, respectively [13]. On average 50 % of the patients who underwent gastric banding, 80 % of those who underwent RYGB and 95 % of those who underwent biliopancreatic diversion experienced remission of diabetes [13]. Noteworthy, in the meta-analysis of Buchwald et al. the data are retrospective and uncontrolled with heterogeneity between the procedures analysed and with unsatisfactory follow-up in many studies [13]. Only one properly designed study with long-term follow-up has been performed primarily using laparoscopic gastric banding procedure [51]. In this study about 25 % of participants had type 2 diabetes at baseline [148]. After 2 years 73 % of subjects in the surgical group and 13 % of subjects in the control group were in treatment free remission, but after 10 years follow-up 9 % of the patients, who had undergone gastric bypass and 25 % of those treated with gastric banding, had regained most of the weight they had lost, and diabetes had occurred in 50 % of patients in whom the condition initially resolved [52]. Whether bariatric surgery cures diabetes or the remission is transient is at present poorly investigated, but surgery is a way of "buying" time with normal glucose levels and less use of antidiabetic agents.

The American Diabetes Association recently defined remission of type 2 diabetes as a return to normal glucose metabolism with a HbA1c <6.0 % and fasting plasma glucose less than 5.6 mmol/l at least 1 year after bariatric surgery without hypoglycaemic medications [78]. The remission rates after bariatric procedures are much lower using the new definition and are in the range of 10–50 % and lowest after gastric banding [78–80]. Expectations of both patients and clinicians may have to be adjusted as regards remission and should focus on improved control and less use of antidiabetic medications. Another question needing investigation in a randomised trial design is whether bariatric surgery is suitable for patients with type 2 diabetes and lower body weight than 35 kg/m^2 or even normal weight [22, 25, 83–85, 147].

Some of the benefits are independent of weight loss [27], and after gastric bypass the remission of type 2 diabetes is observed a few days after operation and depends on changes in gut hormone secretion, especially GLP-1 and caloric restriction after the operation. After gastric banding the metabolic improvement is less immediate and may depend more directly on weight loss [27].

In epidemiological studies weight loss has paradoxically been associated with an increased incidence of cardiovascular events even in patients, who were overweight. Lifestyle intervention in people with prediabetes has not prevented cardiovascular events, even after 10–20 years follow-up [149, 150]. The "Look AHEAD study" using intensive lifestyle intervention in type 2 diabetes has been stopped after a decade. The group treated with intensive counselling lost an average 5 % of starting weight and improved physical fitness levels compared with 1 % weight loss in the less intensively treated arm, but after up to 11 years follow-up, there were no differences between the groups in the rate of cardiovascular events including stroke. The benefits of modest weight loss—if it exists—were too small to see in people with type 2 diabetes, who are already getting good medical care [151].

In the SOS study bariatric surgery was associated with a reduction in total mortality, cardiovascular mortality and a number of cardiovascular events. A higher baseline plasma insulin concentration was associated with a more favourable outcome of bariatric surgery in relation to cardiovascular events [54]. No association was demonstrated with regard to BMI at baseline or changes in BMI during follow-up, suggesting that high insulin may be better selection criteria for bariatric surgery than high BMI as far as cardiovascular events are concerned. Insulin resistance presented as high plasma insulin levels is a well-known risk factor for cardiovascular events during long-term follow-up [152].

On average obese patients have increased mortality, but in people without diabetes or other risk factors the life span is only minimally reduced. Therefore, it is important not to consider the obese population as homogenous with regard to health. The obese population presents a wide spectrum with regard to glucose homeostasis and risk factors as the metabolic syndrome compared with people without comorbidities [153]. One pathophysiological explanation is that some people in response to overeating preferentially accumulate truncal rather than central obesity, which may prevent development of the metabolic syndrome. When the ability to accumulate subcutaneous fat is limited overeating results in central obesity in combination with ectopic fat in the muscles, heart and liver causing insulin resistance, followed by the metabolic syndrome, diabetes and cardiovascular diseases [3–5]. As a result body composition and not overall fatness is the major determinate of the health risk of obesity. BMI may be a misleading indicator of health risk since it does not always reflect body composition, and the reduced mortality, cancers, myocardial infarctions, strokes and prevention of diabetes in the SOS study were unrelated to weight loss and BMI at baseline [53, 54, 58, 103]. We need to acknowledge that it may be time for updating the present guidelines for undergoing bariatric surgery based primarily on BMI, since bariatric surgery is performed to improve the health status and longevity of the patient. Possibly the occurrence of the metabolic syndrome or a high risk score using, i.e., Framingham Risk Score will better predict benefits from surgery.

Notably, the relative risk reduction in mortality is high after bariatric surgery compared with conventional treatment, but the absolute reduction in mortality was only 1.4 % in the study from Adams et al. (2.7 % vs. 4.1 %) and 1.3 % in the SOS study (5.0 % vs. 6.3 %) after 7–13 years follow-up, respectively [54, 58, 101]. Such improvements need to be balanced with surgical risk and safety and should be studied in large randomised, controlled trials with long-term follow-up of people with and without type 2 diabetes.

One meta-analysis revealed a 30 days mortality of 0.1 % after gastric banding, 0.5 % after gastric bypass and 1.1 % after biliopancreatic diversion procedures [13]. The main short-term causes of death are thromboembolism and cardiovascular diseases [13]. Intestinal nutritional malabsorption after biliopancreatic diversion and gastric bypass increases the incidence of complications such as anaemia, hypoalbuminaemia and deficiencies in vitamins and minerals, even in people treated with vitamin and mineral supplementation [55, 124]. About 25 % of the patients will need plastic surgery to provide symptomatic or cosmetic relief from excessive skin tissue, which is often more expensive than the bariatric surgery. Nonetheless, bariatric surgery is cost-effective, especially in patients with type 2 diabetes, saves healthcare costs and generates health benefits [89].

Further examination of the mechanisms of action of RYGB will likely improve our understanding of the regulation of body weight and pathophysiology of type 2 diabetes, which may facilitate the development of novel therapies for obesity and diabetes. Such information will also be important in relation to identification of persons, who are most appropriate candidates for bariatric surgery.

References

1. Field AE, Coakley EH, Must A et al (2001) Impact of overweight on the risk of developing common chronic diseases during a 10-year period. Arch Intern Med 161:1581–1586
2. Willett WC, Dietz WH, Colditz GA (1999) Guidelines for healthy weight. N Engl J Med 341: 427–434
3. Despres JP, Lemieux I (2006) Abdominal obesity and metabolic syndrome. Nature 444: 881–887
4. Despres JP (2011) Excess visceral adipose tissue/ectopic fat the missing link in the obesity paradox? J Am Coll Cardiol 57:1887–1889
5. Despres JP (2012) What is "metabolically healthy obesity"?: from epidemiology to pathophysiological insights. J Clin Endocrinol Metab 97:2283–2285
6. Haffner SM (2003) Insulin resistance, inflammation, and the prediabetic state. Am J Cardiol 92:18J–26J

7. Bays H, Mandarino L, DeFronzo RA (2004) Role of the adipocyte, free fatty acids, and ectopic fat in pathogenesis of type 2 diabetes mellitus: peroxisomal proliferator-activated receptor agonists provide a rational therapeutic approach. J Clin Endocrinol Metab 89: 463–478
8. Dixon JB, Bhathal PS, O'Brien PE (2001) Nonalcoholic fatty liver disease: predictors of nonalcoholic steatohepatitis and liver fibrosis in the severely obese. Gastroenterology 121: 91–100
9. Glueck CJ, Papanna R, Wang P, Goldenberg N, Sieve-Smith L (2003) Incidence and treatment of metabolic syndrome in newly referred women with confirmed polycystic ovarian syndrome. Metabolism 52:908–915
10. Must A, Spadano J, Coakley EH, Field AE, Colditz G, Dietz WH (1999) The disease burden associated with overweight and obesity. JAMA 282:1523–1529
11. Derosa G, Maffioli P (2012) Anti-obesity drugs: a review about their effects and their safety. Expert Opin Drug Saf 11:459–471
12. Buchwald H, Oien DM (2009) Metabolic/bariatric surgery Worldwide 2008. Obes Surg 19: 1605–1611
13. Buchwald H, Avidor Y, Braunwald E et al (2004) Bariatric surgery: a systematic review and meta-analysis. JAMA 292:1724–1737
14. Fontaine KR, Redden DT, Wang C, Westfall AO, Allison DB (2003) Years of life lost due to obesity. JAMA 289:187–193
15. Hollenbeak CS, Rogers AM, Barrus B, Wadiwala I, Cooney RN (2008) Surgical volume impacts bariatric surgery mortality: a case for centers of excellence. Surgery 144:736–743
16. McTigue KM, Harris R, Hemphill B et al (2003) Screening and interventions for obesity in adults: summary of the evidence for the U.S. Preventive Services Task Force. Ann Intern Med 139:933–949
17. Pories WJ (2008) Bariatric surgery: risks and rewards. J Clin Endocrinol Metab 93:S89–S96
18. Waseem T, Mogensen KM, Lautz DB, Robinson MK (2007) Pathophysiology of obesity: why surgery remains the most effective treatment. Obes Surg 17:1389–1398
19. Woodard GA, Peraza J, Bravo S, Toplosky L, Hernandez-Boussard T, Morton JM (2010) One year improvements in cardiovascular risk factors: a comparative trial of laparoscopic Roux-en-Y gastric bypass vs. adjustable gastric banding. Obes Surg 20:578–582
20. Mason EE, Ito C (1967) Gastric bypass in obesity. Surg Clin North Am 47:1345–1351
21. Ashrafian H, Bueter M, Ahmed K et al (2010) Metabolic surgery: an evolution through bariatric animal models. Obes Rev 11:907–920
22. Cohen RV, Schiavon CA, Pinheiro JS, Correa JL, Rubino F (2007) Duodenal-jejunal bypass for the treatment of type 2 diabetes in patients with body mass index of 22–34 kg/m^2: a report of 2 cases. Surg Obes Relat Dis 3:195–197
23. Depaula AL, Macedo AL, Mota BR, Schraibman V (2008) Laparoscopic ileal interposition associated to a diverted sleeve gastrectomy is an effective operation for the treatment of type 2 diabetes mellitus patients with BMI 21–29. Surg Endosc 23:1313–20
24. Depaula AL, Stival AR, DePaula CC, Halpern A, Vencio S (2010) Impact on dyslipidemia of the laparoscopic ileal interposition associated to sleeve gastrectomy in type 2 diabetic patients. J Gastrointest Surg 14:1319–1325
25. Depaula AL, Stival AR, DePaula CC, Halpern A, Vencio S (2012) Surgical treatment of type 2 diabetes in patients with BMI below 35: mid-term outcomes of the laparoscopic ileal interposition associated with a sleeve gastrectomy in 202 consecutive cases. J Gastrointest Surg 16:967–976
26. Strader AD, Clausen TR, Goodin SZ, Wendt D (2009) Ileal interposition improves glucose tolerance in low dose streptozotocin-treated diabetic and euglycemic rats. Obes Surg 19: 96–104
27. Dirksen C, Jorgensen NB, Bojsen-Moller KN et al (2012) Mechanisms of improved glycaemic control after Roux-en-Y gastric bypass. Diabetologia 55:1890–1901

28. Patti ME, Houten SM, Bianco AC et al (2009) Serum bile acids are higher in humans with prior gastric bypass: potential contribution to improved glucose and lipid metabolism. Obesity (Silver Spring) 17:1671–1677
29. Pournaras DJ, Glicksman C, Vincent RP et al (2012) The role of bile after Roux-en-Y gastric bypass in promoting weight loss and improving glycaemic control. Endocrinology 153: 3613–3619
30. Hussain SS, Bloom SR (2012) The regulation of food intake by the gut-brain axis: implications for obesity. Int J Obes (Lond) 2012 Jun. [Epub ahead of print]
31. le Roux CW, Welbourn R, Werling M et al (2007) Gut hormones as mediators of appetite and weight loss after Roux-en-Y gastric bypass. Ann Surg 246:780–785
32. le Roux CW, Bueter M, Theis N et al (2011) Gastric bypass reduces fat intake and preference. Am J Physiol Regul Integr Comp Physiol 301:R1057–R1066
33. Jacobsen SH, Olesen SC, Dirksen C et al (2012) Changes in gastrointestinal hormone responses, insulin sensitivity, and beta-cell function within 2 weeks after gastric bypass in non-diabetic subjects. Obes Surg 22:1084–1096
34. Jorgensen NB, Jacobsen SH, Dirksen C et al (2012) Acute and long-term effects of Roux-en-Y gastric bypass on glucose metabolism in subjects with Type 2 diabetes and normal glucose tolerance. Am J Physiol Endocrinol Metab 303:E122–E131
35. Laferrere B, Teixeira J, McGinty J et al (2008) Effect of weight loss by gastric bypass surgery versus hypocaloric diet on glucose and incretin levels in patients with type 2 diabetes. J Clin Endocrinol Metab 93:2479–2485
36. le Roux CW, Aylwin SJ, Batterham RL et al (2006) Gut hormone profiles following bariatric surgery favor an anorectic state, facilitate weight loss, and improve metabolic parameters. Ann Surg 243:108–114
37. Morinigo R, Vidal J, Lacy AM, Delgado S, Casamitjana R, Gomis R (2008) Circulating peptide YY, weight loss, and glucose homeostasis after gastric bypass surgery in morbidly obese subjects. Ann Surg 247:270–275
38. Rodieux F, Giusti V, D'Alessio DA, Suter M, Tappy L (2008) Effects of gastric bypass and gastric banding on glucose kinetics and gut hormone release. Obesity (Silver Spring) 16: 298–305
39. Strader AD, Woods SC (2005) Gastrointestinal hormones and food intake. Gastroenterology 128:175–191
40. Laferrere B, Swerdlow N, Bawa B et al (2010) Rise of oxyntomodulin in response to oral glucose after gastric bypass surgery in patients with type 2 diabetes. J Clin Endocrinol Metab 95:4072–4076
41. Badman MK, Flier JS (2005) The gut and energy balance: visceral allies in the obesity wars. Science 307:1909–1914
42. Murphy KG, Bloom SR (2006) Gut hormones and the regulation of energy homeostasis. Nature 444:854–859
43. Bueter M, Lowenstein C, Olbers T et al (2010) Gastric bypass increases energy expenditure in rats. Gastroenterology 138:1845–1853
44. Stylopoulos N, Hoppin AG, Kaplan LM (2009) Roux-en-Y gastric bypass enhances energy expenditure and extends lifespan in diet-induced obese rats. Obesity (Silver Spring) 17: 1839–1847
45. Carrasco F, Papapietro K, Csendes A et al (2007) Changes in resting energy expenditure and body composition after weight loss following Roux-en-Y gastric bypass. Obes Surg 17: 608–616
46. Das SK, Roberts SB, McCrory MA et al (2003) Long-term changes in energy expenditure and body composition after massive weight loss induced by gastric bypass surgery. Am J Clin Nutr 78:22–30
47. Olbers T, Bjorkman S, Lindroos A et al (2006) Body composition, dietary intake, and energy expenditure after laparoscopic Roux-en-Y gastric bypass and laparoscopic vertical banded gastroplasty: a randomized clinical trial. Ann Surg 244:715–722

48. Menzies J (2012) My brain made me do it, and my gut didn't help. J Neuroendocrinol 24: 1272–1273
49. Berthoud HR, Zheng H, Shin AC (2012) Food reward in the obese and after weight loss induced by calorie restriction and bariatric surgery. Ann N Y Acad Sci 1264:36–48
50. Hickey MS, Pories WJ, MacDonald KG Jr et al (1998) A new paradigm for type 2 diabetes mellitus: could it be a disease of the foregut? Ann Surg 227:637–643
51. Sjostrom L, Larsson B, Backman L et al (1992) Swedish obese subjects (SOS). Recruitment for an intervention study and a selected description of the obese state. Int J Obes Relat Metab Disord 16:465–479
52. Sjostrom L, Lindroos AK, Peltonen M et al (2004) Lifestyle, diabetes, and cardiovascular risk factors 10 years after bariatric surgery. N Engl J Med 351:2683–2693
53. Sjostrom L, Narbro K, Sjostrom CD et al (2007) Effects of bariatric surgery on mortality in Swedish obese subjects. N Engl J Med 357:741–752
54. Sjostrom L, Peltonen M, Jacobson P et al (2012) Bariatric surgery and long-term cardiovascular events. JAMA 307:56–65
55. Heber D, Greenway FL, Kaplan LM, Livingston E, Salvador J, Still C (2010) Endocrine and nutritional management of the post-bariatric surgery patient: an Endocrine Society Clinical Practice Guideline. J Clin Endocrinol Metab 95:4823–4843
56. Hinojosa MW, Varela JE, Smith BR, Che F, Nguyen NT (2009) Resolution of systemic hypertension after laparoscopic gastric bypass. J Gastrointest Surg 13:793–797
57. Pajecki D, Dalcanalle L, Souza de Oliveira CP et al (2007) Follow-up of Roux-en-Y gastric bypass patients at 5 or more years postoperatively. Obes Surg 17:601–607
58. Sjostrom L (2008) Bariatric surgery and reduction in morbidity and mortality: experiences from the SOS study. Int J Obes (Lond) 32(Suppl 7):S93–S97
59. Dixon JB, O'Brien PE (2002) Lipid profile in the severely obese: changes with weight loss after lap-band surgery. Obes Res 10:903–910
60. Segal JB, Clark JM, Shore AD et al (2009) Prompt reduction in use of medications for comorbid conditions after bariatric surgery. Obes Surg 19:1646–1656
61. Athyros VG, Mikhailidis DP, Didangelos TP et al (2006) Effect of multifactorial treatment on non-alcoholic fatty liver disease in metabolic syndrome: a randomised study. Curr Med Res Opin 22:873–883
62. Soderberg C, Stal P, Askling J et al (2010) Decreased survival of subjects with elevated liver function tests during a 28-year follow-up. Hepatology 51:595–602
63. Mattar SG, Velcu LM, Rabinovitz M et al (2005) Surgically-induced weight loss significantly improves nonalcoholic fatty liver disease and the metabolic syndrome. Ann Surg 242: 610–617
64. Barker KB, Palekar NA, Bowers SP, Goldberg JE, Pulcini JP, Harrison SA (2006) Non-alcoholic steatohepatitis: effect of Roux-en-Y gastric bypass surgery. Am J Gastroenterol 101:368–373
65. Clark JM, Alkhuraishi AR, Solga SF, Alli P, Diehl AM, Magnuson TH (2005) Roux-en-Y gastric bypass improves liver histology in patients with non-alcoholic fatty liver disease. Obes Res 13:1180–1186
66. Liu X, Lazenby AJ, Clements RH, Jhala N, Abrams GA (2007) Resolution of nonalcoholic steatohepatits after gastric bypass surgery. Obes Surg 17:486–492
67. Ashrafian H, le Roux CW, Rowland SP et al (2012) Metabolic surgery and obstructive sleep apnoea: the protective effects of bariatric procedures. Thorax 67:442–449
68. Fritscher LG, Canani S, Mottin CC et al (2007) Bariatric surgery in the treatment of obstructive sleep apnea in morbidly obese patients. Respiration 74:647–652
69. Marshall NS, Delling L, Grunstein RR et al (2011) Self-reported sleep apnoea and mortality in patients from the Swedish Obese Subjects study. Eur Respir J 38:1349–1354
70. Gaede P, Lund-Andersen H, Parving HH, Pedersen O (2008) Effect of a multifactorial intervention on mortality in type 2 diabetes. N Engl J Med 358:580–591

71. DeFronzo RA (1992) Pathogenesis of type 2 (non-insulin dependent) diabetes mellitus: a balanced overview. Diabetologia 35:389–397
72. Pi-Sunyer X, Blackburn G, Brancati FL et al (2007) Reduction in weight and cardiovascular disease risk factors in individuals with type 2 diabetes: one-year results of the look AHEAD trial. Diabetes Care 30:1374–1383
73. Pories WJ, Swanson MS, Macdonald KG et al (1995) Who would have thought it? An operation proves to be the most effective therapy for adult-onset diabetes mellitus. Ann Surg 222:339–350
74. Carlsson LM, Peltonen M, Ahlin S et al (2012) Bariatric surgery and prevention of type 2 diabetes in Swedish obese subjects. N Engl J Med 367:695–704
75. Dixon JB, O'Brien PE, Playfair J et al (2008) Adjustable gastric banding and conventional therapy for type 2 diabetes: a randomized controlled trial. JAMA 299:316–323
76. Mingrone G, Panunzi S, De GA et al (2012) Bariatric surgery versus conventional medical therapy for type 2 diabetes. N Engl J Med 366:1577–1585
77. Schauer PR, Kashyap SR, Wolski K et al (2012) Bariatric surgery versus intensive medical therapy in obese patients with diabetes. N Engl J Med 366:1567–1576
78. Buse JB, Caprio S, Cefalu WT et al (2009) How do we define cure of diabetes? Diabetes Care 32:2133–2135
79. Chikunguwo SM, Wolfe LG, Dodson P et al (2010) Analysis of factors associated with durable remission of diabetes after Roux-en-Y gastric bypass. Surg Obes Relat Dis 6: 254–259
80. Pournaras DJ, Aasheim ET, Sovik TT et al (2012) Effect of the definition of type II diabetes remission in the evaluation of bariatric surgery for metabolic disorders. Br J Surg 99:100–103
81. Schauer PR, Burguera B, Ikramuddin S et al (2003) Effect of laparoscopic Roux-en Y gastric bypass on type 2 diabetes mellitus. Ann Surg 238:467–484
82. Renard E (2009) Bariatric surgery in patients with late-stage type 2 diabetes: expected beneficial effects on risk ratio and outcomes. Diabetes Metab 35:564–568
83. Dixon JB, Zimmet P, Alberti KG, Rubino F (2011) Bariatric surgery: an IDF statement for obese Type 2 diabetes. Arq Bras Endocrinol Metabol 55:367–382
84. de Sa VC, Ferraz AA, Campos JM, Ramos AC, Araujo JG Jr, Ferraz EM (2011) Gastric bypass in the treatment of type 2 diabetes in patients with a BMI of 30 to 35 kg/m^2. Obes Surg 21:283–287
85. Garcia-Caballero M, Valle M, Martinez-Moreno JM et al (2012) Resolution of diabetes mellitus and metabolic syndrome in normal weight 24–29 BMI patients with One Anastomosis Gastric Bypass. Nutr Hosp 27:623–631
86. Cremieux PY, Ghosh A, Yang HE, Buessing M, Buchwald H, Shikora SA (2008) Return on investment for bariatric surgery. Am J Manag Care 14:e5–e6
87. Hoerger TJ, Zhang P, Segel JE, Kahn HS, Barker LE, Couper S (2010) Cost-effectiveness of bariatric surgery for severely obese adults with diabetes. Diabetes Care 33:1933–1939
88. Keating CL, Dixon JB, Moodie ML et al (2009) Cost-effectiveness of surgically induced weight loss for the management of type 2 diabetes: modeled lifetime analysis. Diabetes Care 32:567–574
89. Keating CL, Dixon JB, Moodie ML, Peeters A, Playfair J, O'Brien PE (2009) Cost-efficacy of surgically induced weight loss for the management of type 2 diabetes: a randomized controlled trial. Diabetes Care 32:580–584
90. Keating CL, Moodie ML, Bulfone L, Swinburn BA, Stevenson CE, Peeters A (2012) Healthcare utilization and costs in severely obese subjects before bariatric surgery. Obesity (Silver Spring) 20:2412–9
91. Chen SB, Lee YC, Ser KH et al (2009) Serum C-reactive protein and white blood cell count in morbidly obese surgical patients. Obes Surg 19:461–466
92. Ay L, Kopp HP, Brix JM et al (2010) Thrombin generation in morbid obesity: significant reduction after weight loss. J Thromb Haemost 8:759–765

93. Habib P, Scrocco JD, Terek M, Vanek V, Mikolich JR (2009) Effects of bariatric surgery on inflammatory, functional and structural markers of coronary atherosclerosis. Am J Cardiol 104:1251–1255
94. Algahim MF, Sen S, Taegtmeyer H (2012) Bariatric surgery to unload the stressed heart: a metabolic hypothesis. Am J Physiol Heart Circ Physiol 302:H1539–H1545
95. Algahim MF, Lux TR, Leichman JG et al (2010) Progressive regression of left ventricular hypertrophy two years after bariatric surgery. Am J Med 123:549–555
96. Vogel JA, Franklin BA, Zalesin KC et al (2007) Reduction in predicted coronary heart disease risk after substantial weight reduction after bariatric surgery. Am J Cardiol 99: 222–226
97. Batsis JA, Sarr MG, Collazo-Clavell ML et al (2008) Cardiovascular risk after bariatric surgery for obesity. Am J Cardiol 102:930–937
98. Torquati A, Wright K, Melvin W, Richards W (2007) Effect of gastric bypass operation on Framingham and actual risk of cardiovascular events in class II to III obesity. J Am Coll Surg 204:776–782
99. Romeo S, Maglio C, Burza MA et al (2012) Cardiovascular events after bariatric surgery in obese subjects with type 2 diabetes. Diabetes Care 35:2613–2617
100. Christou NV, Sampalis JS, Liberman M et al (2004) Surgery decreases long-term mortality, morbidity, and health care use in morbidly obese patients. Ann Surg 240:416–423
101. Adams TD, Gress RE, Smith SC et al (2007) Long-term mortality after gastric bypass surgery. N Engl J Med 357:753–761
102. Renehan AG, Tyson M, Egger M, Heller RF, Zwahlen M (2008) Body-mass index and incidence of cancer: a systematic review and meta-analysis of prospective observational studies. Lancet 371:569–578
103. Sjostrom L, Gummesson A, Sjostrom CD et al (2009) Effects of bariatric surgery on cancer incidence in obese patients in Sweden (Swedish Obese Subjects Study): a prospective, controlled intervention trial. Lancet Oncol 10:653–662
104. Christou NV, Sampalis JS, Liberman M et al (2004) Surgery decreases long-term mortality, morbidity, and health care use in morbidly obese patients. Ann Surg 240:416–423
105. Christou NV, Lieberman M, Sampalis F, Sampalis JS (2008) Bariatric surgery reduces cancer risk in morbidly obese patients. Surg Obes Relat Dis 4:691–695
106. Adams TD, Stroup AM, Gress RE et al (2009) Cancer incidence and mortality after gastric bypass surgery. Obesity (Silver Spring) 17:796–802
107. Ocon BJ, Garcia B, Benito P, Gimeno S, Garcia R, Lopez P (2010) Effect of gastric bypass on the metabolic syndrome and on cardiovascular risk]. Nutr Hosp 25:67–71
108. Batsis JA, Romero-Corral A, Collazo-Clavell ML, Sarr MG, Somers VK, Lopez-Jimenez F (2008) Effect of bariatric surgery on the metabolic syndrome: a population-based, long-term controlled study. Mayo Clin Proc 83:897–907
109. Inabnet WB III, Winegar DA, Sherif B, Sarr MG (2012) Early outcomes of bariatric surgery in patients with metabolic syndrome: an analysis of the bariatric outcomes longitudinal database. J Am Coll Surg 214:550–556
110. Alexandrides TK, Skroubis G, Kalfarentzos F (2007) Resolution of diabetes mellitus and metabolic syndrome following Roux-en-Y gastric bypass and a variant of biliopancreatic diversion in patients with morbid obesity. Obes Surg 17:176–184
111. Ballantyne GH, Svahn J, Capella RF et al (2004) Predictors of prolonged hospital stay following open and laparoscopic gastric bypass for morbid obesity: body mass index, length of surgery, sleep apnea, asthma, and the metabolic syndrome. Obes Surg 14:1042–1050
112. Coppini LZ, Bertevello PL, Gama-Rodrigues J, Waitzberg DL (2006) Changes in insulin sensitivity in morbidly obese patients with or without metabolic syndrome after gastric bypass. Obes Surg 16:1520–1525
113. Gazzaruso C, Giordanetti S, La MA et al (2002) Weight loss after Swedish Adjustable Gastric Banding: relationships to insulin resistance and metabolic syndrome. Obes Surg 12:841–845

114. Madan AK, Orth W, Ternovits CA, Tichansky DS (2006) Metabolic syndrome: yet another co-morbidity gastric bypass helps cure. Surg Obes Relat Dis 2:48–51
115. Scopinaro N, Papadia F, Marinari G, Camerini G, Adami G (2007) Long-term control of type 2 diabetes mellitus and the other major components of the metabolic syndrome after biliopancreatic diversion in patients with BMI <35 kg/m^2. Obes Surg 17:185–192
116. Freedman DM, Ron E, Ballard-Barbash R, Doody MM, Linet MS (2006) Body mass index and all-cause mortality in a nationwide US cohort. Int J Obes (Lond) 30:822–829
117. Price GM, Uauy R, Breeze E, Bulpitt CJ, Fletcher AE (2006) Weight, shape, and mortality risk in older persons: elevated waist-hip ratio, not high body mass index, is associated with a greater risk of death. Am J Clin Nutr 84:449–460
118. van Dam RM, Willett WC, Manson JE, Hu FB (2006) The relationship between overweight in adolescence and premature death in women. Ann Intern Med 145:91–97
119. Pamuk ER, Williamson DF, Serdula MK, Madans J, Byers TE (1993) Weight loss and subsequent death in a cohort of U.S. adults. Ann Intern Med 119:744–748
120. Higgins M, D'Agostino R, Kannel W, Cobb J, Pinsky J (1993) Benefits and adverse effects of weight loss. Observations from the Framingham Study. Ann Intern Med 119:758–763
121. Batsis JA, Lopez-Jimenez F, Collazo-Clavell ML, Clark MM, Somers VK, Sarr MG (2009) Quality of life after bariatric surgery: a population-based cohort study. Am J Med 122:1055
122. Gripeteg L, Lindroos AK, Peltonen M, Sjostrom L, Narbro K (2012) Effects of bariatric surgery on disability pension in Swedish obese subjects. Int J Obes (Lond) 36:356–362
123. Karlsson J, Taft C, Ryden A, Sjostrom L, Sullivan M (2007) Ten-year trends in health-related quality of life after surgical and conventional treatment for severe obesity: the SOS intervention study. Int J Obes (Lond) 31:1248–1261
124. Bal BS, Finelli FC, Shope TR, Koch TR (2012) Nutritional deficiencies after bariatric surgery. Nat Rev Endocrinol 8:544–556
125. Ziegler O, Sirveaux MA, Brunaud L, Reibel N, Quilliot D (2009) Medical follow up after bariatric surgery: nutritional and drug issues. General recommendations for the prevention and treatment of nutritional deficiencies. Diabetes Metab 35:544–557
126. Deitel M (2008) The change in the dumping syndrome concept. Obes Surg 18:1622–1624
127. Patti ME, Goldfine AB (2010) Hypoglycaemia following gastric bypass surgery–diabetes remission in the extreme? Diabetologia 53:2276–2279
128. Service GJ, Thompson GB, Service FJ, Andrews JC, Collazo-Clavell ML, Lloyd RV (2005) Hyperinsulinemic hypoglycemia with nesidioblastosis after gastric-bypass surgery. N Engl J Med 353:249–254
129. Goldfine AB, Mun EC, Devine E et al (2007) Patients with neuroglycopenia after gastric bypass surgery have exaggerated incretin and insulin secretory responses to a mixed meal. J Clin Endocrinol Metab 92:4678–4685
130. Abellan P, Camara R, Merino-Torres JF et al (2008) Severe hypoglycemia after gastric bypass surgery for morbid obesity. Diabetes Res Clin Pract 79:e7–e9
131. Meier JJ, Butler AE, Galasso R, Butler PC (2006) Hyperinsulinemic hypoglycemia after gastric bypass surgery is not accompanied by islet hyperplasia or increased beta-cell turnover. Diabetes Care 29:1554–1559
132. Marsk R, Jonas E, Rasmussen F, Naslund E (2010) Nationwide cohort study of post-gastric bypass hypoglycaemia including 5,040 patients undergoing surgery for obesity in 1986–2006 in Sweden. Diabetologia 53:2307–2311
133. Gregg EW, Cheng YJ, Cadwell BL et al (2005) Secular trends in cardiovascular disease risk factors according to body mass index in US adults. JAMA 293:1868–1874
134. Norris SL, Zhang X, Avenell A et al. (2005) Long-term non-pharmacologic weight loss interventions for adults with type 2 diabetes. Cochrane Database Syst Rev. CD004095.
135. Padwal RS, Majumdar SR (2007) Drug treatments for obesity: orlistat, sibutramine, and rimonabant. Lancet 369:71–77
136. Cummings DE, Weigle DS, Frayo RS et al (2002) Plasma ghrelin levels after diet-induced weight loss or gastric bypass surgery. N Engl J Med 346:1623–1630

137. Leibel RL (2008) Molecular physiology of weight regulation in mice and humans. Int J Obes (Lond) 32(Suppl 7):S98–108
138. Sumithran P, Prendergast LA, Delbridge E et al (2011) Long-term persistence of hormonal adaptations to weight loss. N Engl J Med 365:1597–1604
139. Tsai AG, Wadden TA (2005) Systematic review: an evaluation of major commercial weight loss programs in the United States. Ann Intern Med 142:56–66
140. Pi-Sunyer FX (1996) A review of long-term studies evaluating the efficacy of weight loss in ameliorating disorders associated with obesity. Clin Ther 18:1006–1035
141. Pi-Sunyer FX (2006) Use of lifestyle changes treatment plans and drug therapy in controlling cardiovascular and metabolic risk factors. Obesity (Silver Spring) 14(Suppl 3):135S–142S
142. Blackburn G (1995) Effect of degree of weight loss on health benefits. Obes Res 3(Suppl 2): 211s–216s
143. Douketis JD, Macie C, Thabane L, Williamson DF (2005) Systematic review of long-term weight loss studies in obese adults: clinical significance and applicability to clinical practice. Int J Obes (Lond) 29:1153–1167
144. Poobalan A, Aucott L, Smith WC et al (2004) Effects of weight loss in overweight/obese individuals and long-term lipid outcomes–a systematic review. Obes Rev 5:43–50
145. Sjostrom CD, Lystig T, Lindroos AK (2011) Impact of weight change, secular trends and ageing on cardiovascular risk factors: 10-year experiences from the SOS study. Int J Obes (Lond) 35:1413–1420
146. Inzucchi SE, Bergenstal RM, Buse JB et al (2012) Management of hyperglycaemia in type 2 diabetes: a patient-centered approach. Position statement of the American Diabetes Association (ADA) and the European Association for the Study of Diabetes (EASD). Diabetologia 55:1577–1596
147. Rubino F, Kaplan LM, Schauer PR, Cummings DE (2010) The Diabetes Surgery Summit consensus conference: recommendations for the evaluation and use of gastrointestinal surgery to treat type 2 diabetes mellitus. Ann Surg 251:399–405
148. Hofso D, Jenssen T, Hager H, Roislien J, Hjelmesaeth J (2010) Fasting plasma glucose in the screening for type 2 diabetes in morbidly obese subjects. Obes Surg 20:302–307
149. Uusitupa M, Peltonen M, Lindstrom J et al (2009) Ten-year mortality and cardiovascular morbidity in the Finnish Diabetes Prevention Study–secondary analysis of the randomized trial. PLoS One 4:e5656
150. Yamaoka K, Tango T (2005) Efficacy of lifestyle education to prevent type 2 diabetes: a meta-analysis of randomized controlled trials. Diabetes Care 28:2780–2786
151. Wing RR (2010) Long-term effects of a lifestyle intervention on weight and cardiovascular risk factors in individuals with type 2 diabetes mellitus: four-year results of the Look AHEAD trial. Arch Intern Med 170:1566–1575
152. Jeppesen J, Hansen TW, Rasmussen S, Ibsen H, Torp-Pedersen C, Madsbad S (2007) Insulin resistance, the metabolic syndrome, and risk of incident cardiovascular disease: a population-based study. J Am Coll Cardiol 49:2112–2119
153. Perugini RA, Quarfordt SH, Baker S, Czerniach DR, Litwin DE, Kelly JJ (2007) Metabolic characterization of nondiabetic severely obese patients undergoing Roux-en-Y gastric bypass: preoperative classification predicts the effects of gastric bypass on insulin-glucose homeostasis. J Gastrointest Surg 11:1083–1090

Treatment of the Metabolic Syndrome in Daily Clinical Practice: Algorithms

15

Henning Beck-Nielsen

15.1 How to Treat Patients with Metabolic Syndrome in Daily Clinical Practice

All clinicians must have a measuring tape on their desk. This is as important as having a blood pressure metre and scales in their office. If the metabolic syndrome is suspected, waist circumference must be measured. This must be done in patients at high risk, see Fig. 15.1. If increased waist circumference is measured, serum triglyceride, high-density lipoprotein (HDL) cholesterol, low-density lipoprotein (LDL) cholesterol and fasting plasma glucose must also be measured. Based on these measurements, the diagnosis "metabolic syndrome" can be made, and a formal basis for intervention is obtained. The International Diabetes Federation (IDF) has recently formulated a definition of the metabolic syndrome, and we recommend using this definition in clinical practice [1].

In patients with metabolic syndrome, the following measurements may also be considered in addition to the above-mentioned measurements: measurement of the liver function—among others serum alanine aminotransferase and serum urate—and androgen status for both genders and oestrogen status in women.

Figure 15.1 presents a flowchart for diagnosis of the metabolic syndrome in daily clinical practice.

15.2 Treatment of Patients with Metabolic Syndrome

The whole point of diagnosing the metabolic syndrome is that it becomes possible to intervene against the syndrome itself, i.e. against insulin resistance, hyperinsulinism and visceral obesity. The pathophysiological model presented in Fig. 1.1 (Chap. 1) indicates that primarily energy intake must be reduced and weight loss induced.

H. Beck-Nielsen (✉)
Department of Endocrinology M, Odense University Hospital, Kloevervaenget 6, 4th floor, 5000 Odense C, Denmark
e-mail: henning.beck-nielsen@ouh.regionsyddanmark.dk

H. Beck-Nielsen (ed.), *The Metabolic Syndrome*,
DOI 10.1007/978-3-7091-1331-8_15, © Springer-Verlag Wien 2013

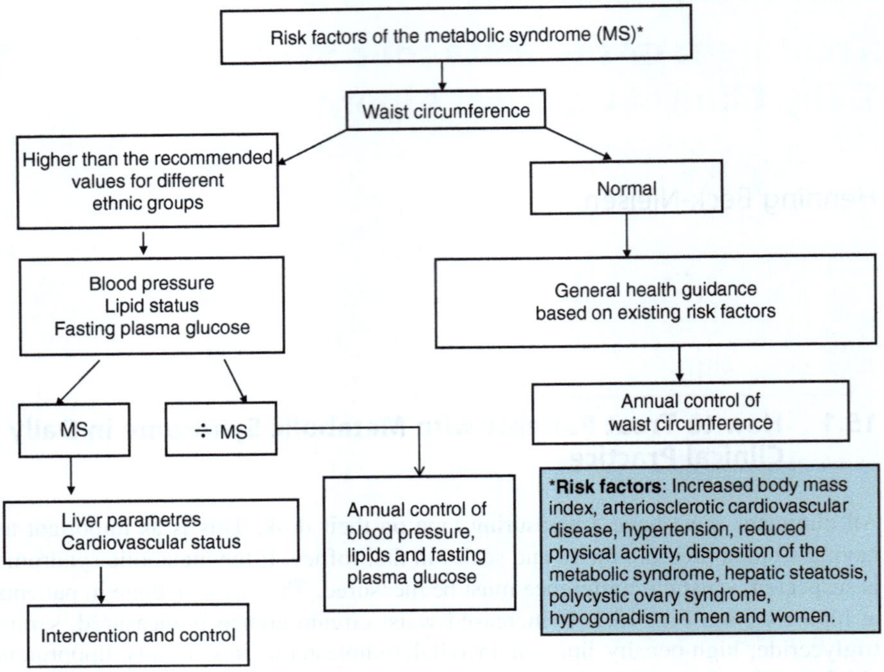

Fig 15.1 Plan of action for examination and treatment of patients at risk of the metabolic syndrome in daily clinical practice

15.2.1 Lifestyle Intervention

The first steps to be taken when treating the metabolic syndrome are to ensure a lifestyle reducing energy intake and/or increasing energy consumption (see Chap. 7) [2]. This can be done as follows:

- Stimulation of weight loss; a reduction of about 10 % will have significant effect on metabolism.
- Increased physical activity, at least half an hour a day (interval walk is effective).
- Reduction of the amount of saturated fat and sugar in the diet.
- Cessation of smoking.
- Control of alcohol consumption (reduction of energy intake).

The above-mentioned interventions have shown to reduce the incidence of the metabolic syndrome by some 40 % and the risk of developing type 2 diabetes and cardiovascular disease (CVD) [3–5].

15.2.2 Pharmacological Treatment

Pharmacological treatment is another modality for reducing the risk of complications of the metabolic syndrome when lifestyle intervention is insufficient.

Obviously, the primary causes such as insulin resistance, hyperinsulinism and visceral obesity must be treated first. The treatment is, however, experimental since no clinical guidelines exist for treating patients with metabolic syndrome only. A number of intervention studies, however, underline the value of early pharmacological treatment against the individual components (see international guidelines for treatment of hypertension, dyslipidaemia and hyperglycaemia).

Metformin is the most commonly used antidiabetic drug worldwide and has especially proved to reduce the risk of myocardial infarction and early death in obese patients with type 2 diabetes (and thereby the metabolic syndrome) [6].

Metformin especially increases insulin sensitivity in the liver and has only limited effect on dyslipidaemia and blood pressure, but it has an anorectic effect and intervenes early in pathophysiology. Metformin has also shown to prevent the development of type 2 diabetes in patients with impaired glucose tolerance. As most patients with metabolic syndrome also suffer from glucose intolerance, metformin is a natural first choice for treatment of the metabolic syndrome as evidence indicates that this drug may reduce the development of CVD (see Chap. 8).

Glucagon-like peptide-1 (GLP-1) agonists. These drugs are new on the market and are registered only for treatment of hyperglycaemia, but they may also be registered with the indication obesity alone. They are efficient for reducing body weight, and since they may reduce the risk of CVD they seem to be a logical choice, specifically in subjects with metabolic syndrome showing increased blood glucose levels and obesity (see Chap. 12).

Glitazones. These drugs would be the natural first choice as they have a specific effect on insulin resistance. They reduce blood glucose, increase HDL cholesterol, reduce triglycerides and blood pressure and inhibit the chronic inflammation characterising patients with metabolic syndrome. This is, however, an experimental treatment, which cannot yet be recommended, mainly due to the side-effects mentioned. However, they may be the drugs of choice in patients with NAFLD and severe insulin resistance (see Chap. 9).

Anorectic drugs. A few drugs exist on the market: Sibutramin, which has an appetite-suppressing effect, and orlistat, which reduces fat uptake in the intestine. Sibutramin may have serious side-effects, such as increased blood pressure. Caution must therefore still be exercised when using this drug. Four-year data on orlistat are now available with regard to treatment of obesity, and a continuous (but modest) weight loss is demonstrated. Furthermore, orlistat may prevent development of type 2 diabetes. This drug is therefore the most obvious drug, if anorectic treatment is to be considered. However, for both drugs no long-term data exist [7].

Fibrates. They are peroxisome proliferator-activated receptor (PPAR)-alpha activators reducing especially triglyceride levels and increasing HDL cholesterol values. They are only registered for treatment of hypertriglyceridaemia. Gemfibrozil has demonstrated to reduce the risk of CVD [8].

Statins. They have plentifully proved their effect against elevated LDL cholesterol values, but they may also increase HDL and reduce triglycerides. They must therefore always be considered and can be combined with fibrates, but this will increase the risk of complications (see Chap. 10).

Aspirin. The use of antithrombotic drugs in patients with metabolic syndrome only results in risk modification in patients with diabetes. Thus, aspirin treatment seems to be recommended only in patients with metabolic syndrome if these patients are hyperglycaemic or present cardiovascular risk factors. On the other hand, patients with type 2 diabetes with more than one cardiovascular risk factor and an age >50 years are recommended aspirin prophylactically if there is no contraindication due to increased risk of specifically gastrointestinal bleeding [9].

15.2.3 Surgical Intervention

Visceral obesity is primarily treated with lifestyle changes, as mentioned above, but this kind of treatment is often insufficient, and surgical intervention is therefore a possibility. Gastric bypass surgery is very efficient with regard to reducing the components of the metabolic syndrome, but it is naturally still associated with a certain surgical mortality. A recent study demonstrated that around 95 % of the patients were cured of the metabolic syndrome within a year after surgery. However, diabetes returned in about two-thirds after 10 years. Bariatric surgery must therefore be strongly considered in treatment resistant cases (see Chap. 14).

15.3 Treatment of the Specific Diseases of the Syndrome

If intervention against the primary causes, such as insulin resistance and hyperinsulinism, and the risk components (elevated blood pressure, lipid and glucose levels) does not succeed in normalising metabolism, the specific diseases caused by the syndrome must be treated, i.e. type 2 diabetes, arterial hypertension, non-alcoholic fatty liver disease/non-alcoholic steatohepatitis and polycystic ovary syndrome. The international clinical guidelines must be followed and are therefore referred to.

15.4 Treatment Algorithm

Reduce energy intake and induce weight loss:

- Low energy diet.
- Consider gastric bypass surgery if body mass index is >35 kg/m^2.
- Consider anorectic drugs: GLP-1 agonists, sibutramin or orlistat.

Treat—if necessary:

- Hyperglycaemia by metformin and in accordance with international guidelines.
- Dyslipidaemia with statins if the cardiovascular risk is increased and/or fibrates (if triglyceride levels are >5 mmol/l).
- Blood pressure ≥140/90 mmHg with angiotensin-converting enzyme inhibitors primarily (follow guidelines).
- With aspirin in patients with metabolic syndrome and hyperglycaemia and/or increased cardiovascular risk.

References

1. Alberti KGMM, Zimmet P, Shaw J (2006) Metabolic syndrome—a new world-wide definition A Consensus Statement from the International Diabetes Federation. Diabet Med 23:469–480
2. Beck-Nielsen H, Pedersen O, Lindskov HO (1979) Normalization of the insulin sensitivity and the cellular insulin binding during treatment of obese diabetics for one year. Acta Endocrinol (Copenh) 90:103–112
3. Lindstrom J, Louheranta A, Mannelin M, Rastas M, Salminen V, Eriksson J, Uusitupa M, Tuomilehto J (2003) The Finnish Diabetes Prevention Study (DPS). Diabetes Care 26:3230–3236
4. Orchard TJ, Temprosa M, Goldberg R, Haffner S, Ratner R, Marcovina S, Fowler S (2005) The effect of metformin and intensive lifestyle intervention on the metabolic syndrome: the Diabetes Prevention Program randomized trial. Ann Intern Med 142:611–619
5. Tuomilehto J, Lindstrom J, Eriksson JG, Valle TT, Hamalainen H, Ilanne-Parikka P, Keinanen-Kiukaanniemi S, Laakso M, Louheranta A, Rastas M, Salminen V, Uusitupa M, Aunola S, Cepaitis Z, Moltchanov V, Hakumaki M, Mannelin M, Martikkala V, Sundvall J (2001) Prevention of type 2 diabetes mellitus by changes in lifestyle among subjects with impaired glucose tolerance. N Engl J Med 344:1343–1350
6. Knowler WC, Barrett-Connor E, Fowler SE, Hamman RF, Lachin JM, Walker EA, Nathan DM (2002) Reduction in the incidence of type 2 diabetes with lifestyle intervention or metformin. N Engl J Med 346:393–403
7. Richelsen B (2007) Obesity and pharmacological treatment. In: Mogensen CE (ed) Pharmacotherapy of diabetes: new developments. Springer, New York, pp 167–172
8. Reaven GM (2007) The insulin resistance syndrome: concept and therapeutic approaches. In: Mogensen CE (ed) Pharmacotherapy of diabetes: new developments. Springer, New York, pp 19–30
9. Laakso M, Lehto S (1997) Epidemiology of macrovascular disease in diabetes. Diabetes Rev 5:294–315

Index

A
Acetylsalicylic acid (aspirin), 156
Acute coronary syndrome (ACS), 44, 155–160, 162
A Diabetes Outcome Progression Trial (ADOPT), 122–124, 127–129, 134, 135
Adipose tissue, 17–19, 21, 23, 25–27, 31, 35, 37, 56, 118, 119, 131, 167, 174, 176
Ageing, 10
Alternative healthy eating index (AHEI), 66
Angiotensin-converting enzyme inhibitors (ACEi), 186–188
Angiotensin II-AT1 receptor blockers (ARB), 186, 188
Anticoagulants, 157, 162
Antiplatelet therapy, 156, 158, 162
Antithrombotic primary prophylaxis, 155–162
Atherosclerotic disease, 160–161
Atherothrombotic disease, 161
Atrial fibrillation, 162

B
Biochemical parameters, 77
Bladder cancer, 135–136
Blood pressure, 71–72, 125, 167–169, 171–173, 177–181, 192, 196, 209, 210
Blood pressure levels, 149–150
Body fat distribution, 128–129
Body weight, 166–168, 170, 171, 173–176, 181
Bone fractures, 134–135

C
CAD. *See* Coronary artery disease (CAD)
Cancer, 55–59
Carbohydrate intake, 65
Carbohydrates, 89, 91–93
Carcinogenesis, 56
Cardiovascular, 102, 107–109, 111
Cardiovascular disease (CVD), 191, 192, 194, 197, 204, 209, 211, 212
abnormal glucose tolerance, 46–48
low-carbohydrate diet, 65
prediction of, 11–12
risk factors, 8, 12–13, 63–64
Cardiovascular risk factor, 47–49
Cardiovascular side effects, 132–133
Clinical management, 64
Clinical practice, 12–13
Clinical uses, 104–106
Congestive heart failure, 133–134
Coronary artery disease (CAD), 155, 159, 161
Coronary heart disease (CHD), 43–44
CVD. *See* Cardiovascular disease (CVD)

D
Diabetes, 11, 99, 104, 106, 108–111
Diabetes in Germany study (DIG), 48
Diabetes mellitus, 155, 156, 158–162
Diabetes prevention program (DPP), 108–111
Diabetes reduction assessment with ramipril and rosiglitazone medication (DREAM), 120, 121, 128
Dietary fat intake, 64–65
Dietary recommendations, 66
Dimethylbiguanide, 99
DPP-4 inhibitors, 58
DPS intervention, 73, 74
DREAM. *See* Diabetes reduction assessment with ramipril and rosiglitazone medication (DREAM)
Dysglycaemia, 47
Dyslipidaemia, 19, 21, 37, 102, 108, 150–151

E
Endothelium, 103
Energy expenditure, 194, 209

H. Beck-Nielsen (ed.), *The Metabolic Syndrome*,
DOI 10.1007/978-3-7091-1331-8, © Springer-Verlag Wien 2013

Energy intake, 89
Epidemiology, 7–13, 55
European Group for the Study of Insulin Resistance (EGIR), 9, 10
Ezetimibe, 57

F

Fasting plasma glucose, 169, 171, 173, 180
Fat, 92–93
Fibrinogen, 101, 103
Fluid retention, 133–134

G

GIP. *See* Glucose-dependent insulinotropic polypeptide (GIP)
GLP-1 receptor agonists, 168–182
Glucagon-like peptide, 165, 167, 170, 177–180
Glucose, 100, 101, 107, 108, 110, 111
Glucose-dependent insulinotropic polypeptide (GIP), 165–167
Glyburide, 122–124, 127–130, 135
Glycaemic index (GI), 91, 93
Glycation, 104

H

HbA1c, 88, 123–125, 134
Heart rate, 172
High-density lipoprotein (HDL), 176, 177
  cholesterol, 69, 70, 72, 74, 77, 79, 88, 90, 93, 147, 150
3-Hydroxy-3-methyl-glutaryl-CoA (HMGCoA), 147
Hyperglycaemia, 26
Hyperinsulinaemia, 58, 101, 108, 111
Hypertension, 19, 21–23, 31, 47, 125, 130, 185–189
Hypoglycaemia, 171

I

Impaired fasting glucose (IFG), 107, 108
Impaired glucose tolerance (IGT), 101, 107–111
Incretin, 165–168, 172, 180, 181
  effect, 165–167
Inflammation, 19, 25, 31, 35, 38, 56
Inflammatory markers, 129–130
Insulin, 99, 101, 104–108, 111
  receptor, 107
  resistance, 7, 18–22, 24–27, 31–38, 50, 67–69, 74, 76, 78, 100, 101, 103, 108, 111, 119–125, 129–131, 136, 166, 167, 174, 176, 180
  secretion, 89
Insulin-like growth factor (IGF), 56
Intensive lifestyle counselling, 71
Intima-media thickness (IMT), 46

L

Lactic acidosis, 99, 105, 106
Left ventricular diastolic dysfunction (LVDD), 45
Leisure time physical activity (LTPA), 67–68, 70, 71, 78–80
Lifestyle, 100, 104, 107–108, 111
Lifestyle intervention, 63–81
Lipids, 101, 102, 111, 118, 125–128, 167, 173, 174, 176–177, 181, 196–199, 202, 203
  management, 71–72
Lipolysis, 18, 19, 35, 37
Liver, 18–22, 25, 32–33, 35, 37
Low-carbohydrate diets, 87–93
Low-density lipoprotein (LDL), 176, 177
  cholesterol, 147, 148, 150, 151
LTPA. *See* Leisure time physical activity (LTPA)
LVDD. *See* Left ventricular diastolic dysfunction (LVDD)

M

Mechanism of action, 106–107
Mediterranean diet, 89
Metabolic effects, 90, 119
Metabolic flexibility, 20–21
Metabolic syndrome, 165–182, 191–212
Metabolomics, 20, 35–38
Metformin, 59, 99–111
Mitochondria, 20, 32–34, 38
Mortality, 192, 195, 197, 204–209, 211, 212
Muraglitazar, 118

N

National Cholesterol Education Program Adult Treatment Panel III (NCEP-ATP-III), 10, 11
Non-alcoholic fatty liver disease (NAFLD), 130–132
Non-alcoholic steatohepatitis (NASH), 130, 131

O
Obesity, 17–19, 23, 26–28, 31, 33–38
Oedema, 133–134
Oral glucose tolerance test (OGTT), 69–70

P
PAD. *See* Peripheral arterial disease (PAD)
Pancreatitis, 172
Pathophysiology, 17–38
Patient-centred treatment, 51
Peripheral arterial disease (PAD), 155, 158, 160–162
Peroxisome proliferator-activated receptor (PPAR)-gamma agonists, 117, 118, 131, 133–135
Pharmacokinetic, 104, 105
Pioglitazone, 118, 121, 125–129, 131–136
Plasminogen activator inhibitor-1, 101, 102
Platelet dysfunction, 156
Polycystic ovary syndrome (PCOS), 106, 111

R
Region-specific cut-points, 8
Renal function, 106
Resistance training, 68
Resolution, 76, 78–79
Risk of bariatric surgery, 208–209
Risk prediction, 12–13

S
Secondary prophylaxis, 160–161
Sedentary lifestyle, 68–69
Statins, 57, 147–151
Swedish obesity study (SOS), 195–198, 201, 204, 207–209, 211, 212

T
Thiazolidinediones, 117–136
Thromboembolic complications, 155–162
Ticagrelor, 157, 159, 162
Troglitazone, 118, 121, 133
Type 2 diabetes, 7, 11, 47, 63, 65–70, 80, 99–108, 110, 111, 120–125, 166–170, 172–174, 176, 177, 180, 181, 191–199, 201, 204, 207, 208, 210–212

U
Unfractionated heparin (UFH), 157, 160

V
Vascular, 101–104

W
Waist circumference, 173–176
Weight, 101–103, 105, 107–111
  gain, 134
  loss, 64, 65, 67–69, 71, 73, 74, 76, 78, 87–93, 191–195, 197–199, 201, 204, 206, 207, 209–212

MIX
Papier aus verantwortungsvollen Quellen
Paper from responsible sources
FSC® C105338

If you have any concerns about our products,
you can contact us on
ProductSafety@springernature.com

In case Publisher is established outside the EU,
the EU authorized representative is:
Springer Nature Customer Service Center GmbH
Europaplatz 3, 69115 Heidelberg, Germany

Printed by Libri Plureos GmbH
in Hamburg, Germany